Penguin Health
Encyclopaedia of Nutrition

John Yudkin was Professor of Nutrition and Dietetics at the University of London from 1954 to 1971 and is now Emeritus Professor. Born in 1910 he proceeded from Christ's College, Cambridge, to the London Hospital and later did research work in the Biochemical Laboratory and the Nutritional Laboratory at Cambridge, where he was also Director of Medical Studies at Christ's College. His degrees include M.A., Ph.D., M.D. (Cantab.), F.R.C.P. and F.R.S.C. From 1945 to 1954 he was Professor of Physiology at Queen Elizabeth College, University of London. He has published some 300 articles on biochemistry and nutrition in learned journals, and his books include *This Slimming Business* (1958), *Pure, White and Deadly* (1972), *This Nutrition Business* (1976) and *The A–Z of Slimming* (1977).

D0130171

JOHN YUDKIN

The Penguin Encyclopaedia of Nutrition

PENGUIN BOOKS

Penguin Books Ltd, Harmondsworth, Middlesex, England
Viking Penguin Inc., 40 West 23rd Street, New York, New York 10010, U.S.A.
Penguin Books Australia Ltd, Ringwood, Victoria, Australia
Penguin Books Canada Limited, 2801 John Street, Markham, Ontario, Canada L3R 1B4
Penguin Books N.Z.) Ltd, 182–190 Wairau Road, Auckland 10, New Zealand

First published by Viking 1985
Published in Penguin Books 1986

Made and printed in Great Britain by
Richard Clay (The Chaucer Press) Ltd,
Bungay, Suffolk
Typeset in Photina

To Muni

I am grateful to Dr Jean Watkins and to Biddy Martin for their constant, friendly and efficient help in the preparation of this book.

INTRODUCTION

Nutrition concerns everybody. All the living processes of the body require the supply of materials that provide both energy and the wherewithal for growth and repair of the body's tissues. Apart from oxygen, all of these are provided by what we eat and drink. One thing then that you would expect to find in an encyclopaedia of nutrition is a description of those items in our foods that the body is using. You would also wish to know what functions these items perform, that is, how the body uses them and for what purpose. This leads to several questions. How much does the body use of each? In what circumstances does this requirement change? What happens when too much is taken, or too little, of these items? In which foods are particular nutritional components found? Where do the foods themselves come from, and are they available to everyone? If not, is it because some people are too poor, or is it because food production does not keep up with population growth, or are there other reasons?

These sorts of questions soon make it evident that nutrition is not simply a description of such matters as protein, vitamins and minerals, and their effects in the body. It is concerned with the total relationship between people and their food. That is why this encyclopaedia touches on such subjects as food rationing, population growth, novel foods, and food preservatives and additives. It points out that the relationship between nutrition and disease is not confined to obvious conditions such as scurvy and rickets, but includes other diseases such as diabetes, coronary heart disease and perhaps some sorts of cancer. It seemed necessary too to explain terms such as epidemiology, remissions, osmotic pressure and pH, in order to make clear some of the concepts used by nutritionists, and to remove some of the common misunderstandings between nutritionists and non-nutritionists.

In all branches of knowledge, the accumulation of both hypotheses and facts is determined both by the insight of a succession of keen and observant minds, and by the discussion – not to say argument – that they elicit. I therefore thought that it would be of interest for the reader to have available the brief biographies of twenty-five or so scientists who have made notable contributions to what we now know as nutrition. Instead of showing their portraits, which I believe tell us little more about them, I have chosen to show the title pages of a few of the most important books they published. I have not included the biography of any living nutritionist; to have done so might have provoked even more dissension than will understandably be aroused because of those I have in fact included, or omitted.

The individual foods that I have chosen to describe fall into three categories. They are those that are a major part of the diet for many people, or they are commonly found in Western diets though in small quantity, or they are found infrequently in Western diets yet have some especially interesting quality. The table of nutritional values that appears lists only a few of the foods mentioned in the encyclopaedia; if information is required for other foods, it will be found in one of the many specialized publications, beginning with that great compilation, McCance and Widdowson's *The Composition of Foods*, revised by Paul and Southgate.

I have attempted to make each entry complete in itself, but not necessarily exhaustive. Thus, on the one hand, some of the information in one entry may be repeated in another; on the other hand, more information, which is relevant but not essential, will be given in other entries, and these are indicated as items designated 'See also'.

As with all other sciences, our knowledge of the science of nutrition is not complete, as the hundreds of research workers around the world would testify. But if we wish to know what sorts of foods we should be eating, we must take the limited knowledge we have and supply what is missing as best we can. For this purpose, we rely on the experience and judgement of the nutritionists who are involved in research. But it is understandable that different nutritionists may make different extrapolations from the known into the unknown. Thus, there is still disagreement about the role of diet in causing heart disease, and about the importance of dietary fibre in preventing or curing obesity. In dealing with this problem, I have attempted to distinguish between the certainties of the facts and the uncertainties of their extrapolation.

I am aware that I have not always avoided error, both of commission and of omission. As Samuel Johnson said in the preface to his *Dictionary of the English Language*, 'The work, whatever proofs of diligence and attention it may exhibit, is yet capable of many improvements.'

John Yudkin
London, 1984

A

Absorption

In order that food enter and affect the body, it has to be absorbed into the bloodstream. The inside of the alimentary canal, from the mouth to the anus, is in effect 'outside' the body; so long as food remains within the alimentary canal, its nutrients are no more available to the body than if the food were being clutched in the palm of the hand. The nutritional components 'reach' the body only when the food has been digested and absorbed across the wall of the gut into the blood.

Some digestion takes place in the mouth, where starch begins to be broken down to the sugar maltose. In the stomach and small intestine the digestion of starch continues, and the digestion of fat and protein begins. Nothing except alcohol is absorbed in the stomach; the absorption of the products of digestion occurs mainly in the small intestine, where they pass into the blood vessels in the tiny villi that project from the lining of the intestine like the pile on velvet. The large intestine absorbs a great part of the water and some of the salts; mostly it is a place where vast numbers of bacteria and other micro-organisms exist. These break down some of the materials that have escaped digestion higher up in the gut, including some small part of the dietary fibre. The activity of the micro-organisms may also produce some vitamins, and it is possible that to some extent these can be absorbed by the large intestine.

Because of the large quantity of digestive juices manufactured from the blood by the salivary glands, and by the stomach, pancreas, liver and small intestine, there is very much more to absorb than that which enters the mouth. The total volume of water alone that enters the alimentary canal during an average day is about 7 litres, compared with an average consumption of perhaps $1\frac{1}{2}$ litres. The amount of salt (sodium chloride) is also four times or so that which is usually taken by mouth, and the amount of protein, partly from the digestive enzymes and partly from the protein in the dead cells of the lining of the alimentary canal, is about equal to that taken by mouth.

Interference with absorption can therefore have serious or even fatal effects. Severe vomiting and diarrhoea can soon cause dehydration of the body, particularly serious in infancy and early childhood. There may be important loss of sodium and potassium, or even protein. Sometimes, there is impairment of the absorption of specific foods. For example, fat absorption is reduced in coeliac disease; this results in reduced absorption also of the fat-soluble vitamins.

See also: Absorption of fat; Digestibility; Digestive juices; Water

Absorption of fat

Fat is absorbed by the intestinal villi, the tiny threadlike projections of the lining membrane (mucosa) of the small intestine. They contain blood vessels that run from the base of each villus towards its tip and then back again. In addition, the villus contains a lymph vessel with its blind end near the tip.

The fat (triglyceride) in the intestine has been emulsified with the aid of the bile salts, and then hydrolysed so as to yield monoglycerides, diglycerides, fatty acids and glycerol. These products are absorbed through the wall of the villi, where they are re-synthesized into triglycerides, in which the fatty acids are rearranged on the glycerol so that the resulting fat is chemically nearer to that of the human body. The fat now appears in the lacteal as tiny droplets called chylomicrons, and is passed along the lymphatic system as chyle, and so into the subclavian veins.

See also: Bile; Hydrolysis

Acidosis

A change towards acidity in the normal balance between acidity and alkalinity in the blood and tissues of the body, acidosis should not be confused with acidity. The balance is normally very slightly alkaline, that is, just on the alkaline side of being neutral. This can best be expressed in terms of pH. A pH of 7.0 is exactly neutral; anything below 7.0 is acid, and anything above 7.0 is alkaline. The normal pH of the blood is 7.4, and there are very sensitive systems in the body that keep it at, or very near, that level by adjusting the amount of carbon dioxide (which is acid) and of bicarbonate (which is alkaline) in the blood.

Acid is formed when protein-rich foods are metabolized, and alkaline when fruit or vegetables are metabolized. This is true even if acid fruits are eaten, which contain one or more of a variety of acids and their salts. Oranges, lemons, grapefruit, pineapple and many berries contain citric acid; apples and plums malic acid; strawberries, rhubarb and tomatoes oxalic acid; grapes tartaric acid. Tartaric acid and oxalic acid are not well absorbed, and those that are, are readily oxidized in the body. As a result, they do not cause acidosis, but the salts of these acids leave an alkaline residue.

If acids tend to accumulate in the blood, more carbon dioxide (CO_2) than usual is expelled from the lungs, and more acid is excreted in the urine. If there is a tendency for the blood to become alkaline, the opposite occurs. It is mostly in particular disease conditions that the normal compensatory mechanisms are insufficient to prevent a significant reduction in pH, and true acidosis arises with a fall in pH to 7.2 or lower.

The chief acids that cause acidosis are lactic acid, and acetoacetic and beta-hydroxybutyric acids. Lactic acid tends to accumulate after strenuous exercise, and is the chief reason for the continued and rapid deep breathing for a time after the exercise ceases; the extra carbon dioxide expired in this way helps to bring the body's pH back to normal. Importantly, however, lactic acid occurs in severe heart failure, when the body is unable to get enough oxygen to the tissues.

The accumulation of acetoacetic acid and beta-hydroxybutyric acids occurs during the incomplete metabolism of fat, and is thus associated with ketosis.

See also: Ketosis; pH

Acne

The common form that mostly affects adolescents is *acne vulgaris*. It is an extremely common skin condition, showing itself mostly on the face and chest. Usually it appears in a mild form, consisting of so-called blackheads (comedos) in the middle of a small circle of slightly raised or reddened skin. The blackhead is composed of a plug of the oily sebum from the sebaceous gland in a hair follicle, covered with some keratin, the dry outer layer of the skin. Occasionally these areas become infected, and may then leave permanent scars. Even when the condition is only mild, many young people feel that it is disfiguring. It usually disappears when puberty and growth are complete.

There is a common belief that acne is caused or aggravated by particular foods. Sweets and especially chocolate are the items mostly incriminated, but this has little scientific support. However, since any sensible dietary recommendation for health would include a low consumption of these items, it is certainly appropriate to recommend it for the acne sufferer.

See also: Skin

Acute

Of rapid onset, and usually lasting a short time: the opposite of chronic. This is a term mostly used in relation to illness. It does not refer to severity, although it is often used colloquially to mean 'severe'.

Addiction

True addiction for a substance, usually a drug, has four characteristics:

(1) an uncontrollable desire or craving;
(2) increasing tolerance, so that more and more is necessary in order to produce the same effects;
(3) physical or psychological dependence;
(4) harmful effects on the individual and on society.

The craving may be so great as to tempt the addict into crime in order to obtain the material. The increasing tolerance may eventually lead to the intake of an amount of a drug that would be more than enough to kill a non-addict. Dependence occurs because the body's chemistry is changed, so that the chemical balance is disturbed when the material is no longer taken. This leads to withdrawal symptoms which may be extremely unpleasant. The harmful effects of addiction can be both on the physical health of the individual, and on his personality.

'Addiction' is sometimes used to refer to a strong desire for taking sugar, or caffeine in tea or coffee, or alcohol. However, the craving for an item in which some but not all of the features of addiction are present is more correctly described as habituation. But the demarcation is not always clear. For example, the craving for the caffeine in tea or coffee, or in cola nuts or maté, does not ordinarily result in withdrawal symptoms, although there are reports that people who drink as many as 12 or 15 cups of strong coffee a day do suffer from headaches and sleepiness for a week or so if they suddenly stop taking coffee.

Whether a craving is habituation or addiction depends partly on the individual as well as on the substance. The best known example of the former is with alcohol. Some people drink only when a companion does so. Others, who are in the habit of 'taking a drink' each evening, may be a little unhappy if they do not get it; nevertheless, they do not suffer unbearably without it. At the other extreme, there are those who are defined as alcoholics, who insist on drinking a great deal each day and suffer badly if they suddenly stop drinking.

Whereas this whole range of individual reactions occurs with alcohol, it does not occur with morphine or heroin. Anyone who has either of these regularly for quite a short while will become an addict. A craving for sugar is probably in most people habituation, although the recent evidence that sugar may in some people produce significantly increased secretion of hormones may point to a degree of true addiction in such susceptible individuals.

See also: Alcoholism; Caffeine; Sugar

Adrenal glands

These are also called suprarenal glands or suprarenal capsules. They are two small bodies, one situated on top of each kidney. Each gland is made up of two quite different tissues. The inner part is the adrenal medulla, and is really part of the involuntary nervous system, the autonomic system. It produces two hormones, adrenaline and noradrenaline. (In the US, these are called epinephrine and norepinephrine.) The outer part of each gland is the adrenal cortex, which has nothing to do with the nervous system. This produces three groups of hormones:

(1) cortico-steroids, the best known being hydrocortisone;
(2) aldosterones, concerned chiefly with the balance between body water and salt;
(3) male and female sex hormones, although these are produced in far greater quantities by the testes and the ovaries.

See also: Hormones

Aerobic/Anaerobic

In the body, energy is ultimately produced by aerobic means, in which materials such as glucose and fat are oxidized by the oxygen brought to the cells from the lungs by the blood. However, the first stages of energy release are anaerobic, consisting chiefly of the conversion of glucose to lactic acid which requires no oxygen. This is followed by the aerobic phase, in which the lactic acid is oxidized.

During strenuous physical activity, the anaerobic phase proceeds fast enough to lead to an accumulation of lactic acid; when this activity ceases, the aerobic phase continues. It is this that is responsible for the continuing deep and rapid breathing during recovery from strenuous exercise. In other words, the exercise is accompanied by the building up of an oxygen debt, which is repaid during the period when increased respiration continues after the activity.

Another use of the words 'aerobic' and 'anaerobic' is in referring to the lifestyle of bacteria and other micro-organisms. Some require oxygen for their growth, and these are called aerobic. Those that can live without oxygen are anaerobic; they may be strict anaerobes, so that they cannot survive in the presence of oxygen, or they may be facultative anaerobes which can live with or without oxygen. Food which is not protected in some way will become infected with bacteria and yeast; the extent to which these are aerobes or strict or facultative anaerobes depends on the extent to which the food is exposed to the air rather than being tightly covered.

See also: Acidosis; Bacteria; Fermentation

Aflatoxins

These are highly poisonous substances formed by the growth of moulds, usually *Aspergillus flavus*, on groundnuts, cereals and some other foods, when these are harvested and stored in humid conditions. They were first recognized in 1960 in the UK, following an outbreak of fatal liver disease in turkey poults fed with contaminated groundnuts. In 1974 an outbreak of acute jaundice, with a high mortality, occurred among the inhabitants of some Indian villages, and this was attributed to the consumption of contaminated maize. It has been suggested that aflotoxins may be a cause of primary cancer of the liver, which is seen in Africa and Asia; this condition is rare in other parts of the world, where cancer of the liver is usually caused by secondary deposits originating elsewhere in the body.

See also: Food spoilage; Fungi; Poisons in food

Agar

Also known as agar-agar, this is produced from some species of seaweed and used as a vegetable gelling agent. Like gelatin, it dissolves in hot water and sets when it cools, so long as its concentration is above 0.5%. It is used as an alternative to gelatin in many of the same foods, that is, in jams, jellies, sweets and other foods where a jelly is required, or in ice cream, mayonnaise and soups, where only thickening is needed. Since, unlike gelatin, it is not derived from an animal source, agar is especially sought after by vegetarians and by observant Jews.

Chemically, it is a polysaccharide called a galactan, i.e. a polymer made up of galactose units. It is not digested in the alimentary canal, although some very small quantities might be broken down by the bacteria in the large intestine and release some galactose which can be absorbed; for this reason, it may cause symptoms in people with galactosaemia.

Agar is used in microbiological laboratories in making culture media that set, and on which bacterial colonies may be grown.

See also: Alginates; Gelatin

Ageing

Ageing of flour: Freshly milled flour does not make very good bread. When it is stored for some weeks, the flour becomes whiter and the bread made from it rises more; the technical term for these changes is that the flour is 'bleached' and 'improved'. Commercially, it is disadvantageous to have to wait for several weeks for this to happen, because this would necessitate having a large stock of flour carefully stored. However, the process can be accelerated by the addition of chlorine dioxide, which both bleaches and improves the flour.

Nitrogen trichloride, known as agene, was previously the most commonly used bleach and improver. It was, however, banned after it was discovered that dogs fed flour treated with large amounts of agene developed a neurological condition known as canine hysteria. It later turned out that dogs are much more susceptible to agenized flour than are human beings and most other species. Nevertheless, agene is still not allowed in the treatment of flour in the UK.

Ageing of wine: In some wines, increased storage time leads to an improvement in acceptability and attractiveness, both in taste and in smell, but this may later proceed to deterioration. The changes are due partly to oxidation, which at first removes some of the harsher taste, and partly to the development of new substances from the alcohol, which change both the bouquet and the taste.

See also: Wine

Albumin

Albumin is a protein that is soluble in water and is coagulated when a solution is boiled. The two best-known albumins are those in egg white and in blood plasma. The former coagulates not only when boiled; it also coagulates when it is beaten in air. It then makes a froth in which tiny air bubbles are enclosed by thin walls of coagulated albumin. The albumin in the blood cannot pass through the walls of the capillaries as can the smaller molecules such as salt and glucose; as a result, the albumin is the chief substance that determines the osmotic pressure of plasma, thus maintaining the blood volume.

Albumin, usually spelt 'albumen', was formerly used as a general word for protein. This usage is now obsolete.

See also: Eggs; Lymphatic system; Osmotic pressure

Alcohol

The alcohols form a group of chemical substances of a similar structure, which for example can combine with acids to make new compounds called esters. Used by itself, the word 'alcohol' refers to ethyl alcohol, also known as ethanol, with the formula C_2H_5OH. It is formed by the fermentation of glucose or other sugars by yeasts. The process of making alcoholic beverages was, it seems, discovered in pre-historic times independently in different parts of the world, presumably by the observation of fermentation that occurred in ripe fruits. Later, fermentation was found to occur also in cooked cereals.

Since the oxidation of alcohol in the body releases energy, it is classed as a food; 1g yields 7 kcal. It has, however, several unusual features. Firstly, it can be absorbed very readily from the stomach; other food constituents are not absorbed until they reach the intestine. Secondly, it is not possible to reduce the rate of absorption except slightly, for example by drinking milk before taking the alcohol. Thirdly, its rate of oxidation and so of energy release is almost constant; it is not affected either by the amount in the blood or by the amount of physical activity. As far as is known, the only way in which the rate of oxidation can be affected is by the consumption of fructose, which may increase it by about 20%. The excretion of the alcohol by the breath and in the urine is small, but since it is proportional to the amount in the blood, the simple measurement of alcohol in breath or urine is a convenient way of assessing the amount of alcohol consumed in a given time.

The rate at which the body oxidizes alcohol depends chiefly on the weight of the individual. An average man of 65kg can oxidize about 6g of alcohol in an hour, so that it will take some 5 hours to oxidize 30ml; as the Table indicates, this is the quantity in 100ml of whisky or other spirits, 300ml of table wine, or 1 litre of average beer.

The oxidation of ethanol in the body cannot be used directly for muscular activity. It does, however, reduce the amount of carbohydrate and fat that needs to be oxidized for other purposes, so that it could contribute to the excessive energy intake that gives rise to obesity.

Although people react in varying ways to the consumption of alcohol, there is measurable impairment in judgement and co-ordination when the blood concentration reaches 40mg/100ml, and obvious intoxication when it reaches 100mg/100ml. The latter would occur if 3 pints of beer were drunk within an hour by a man of 65kg. In the UK, a blood concentration of 80mg/100ml is the legal limit above which a car driver can be prosecuted for being under the influence of alcohol.

As well as its effect on the central nervous system, alcohol causes a dilatation of the skin capillaries, and makes one feel warm. Since, however, this increases the loss of heat from the body, it can be dangerous to take alcohol during exposure to the cold, but it may safely be taken on returning to a warm environment.

The concentration of alcohol in a beverage may be expressed in several ways. The three commonest are volume of alcohol in 100ml beverage, weight of alcohol in 100ml beverage, and percentage of proof spirit. The last method was introduced long before modern methods were available. Proof spirit was defined as a distillate that contained just enough alcohol to allow the ignition of gunpowder mixed with it. In the UK, this is now defined as 57.07% by volume, or 49.24% by weight; in the US, proof spirit is 50% by volume.

Alcohol consumption in the UK has been falling for the last 200–300 years, except for a rise with the prosperity of the late nineteenth century, and a smaller rise since 1950 or so. By 1980 alcohol was supplying on average about 6% of total calories. However, since babies take no alcohol and children and many adults little if any, average figures are not very meaningful.

Fermentation itself produces a concentration of alcohol of at most 13g/100ml; at this concentration the action of yeast is inhibited. Beverages containing more than this amount of alcohol can be made only by distillation, or by the addition of such distilled products to wine or other beverages.

ALCOHOL IN SOME BEVERAGES
(*grams in 100ml*)

Typical values

BEER
Mild ale	3.0
Strong ale	6.5

CIDER
Ordinary cider	3.5
Strong cider	10.0

WINES
Table wine (white or red)	10.0
Fortified wine (port and sherry)	16.0

SPIRITS (*70% UK proof*)
Brandy, gin, whisky	31.0

See also: Absorption; Beer; Fermentation

Alcoholism

Alcoholics may suffer from a variety of clinical conditions. One of the best known is cirrhosis of the liver. Several other conditions, however, are, at least in part, caused by a deficiency of thiamin (vitamin B_1). The association of this deficiency with a prolonged high intake of alcohol is probably due to several factors. One is that the high energy content of the alcohol reduces the intake of other foods, at least some of which would have provided thiamin. A second factor is that, as deficiency of thiamin develops, anorexia is produced, and this is aggravated by the anorexia caused by the chronic gastritis that accompanies high alcohol intake. Thirdly, alcohol itself may cause a higher demand for thiamin, as does dietary carbohydrate.

One or more of the effects of this deficiency are as follows:

(1) The production of straightforward wet or dry beri-beri.
(2) Alcoholic polyneuropathy, sometimes called alcoholic polyneuritis, which affects the motor and sensory nerves of the limbs, especially the legs. This results in pain, sometimes in the form of severe pins and needles, and in addition there is paralysis with muscle wasting.
(3) Wernicke's encephalopathy: this is a neurological condition with weakness of the eye muscles and unsteadiness of gait (ataxia). Chronic alcoholism is not, however, the only cause of Wernicke's encephalopathy. It has also been reported in persons who have undergone prolonged fasting, for example on a hunger strike.
(4) Korsakoff's syndrome: this shows itself as a severe loss of memory for recent events, but not for past events. It responds only slowly and partly to thiamin therapy.

Both Korsakoff's syndrome and Wernicke's encephalopathy are accompanied by severe destruction of brain tissue; which of the two conditions becomes manifest presumably depends on which areas of the brain tissue are most affected.

See also: Alcohol; Beri-beri; Vitamin B_1

Algae (singular: alga)

These are plants that have no differentiated root, stem or leaf. They range from microscopic single-cell organisms to large seaweeds. They contain chlorophyll, but may have other pigments in addition, so that not all of them are green in appearance. Like all plants with chlorophyll, they obtain their energy for growth by photosynthesis. It has been suggested that some of the algae, notably the single-celled varieties *Chlorella* and *Spirulina*, could be used for the production of human protein-rich food, but no successful commercial production has yet emerged.

See also: Alginates; Novel protein

Alginates

These are made from seaweed, and consist of salts of alginic acid with sodium, potassium, calcium, magnesium and other ions. They form viscous solutions and are used by food manufacturers as emulsifiers, thickeners and jelling agents in such foods as salad cream, ice cream, processed cheese, artificial cream and instant puddings. Like cellulose, they are not digested, but pass straight out of the body with the faeces.

See also: Agar; Algae; Food additives

Alkaloid

There is a varied collection of organic substances found in plants that have an action on the body, often a potent action. Although they are all called alkaloids, they have little in common chemically except that they contain nitrogen and are basic, that is, they combine with acids. They are not soluble in water, but are soluble in a variety of organic solvents such as ether and chloroform. The best known examples are nicotine, morphine and strychnine.

See also: Cocoa/Chocolate

Allergy

A person who reacts to a drug or a food or to pollen or dust to a degree that far exceeds the way most other people react is referred to as being hypersensitive. Although many lay people use the word 'allergy' to describe this condition, allergy strictly speaking is a special sort of hypersensitivity in which the offending agent is a protein. Someone who cannot take moderate amounts of milk because of the lactose it contains has lactose intolerance; if, on the other hand, the hypersensitivity to milk is due to its protein, then the individual is likely to be allergic.

The commonest foods to which some people are allergic are milk, eggs, fish (especially shellfish), wheat, strawberries, nuts and chocolate. Some food additives also produce allergic reactions; those most frequently involved are tartrazine (a yellow dye), BHT and BPA (antioxidants), and penicillin and tetracycline (antibiotics). The substance responsible is called an allergen, and is either a protein or is bound to a protein. The adverse effects are caused by a reaction between the allergen and an antibody in the tissues, which releases histamine and other irritant and damaging substances into the bloodstream. Typical allergic reactions include tingling and swelling of the lips, urticaria (nettle rash), asthma, dyspepsia, vomiting and diarrhoea. The reactions, however, vary from person to person; moreover, an individual sensitive to more than one substance may respond differently to each of them.

Sometimes the offending food is obvious, sometimes it is very difficult to discover. A careful record of the diet and of the occurrence of the symptoms may be sufficient; otherwise it may be necessary to use elimination diets, in which likely foods are excluded one by one. Since some people develop a psychological aversion from particular foods, even to the extent of developing symptoms, the elimination tests may have to have the suspected food or the placebo food administered by naso-gastric tube.

Infants often grow out of allergies to the commoner foods. Children and adults should avoid for some years, if possible, the food or foods to which they are allergic, and may then try to take them in small quantities, to see if they have lost their sensitivity. Unlike hay fever, food allergies are not easily cured by desensitization.

It seems that about 5–10% of people show allergy to one or more foods, and that the tendency to develop this condition is to some extent inherited. Claims that a large proportion of the population is affected, and that a large number of foods can produce allergic reactions, have not been substantiated.

There is no acceptable evidence that food allergy is responsible for several sorts of psychological disturbance such as hyperactivity, depression and schizophrenia, as has been suggested.

A detailed research study showed that only 1 in 6 of a group of people claiming to be allergic to one or more foods could be confirmed as having true allergy. Of the remainder, a large proportion was found to have a variety of complaints not known to be associated with allergy. Moreover, carefully controlled tests did not support their belief that they were sensitive to particular foods. Finally, whereas none of those with demonstrable food allergy had any detectable psychiatric symptoms, almost all those in whom food allergy was not confirmed suffered from depression or anxiety or some other neurosis.

See also: Food additives; Lactose intolerance

Aluminium

There is an abundance of aluminium in the soil, but only very little finds its way into plants and animals. As a result, the amount that accumulates in the human body comes to only about 0.1g. Aluminium does not have any known biological function. Because it is so insoluble, practically none is taken up into food that has been cooked in aluminium vessels.

The compound of aluminium, aluminium hydroxide, is used in medicine as an antacid in the treatment of indigestion associated with the presence of an excess of hydrochloric acid in the stomach. Another use of aluminium hydroxide is in the treatment of patients undergoing dialysis. One of the hazards of dialysis is the accumulation of too much phosphate in the blood; this can be prevented if a small amount of aluminium hydroxide is added to the dialysis fluid. This, however, may produce another hazard, since an excessive amount of aluminium may accumulate in the blood and this produces both absorption of bone and damage to the brain.

See also: Dialysis; Mineral elements

Amino-acids

These are chemical compounds that form the constituent units making up a protein. There are 20 common amino-acids. When different numbers of molecules of some or all of them are joined together to make long chains, with the various amino-acids in different positions in the chains, different proteins are formed with a wide range of properties.

The combination of the amino-acids with one another occurs because of their characteristic feature, which is the possession of both an acidic and basic (alkaline) part of their molecules. It is this feature that enables them to join together to form protein, the acid part of one amino-acid molecule joining up with the basic part of another, and the repetition of this to involve from 50 to several hundred amino-acid units.

Animals cannot synthesize the amino group that is one of the characteristic features of all amino-acids; plants do this from the nitrogen they pick up from the soil. What animals can do, however, is to take the amino group from one amino-acid and put it on to some other substance in the body and so manufacture a different amino-acid. They can do this with all but 8 of the amino-acids; these have to be supplied to the body from the proteins in food, and consequently they are called the essential amino-acids. During the rapid growth of infants and children, a ninth amino-acid, histidine, is also needed in the diet since its manufacture in the body does not keep pace with the body's needs.

As well as joining together to form the very many kinds of protein present in the body, some amino-acids have additional characteristics.

Phenylalanine can be converted into the hormones adrenaline and thyroxine.

Tryptophan can be converted into the vitamin nicotinic acid; this conversion is not very efficient, however, so that 60mg of tryptophan produces only 1mg of the vitamin.

There are two amino-acids that contain sulphur in their mole-

AMINO-ACIDS

NON-ESSENTIAL	ESSENTIAL
Alanine	Isoleucine
Arginine	Leucine
Aspartic acid	Lysine
Cysteine	Methionine
Glutamic acid	Phenylalanine
Glycine	Threonine
Hydroxyproline	Tryptophan
Ornithine	Valine
Proline	Histidine*
Serine	
Tyrosine	

* Histidine is essential for infants and children.

cules; these are cysteine and methionine. Methionine is an essential amino-acid, but cysteine is not, since the body can make it from methionine.

Glutamic acid is not an essential amino-acid. It is interesting because its salt, monosodium glutamate, has the property of enhancing the flavours of other goods, as well as having a slight meaty flavour of its own. It is therefore widely used in cooking and in food manufacture. It occurs in meat gravies, but is usually manufactured from wheat gluten or from beet pulp.

See also: Proteins

Anaemia

The normal quantity of haemoglobin, the red pigment in the blood, is about 16g/100ml for men, about 15g/100ml for women, and rather less for children up to the age of 6. According to WHO standards, anaemia is present when the concentrations are below those shown in the Table.

Mild anaemia may be accompanied by few symptoms, except perhaps a degree of lassitude and weakness. More severe anaemia involves more pronounced weakness, with shortness of breath from exertion; the lips and everted eyelid may be extremely pale, and the heart rate is raised. It is, however, misleading to diagnose mild degrees of anaemia by pallor; British children classified as pale were found to have the same concentration of haemoglobin as those who were not noticeably pale.

The haemoglobin is contained entirely within the red blood corpuscles (erythrocytes). These have a limited life of about 120 days, after which they disintegrate. The broken-down components of the erythrocytes are to a large extent conserved and used towards the construction of the new erythrocytes and their haemoglobin, which are constantly being manufactured in the bone marrow.

There are three reasons why anaemia may occur:

(1) Blood may be lost, i.e. haemorrhage may occur.
(2) The red blood cells may be breaking down faster than usual, at a rate greater than that by which they can be replaced.
(3) There may be faults in the manufacture of the erythrocytes, or of the haemoglobin, or of both. Some of these faults may be nutritional.

The amount of haemoglobin in the blood is assessed with an instrument that simply measures the depth of red colour. The number of red blood corpuscles (RBC) is counted under the microscope in a specially graduated chamber; nowadays this is done automatically with an instrument called the Coulter counter.

Nutritional anaemia is caused by deficiency of particular nutrients concerned in the production of the red cells or of haemoglobin. Several nutrients are needed to ensure adequate production of red cells. Impairment is almost always due to deficiency of folate or of vitamin B_{12}. It shows itself in the occurrence of immature blood cells (megaloblasts) and the red cells are larger than usual (macrocytes), as if the bone marrow is putting as much haemoglobin as possible into each of the limited number of red cells. This type of anaemia is therefore usually called megaloblastic, or less commonly macrocytic.

The commonest limitation for the production of haemoglobin is the shortage of iron. Mostly this is a primary iron deficiency, that is, an inadequate dietary intake of iron. Less commonly, it is due to an impairment in the ability to absorb iron from the alimentary canal. The erythrocytes are smaller and paler than normal. They are not always reduced in number; when, however, the anaemia is very severe, with a haemoglobin level of some 8g/100ml or less, there may be a reduction in cell number, as though the bone marrow does not bother to make more cells since there is so little haemoglobin to go into them. These features lead to the condition being called microcytic hypochromic anaemia.

As well as the usual symptoms of shortage of haemoglobin, the anaemia of iron deficiency is usually accompanied by little or no hydrochloric acid in the gastric juice (hypochlorhydria), which, unlike the achlorhydria of pernicious anaemia, is restored when histamine is administered. The nails are sometimes spoon-shaped and the tongue may be exceptionally smooth.

Deficiency of vitamin B_{12} in the diet is rare. More commonly, deficiency occurs because of a failure to absorb the vitamin. This results in pernicious anaemia. Before 1926, the disease was invariably fatal. As well as the extreme anaemia, with haemoglobin values as low as 3g/100ml or even lower, there occurs a neurological condition known as sub-acute combined degeneration of the cord (SACD). This begins with unsteadiness, and with numbness and a sensation of pins and needles in the hands and especially in the feet. There is slow and continuing deterioration until the individual becomes bedridden. It is still not known why deficiency of vitamin B_{12} causes the degeneration of some of the nerve tracts in the spinal cord responsible for this condition, other than that the vitamin is needed for the production and integrity of the myelin sheath of the nerve fibres. The anaemia and the SACD are always accompanied by a complete absence of acid in the gastric secretion (achlorhydria), even after administration of histamine.

In 1926, it was shown that pernicious anaemia could be alleviated by the consumption of liver. It is now known that the vitamin B_{12} that occurs in some foods, notably meat, fish and milk, usually requires for its absorption a substance present in the gastric juice; the former used to be called 'extrinsic factor' and the latter 'intrinsic factor'. Liver contains a high concentration of vitamin B_{12}, and so enough is absorbed, even without the intrinsic factor, to cure pernicious anaemia.

Deficiency of folic acid produces a megaloblastic anaemia exactly similar to that seen in pernicious anaemia, but without the neurological effects.

CONCENTRATION OF HAEMOGLOBIN BELOW WHICH ANAEMIA CAN BE DIAGNOSED

		g/100ml blood
CHILDREN	6 months to 6 years	11
	6 years to 12 years	12
ADULTS	Men	13
	Women	12
	Pregnant women	11

See also: Folic acid; Iron; Liver; Vitamin B_{12}

Anatto

Made from the seed pods of a small plant, *Bixa orellana*, grown in the Caribbean, this yellow substance is chemically similar to carotene. It is permitted as an additive to cheese and butter, but not to margarine in the UK. It is not the same as the dye, butter yellow, which is now not allowed since it has been discovered to cause cancer.

See also: Butter; Carotene; Cheese; Food additives

Anorectic agents

Since overweight is so common in Western countries, and since many people find it difficult to reduce their food intake in order to reduce their body weight, drugs have been introduced for the purpose of reducing the desire for food; these are the anorectic agents or, as they are sometimes called, appetite suppressants.

They fall into two categories:

(1) substances that increase the volume of the stomach contents;
(2) substances that affect the 'appetite' centre in the brain, specifically by inhibiting the activity of the lateral hypothalamus.

The most commonly used 'stomach fillers' are cellulose derivatives such as methylcellulose. Guar gum may also be used; this is a polymer of the sugars galactose and mannose, in the same way that cellulose is a polymer of glucose. Fairly large doses of such materials are needed if they are to be effective – at least 10g a day.

Amphetamines were the first anorectic drugs to be described. The best known is Dexedrine, a brand name for dexamphetamine. This, however, is no longer used to any extent because it is a stimulant and causes irritability and sleeplessness and often leads to dependence. Several derivatives of the original amphetamines are now available, which retain the anorectic effect but have little or no stimulatory effect. Examples are diethylpropion and fenfluramine. There are also some drugs that are not derivatives of amphetamines; one well-known such drug is mazindol. Diethylpropion and mazindol do produce some stimulation of the central nervous system (CNS); fenfluramine on the other hand is mildly sedative.

Anorectic drugs should always be used in conjunction with a diet of reduced caloric content, and it should be stressed to the patient that they are aids to such a diet and not a substitute for it. Patients should be warned too that the anorectic effect of the drugs is likely to diminish after a few weeks; they should therefore consider them as temporary 'crutches' to help them get used to new eating habits, rather than for use as a continuing treatment for their obesity.

See also: Appetite; Guar gum; Obesity

Anorexia nervosa

Anorexia is the technical name for loss of appetite. The first description of the disease anorexia nervosa was given in a book published in Latin by Richard Morton in 1689: it appeared in an English translation in 1694 as *Phthisiologia or, a treatise of consumptions*. As its title indicates, it was concerned largely with what later became known as phthisis or pulmonary tuberculosis, or simply as consumption. Yet the first two cases described, with the chief feature a wasting without fever, were clearly what we now know as anorexia nervosa. One of the two young people described was a man, which is interesting in view of the current much commoner occurrence in young women.

The three features that characterize the disease are the profound fear of becoming fat, excessive loss of weight, and amenorrhoea or loss of libido. The disease occurs mostly in the wealthier countries and in the upper and middle socio-economic groups. Some 90% or more of the cases are girls. There is an abnormal interest in food, expressed for example in a considerable knowledge of nutritional values, and a lively interest in cooking.

The term anorexia, suggesting a loss of appetite, is not entirely appropriate; it is rather that the subject fears the consequences of satisfying her appetite. Her self-image is distorted in that, although obviously thin, she will insist that she is too fat. Characteristically, the subject with anorexia nervosa is of a quiet disposition, somewhat introverted, ambitious, but of low self-esteem.

The thinness is not accompanied by atrophy of the breasts, and there is no loss of pubic or axillary hair; these features distinguish anorexia nervosa from the amenorrhoea of pituitary deficiency.

There is still a great deal of discussion about the cause of the condition. It seems that there is some genetic predisposition, since it is commoner in identical twins than in non-identical. On the other hand, there is no doubt that environmental factors predominate, and especially the interplay of family relationships. The members of the family are often unusually close and interdependent; the mother is somewhat dominant and over-ambitious and demanding of her daughter or son.

Some observers maintain that keeping the body thin expresses a control by the patient that is otherwise excessively in the hands of others, especially her family. Again, it is suggested that the individual with anorexia nervosa seeks to avoid the problems of adolescence and the sometimes traumatic adjustment to becoming adult, by adopting a form of behaviour that helps to delay the physical changes associated with puberty. In other times, and in other cultures, different ways were, and are, adopted in order to postpone or modify the difficult process of adolescence.

It is widely but erroneously believed that anorexia nervosa is a direct result of the now widespread interest and concern in Western cultures about the need to have a slim figure. Many doctors speak of this concern as an obsession, especially of young women. The continual appearance of books and articles about weight reduction, the existence of slimming clubs, the photographs of svelte models, may well suggest a mechanism of escape to the intelligent and ambitious girl of an over-protective family. It is likely that in another age the same girl would have chosen simply to be suffering from chronic neurasthenia, or to have had repeated attacks of the vapours. In this view, the combination of personality and environment that leads to the problems of adjustment in young people is not produced by the obsession about slimming; slimming does, however, offer a convenient and fashionable way of seeking a solution that would otherwise be sought in some other direction.

Treatment is best carried out by psychotherapy, which should include joint sessions with members of the family and especially the mother. Sensible dietary advice must be given at the same time, preferably by co-operation between therapist and dietitian. No special diet is required, but there should be instruction on the sorts of foods, and in what amounts, that will provide nutritional adequacy without caloric excess.

The outlook is usually quite good, although it may take as long as 2–3 years for the individual to be entirely restored to normal dietary habits. In very rare cases, however, the loss of weight continues, and death results, usually from superimposed infection.

See also: Appetite; Obesity; Puberty

Anthropometry

Nutritionists frequently measure body size, such as height and weight, in order to gain information about nutritional status. Although the measurements seem simple, care is necessary in making them. Spring balances not checked and calibrated at weekly intervals may be grossly inaccurate; on the other hand, scales with beams are usually accurate for periods of over a year or more, but must be used with care if reliable readings are to be obtained.

In adults, measurements of height and weight are used mostly to determine whether an individual weighs too little or too much. It should, however, be said that experts do not always agree on the precise standards for weight in relation to height.

Growth of children is determined by several factors, including heredity, repeated acute diseases, chronic infection, and diseases such as hormonal imbalance. Growth is also affected by diet, but nutritional status is unlikely to be revealed for a particular child from measurements made only at one particular time. A useful pointer nevertheless would be that restricted growth in stature could arise from chronic under-nutrition, while an unexpectedly low weight could arise from short-term under-nutrition. But rates of growth, made by measurements repeated at intervals, are better indicators of nutritional status, especially if there is also a record of previous illness. Similarly, comparisons of groups of children of the same age may give useful clues as to different nutritional experiences among the groups.

Children and adults of the poorer countries are on average shorter and lighter than those of the wealthier countries. But the reasons for this are not, or not entirely, genetic. Studies of the descendants of immigrant Japanese now living in Hawaii and the west coast of the US show that they are taller and heavier than their compatriots still living in Japan, indicating that the environment – perhaps the poorer diet and greater exposure to disease – was mostly responsible for their small size in Japan. Meanwhile, the average size of the Japanese in their own homeland has increased during the last quarter of a century, presumably because of improved living standards, including nutrition.

The question is often discussed whether adults are now taller than they were in earlier generations. There are in fact few reliable data; the most revealing are those collected since 1851 on the height of conscripts by the authorities in the Netherlands. These figures suggest that between 1865 and 1975, the average height of 18-year-old conscripts has increased by 15cm (nearly 6 inches). In the first half of this period the increase was chiefly in those of smaller stature, suggesting that it was poor nutrition and other socio-economic conditions that had been at least partly responsible for their small stature; increased prosperity has helped them to grow towards their genetic potential. Since 1900 the increase in stature has affected young men over the whole range of heights to about the same degree. Moreover, average height is still increasing, 2.7cm having been added between 1965 and 1975. The reason for this is not known.

See also: Obesity

Antibiotics

Antibiotics can affect the diet in three ways. Firstly, for reasons that are still not clear, minute amounts of penicillin, terramycin and some other antibiotics in the feed can increase the growth of non-ruminant farm animals, such as chickens and pigs. The residue of antibiotics in the meat of these animals is minute, so that 1kg of their meat would contribute at most 1mg, which is about one thousandth of the daily medicinal dose. Secondly, some antibiotics added to food can act as a preservative; in the UK the only antibiotic permitted to be used in this way is nisin, which is in fact not used in medicine. Thirdly, the treatment of cows with penicillin for mastitis results in some of the antibiotic appearing in the milk, and this may interfere with the growth of the micro-organisms necessary for the souring of the milk in cheesemaking.

See also: Food additives

Anticaking agents

To ensure that powders remain free-flowing, anticaking agents are sometimes added. Examples are calcium silicate added to baking powder or to salt, and disodium hydrogen phosphate added to salt or sugar.

See also: Food additives

Antimycotics

Substances that retard the growth of moulds. They include sorbic acid, proprionic acid, and benzoic acid. In the UK, sorbic acid is allowed in cheese, proprionic acid in bread, and benzoic acid in drinking chocolate and fruit juices.

See also: Food additives

Antioxidants

The quality of some foods is prone to deteriorate through oxidation. It is, then, desirable to add to them substances that prevent or retard the oxidation. These antioxidants fall into two groups: those soluble in water and those soluble in fat. An example of the former is ascorbic acid (vitamin C), which prevents the darkening of peeled vegetables such as potatoes or of cut fruits such as apples, apricots, bananas, peaches or pears. More commonly used are the fat-soluble anti-oxidants, which retard the development of rancidity in fats and oils. A natural antioxidant is tocopherol (vitamin E), which occurs in some vegetable oils but may be added to any food; others are BHT (butylated hydroxyanisole) (E320) and BHA (butylated hydroxytoluene) (E321), which are permitted to be added to any edible oil or fat, except butter sold retail.

Another way in which oxidative rancidity may be retarded is by removing some of the small quantities of salts often present in fats and oils. These salts, usually of copper, molybdenum or nickel, increase the susceptibility of the fat to oxidation, but only when the salts are ionized; ionization can, however, be prevented by what are called sequestrants, or chelating agents. They work by forming a non-ionizable complex with the metal ion. The commonest sequestrants are citric acid and the amino-acid glycine.

Sequester is from a Latin word meaning to hold for safe-keeping; chelate from *chela*, the Greek word for a claw like that of a crab.

See also: Food additives

Antistaling agents

The keeping quality of bread and cakes may be increased by the addition of substances such as glyceryl monostearate or sucrose stearate.

See also: Food additives

Antivitamins

Food sometimes contains substances that significantly reduce the amount of a vitamin in the diet, or significantly increase the amount of the vitamin the body requires. This can happen in several ways, as the following examples show:

(1) In the 1930s, a disease occurred in a silver fox farm in the US owned by a Mr Chastek. It resulted in paralysis and death among the foxes. This was traced to the consumption of the raw fish that constituted a large part of their diet. 'Chastek's paralysis' turned out to be a sort of beri-beri, caused by an enzyme, thiaminase, in the raw fish, which destroyed the thiamin in the diet.

(2) Sweet clover disease in cattle was also described in the US. It was caused by the production in spoiled sweet clover of a substance, coumarin, which acts as an antagonist to vitamin K. Such vitamin K antagonists are used in medicine to reduce an excessive tendency of the blood to clot. They act in a sort of dog-in-the-manger manner. Their molecules are similar to those of vitamin K, so that they get to the part of the cell where the vitamin would go, and prevent the vitamin itself from getting there. But as they do not have exactly the same molecular structure as the vitamin has, they cannot carry out its function.

(3) Biotin is a vitamin for some species of animals, including man. Deficiency of biotin occurs, however, only in the most unusual circumstances, namely when the diet contains large quantities of raw eggs. This is because egg white contains a substance, avidin, which combines with biotin so that the vitamin cannot be absorbed. This property of avidin is lost when eggs are cooked.

See also: Avidin; Beri-beri; Biotin; Vitamin K

Appetite

The word 'appetite' is frequently used as a synonym for hunger, to indicate a general desire for food. For example, experiments with animals, in which damage to special localized parts of the brain result either in a voracious consumption of food or the virtual cessation of eating, are said to demonstrate different parts of the appetite centre. Again, drugs used in the treatment of obesity, which reduce the desire to eat, are called appetite suppressants or anorectic agents.

It is, however, important to distinguish between appetite and hunger, although both represent a drive towards food consumption. Appetite is a pleasant sensation, often accompanied by salivation, aroused by the sight or smell or even the thought of particular foods or drinks. Hunger is an unpleasant or painful sensation, and is directed towards food in general; its arousal does not require the presence of any food, although it is often accompanied by thoughts of food the individual considers attractive or 'appetizing'.

Hunger is an expression of the body's need to replenish its energy supplies; appetite is an expression of the wish to experience the pleasurable sensations that accompany or follow the consumption of specially attractive foods or drinks. Having eaten well by the end of the main course, guests at a sumptuous dinner party may feel they can eat no more, but will still happily take the attractive dessert when it appears; even after this, they may offer no resistance to the brandy or liqueurs offered. The consumption of additional calories in this way is an expression of appetite, and certainly not an expression of hunger.

On the other hand, it is not appetite but hunger that will drive a person during a famine to search the gutters for a crust of mouldy bread, or that drove the people of Paris to eat rats when the city was under siege during the Franco-Prussian war.

Appetite and hunger are not only related qualitatively, in that both represent a desire to take food or drink. They are also related quantitatively, in that the more hungry one is, the less does it matter whether the food is appetizing, that is, the smaller is the role of appetite. On the other hand, the less hungry one is, the more does it matter that the food should appeal to the appetite.

See also: Anorectic agents; Anorexia nervosa; Dietary instinct; Obesity

Apples

The characteristic feature of apples, and of pears, is that the fruit, called a pome, is made up of the considerably enlarged wall of the ovary that contains the seeds. Both apples and pears belong to the large family of Rosaceae, which includes not only roses but plums, peaches, apricots, strawberries and raspberries.

The apple has been called the king of fruits. It is frequently used as a paradigm for an attractive fruit, both in legend and in reality. Paris had to decide to whom to give the apple of discord; the true Bible translation of Eve's offering to Adam is 'the fruit of the tree', not an apple; there is no truth in the story that it was a falling apple that drew Newton's attention to gravity. 'Golden apple' is the translation of the Italian word for tomato, and of the Hebrew words for orange. Again, the French, the Dutch and the Israelis use the phrase 'earth apple' for the potato. The tomato has also been known as the 'love apple' because of its supposed aphrodisiac properties.

It is estimated that there are now more than 6,000 varieties of apple being grown, which vary considerably in size, colour, shape and taste. They are all derived from the wild crab apple, *Malus pumila*, which can be found in Europe, Asia and America. Most of the trees of the crab apple now seen are likely to be reversions to the wild type from cultivated varieties.

Apples grow readily in most of the temperate regions of the world. They were available in Roman times, and were probably introduced into America and the Antipodes when these lands were settled by Europeans. Their popularity was largely dependent on their excellent keeping qualities, so that for centuries they were almost the only fruit available in winter in temperate climates; new methods of preservation and transport have reduced this virtual monopoly. Until the seventeenth century there were only two popular varieties grown in Britain. One of these was the costard apple, the word costard being derived from *costa*, the Latin word for rib, thus referring to the ribbed character of the costard apple. In turn, the word 'costermonger' was originally used for the name of the man who sold his apples from a stall or barrow.

Apples, especially crab apples, contain a large amount of pectin. This is a useful stabilizer and emulsifier, but is chiefly used for its setting property in the making of jams and jellies.

Arachidonic acid

One of the fatty acids that occurs mostly in the fat of animals and fish. It is the form in which the essential fatty acids (EFA) act in the body, for example in producing the prostaglandin hormones, which are concerned in a variety of essential bodily processes. However, arach-

idonic acid is not itself essential in the diet because it can be manufactured in the body from the much more plentiful linoleic acid. Both
arachidonic acid and linoleic acid occur in the membranes of the
body's cells.

See also: Essential; Fatty acids

Arthritis

A wide variety of diseases involving the muscles or joints are referred
to as rheumatism; arthritis is the name given to that group of rheumatic diseases characterized by inflammation of one or more joints.
These are often considered by lay people to be one disease with one
cause, but this is not so. They are quite distinct entities, the best
known of which are gout, osteoarthritis and rheumatoid arthritis.
The precise causes of these diseases are not known, although the
causes are not the same for all of them. There is no evidence, either,
that any of them is caused by nutritional deficiency of any kind. There
is therefore no justification for claims that the administration of particular nutrients, such as pyridoxine or selenium, will relieve the
symptoms of 'arthritis'.

Until the introduction of new and highly effective drugs in the
1950s, the chief treatment for gout was by diet. This consisted of the
avoidance of 'organ meats' such as liver and kidneys, the avoidance of
overeating so as to prevent obesity, and the restriction of alcohol.
Physicians are now less insistent on these dietary changes unless for
any reason drugs are not appropriate. There are no dietary regimes
that can be recommended for other forms of arthritis, except a low-
calorie diet for the excessive weight that often accompanies osteoarthritis, especially of the hip.

Some of the arthritic diseases show episodes of spontaneous remission and relapse. This may confuse the assessment of the efficacy of
treatment.

See also: Gout; Remissions and relapses

Atherosclerosis

A condition that affects the arteries in any part of the body. It consists of atheroma, that is, discrete accumulations of fatty material in the lining of the walls of the arteries, and some thickening of the arterial wall itself. One result is that the arteries become harder, so that atherosclerosis is one of the types of arteriosclerosis, or hardening of the arteries; it is also by far the commonest type.

The atheromatous accumulations are called plaques, and are yellowish and irregular, rather like small curds. The word 'atheroma' is derived from the Greek word for porridge. Atheroma consists of a mixture of cholesterol and other fatty materials, complex carbohydrates, blood and fibrous tissue. The plaques tend to grow and to join together. After a time, the atheroma may begin to calcify, and this will be visible in an X-ray photograph.

The effect of these processes will depend not only on the extent of the atheroma, but also on which particular arteries are affected. The most important arteries are the coronary arteries supplying the heart, the arteries supplying the brain and the femoral artery supplying the legs. The conditions that may be produced from severe atheroma of these arteries are coronary heart disease, a stroke, and peripheral vascular disease.

See also: Blood pressure; Coronary heart disease; Fat; Sucrose; Stroke

Atwater, Wilbur Olin (1844–1907)

Born in New York State, Atwater was trained as an engineer but soon became interested in agricultural chemistry. In 1875, he and Dr S. W. Johnson were responsible for the establishment of the first American agricultural research station, at Middletown, Connecticut, where a few years later he demonstrated the 'fixation' of atmospheric nitrogen by leguminous plants. Atwater was also largely responsible for the Hatch Act of 1887, which required every state to support at least one agricultural research station.

In 1877 Atwater visited Voit and Rubner in Germany, and became interested in calorimetry. On his return to Middletown he collaborated with Ross and Benedict to build a calorimeter, with which he was able to demonstrate that the amount of heat produced by the human body was the same as that produced by the oxidation of the food consumed. With Benedict he prepared an elaborate table of the energy value of many foods, and also studied the energy requirements of people carrying out different tasks. He proposed the values of 4, 4, 9 and 7 kcal for the energy released in the body by 1g of protein, carbohydrate, fat or alcohol, which allowed for the energy lost in the urine and faeces; these figures are still known as the Atwater factors. He estimated protein requirements, which he put at 150g a day. His plans to set up an international research programme, relating diet and labour potential, never reached fruition because of his death at the age of sixty-three.

See also: Benedict; Energy content of food; Rubner; Voit

Availability

Foods may contain nutrients that are not absorbed, or not completely absorbed, into the bloodstream and so may not be adequate for the body's cells. Clearly, what is not absorbed is not available to the body. An example is a food that contains calcium and phytin, or contains calcium and is taken with other foods that contain phytin. Another example is the iron in a vegetable food which is available to the extent of perhaps 75%, but when the food is taken with tea, is available to the extent of perhaps only 25%. Because of these sorts of interaction between food constituents, it cannot always be assumed that the amount of a nutrient in a diet demonstrable by analysis represents the true contribution it makes in supplying that nutrient to the body.

See also: Absorption; Calcium; Iron; Phytic acid

Avidin

A small proportion of the protein in egg white is avidin. It is interesting chiefly because it is an antivitamin, since it combines with biotin and so prevents its absorption in the gut. It is destroyed when heated, so egg white interferes with biotin absorption only if it is eaten raw.

See also: Antivitamins; Biotin; Eggs

B

Bacteria

Lay people sometimes wonder about the different words that are used in connection with some micro-organisms. The following description may help to clarify their meaning.

Bacteria (singular: bacterium) are living organisms, each of a single cell, that can be seen only with a microscope. They reproduce by simple division. They tend to be between one thousandth to one ten-thousandth of a millimetre in size; these dimensions are frequently written as $1\,\mu m$–$0.1\,\mu m$ (micrometres). They are classified according to their shape. Those that are rod-shaped are called bacilli (singular: bacillus); those that are spherical are cocci (coccus), and are called streptococci if they tend to lie in chains and staphylococci if they are in clumps, like bunches of grapes. There are also species of bacteria that are spiral in shape, and these are called spirella.

See also: Intestinal bacteria

Baking

Although the word is used for the cooking of any food by dry heat, and indeed similarly for heating non-food materials such as clay, baking most commonly refers to the whole process by which bread is made. Bread is usually baked from risen dough, but in some parts of the world or for special occasions such as the Jewish Passover, un-leavened bread is baked. The more usual process is that flour is mixed with water to form a dough, while other agents such as yeast or baking powder are added with a variety of substances that may be required by law or are used to accelerate or improve one stage or other of the bread-making process. In earlier times, growing yeast was transferred by adding to the new dough some left over from previous bread-making, and such a transfer continued for successive batches of bread.

The dough is left to rise, in order for the yeast or baking powder to produce carbon dioxide gas. After it has risen for a time, the dough is kneaded and allowed once more to rise, or 'prove'. The kneading stretches and straightens the gluten molecules, so that the dough holds more of the gas produced. If all goes well, a 'bold' loaf is produced, that is, a loaf that is well risen with an evenly porous structure.

In this traditional method of making bread, the flour used has to be 'strong', that is, it needs to have a high protein content. Nowadays, about 75% of bread in the UK is baked by the Chorleywood Bread Process (CBP), in which the dough is mixed very rapidly for about 5 minutes. There are several advantages to this. One is that the process is much quicker than the normal 1–4 hours in the conventional process; it is also possible to use a higher proportion of British flour, which is weaker than the traditional strong imported flour.

Finally, the Chorleywood Process saves an appreciable amount of flour, since the traditional method with yeast uses up about 7% of the flour in providing the carbon dioxide gas that raises the dough.

See also: Baking powder; Bread; Gluten; Yeast

Baking powder

Instead of using the action of living yeast to produce carbon dioxide gas in dough, one may use a mixture of a bicarbonate and an acid. When this mixture is dry, the ingredients do not interact; when they are wetted, they react to produce carbon dioxide. The bicarbonate is sodium bicarbonate (bicarbonate of soda, sometimes known as baking soda). The acid is a weak acid, sometimes in the form of an acid salt. Thus, common baking powder is a mixture of the bicarbonate with tartaric acid and cream of tartar (potassium acid tartrate); when moistened, there is a rapid release of CO_2. Another sort of baking powder has, as the acid, calcium acid phosphate, perhaps with sodium acid pyrophosphate. When this mixture is moistened, there is a slow release of CO_2.

Usually, starch is included in the mixture; it tends to absorb moisture from the air, which prevents the active ingredients from becoming moist, and thus reacting.

See also: Baking

Balanced diet

For the attainment and preservation of optimal health, an essential requirement is a diet that provides adequate amounts of all the nutrients, and an appropriate amount of energy. To achieve the first aim, foods may be classified into groups, with the intention of indicating that eating one or more foods from each of the groups each day would satisfy the body's nutrient requirements. To achieve the second aim, one is told to take each of these foods in moderation, and ensure that body weight is not, and does not become, less or more than it should be.

All those who give dietary advice would agree with this concept of a balanced diet; they would, however, possibly disagree as to how to divide the foods into groups, and even whether it is necessary to do so. Moreover, they would probably differ in their views in regard to the amounts of the dietary items.

As well as ensuring that the diet contains the necessary quantities of the items that the body requires, it is necessary that it does not contain items or amounts of items that are harmful; in other words, the diet must be wholesome as well as adequate.

With the growing belief by many nutritionists that it is unwise to take excessive amounts of fat, especially saturated fat, or of cholesterol or of sugar, injunctions to this effect are added to the general advice about a balanced diet. For example, some people suggest that no more than two eggs a week should be eaten because of their high content of cholesterol. Other suggestions may in practice be far less easy to follow, for example that fat intake should be restricted to the equivalent of no more than 30% of the energy (caloric) content of the diet. This advice would require a reasonably exact assessment of one's average diet, and of the proportion of fat that each item contains; it is unlikely that more than a small minority even of professional nutritionists would be able at once to give this information about their own diets.

A different approach to the problem of how to choose a balanced diet is discussed under Dietary instinct.

See also: Dietary instinct; Food habits

Bananas (*Musa species*)

Their attractive flavour, their sweetness because of their sugar content, and their wide distribution and easy availability have made bananas a particularly popular food, especially with children. The fact that bananas do not cause symptoms in children with coeliac disease was a chance discovery; it was only many years later that the explanation was found to be that the fruit contains no gluten. In fact they contain little protein or vitamins, and marginally higher potassium than other fruits and vegetables. Like other fruits, they are low in sodium, so that bananas are frequently recommended for people requiring a high-potassium, low-sodium diet. This is not very sound advice since the potassium comes with a high energy content; a high-potassium, low-sodium diet is usually prescribed for conditions in which a low-calorie diet is indicated.

As well as the dessert banana, there are some varieties that contain less sugar and more starch. These have to be cooked before they are eaten, and they form a major article of diet in parts of the tropics. They are sometimes called plantains, a name that is also occasionally used for dessert bananas; in East Africa they are called matoke.

The banana plant is unusual in that it is sterile and has a growth habit characteristic of a herb rather than of a shrub or tree. Propagation has to be carried out from pieces cut from its underground rhizome. The fruit grows from the unfertilized flower. Each bunch contains 10 or 12 hands, and each hand contains a dozen or more fruits. The whole bunch will therefore have between 120 and 200 fruits, and can weigh up to 80lb. The plant can go on producing fruit from 5 years to 50 or 60 years, but commonly it is replaced after 20 years. The leaves of the plant are large, and are used to thatch roofs of huts, or for wrapping food or other articles, or as a covering on which food can be set out for a meal.

The banana plant originated in a wide region of the world, stretching from India south-eastwards to New Guinea. It is now cultivated in most tropical countries, but especially in Central America and the Caribbean islands. The fruit is difficult to transport without damage, and thus the large export across the oceans, for example from the Americas to Europe, involves the use of ships specially constructed for the purpose, with the ventilated holds kept at carefully controlled temperatures. The fruit is picked and shipped while it is green, and the ripening that begins on board is continued in special stores in the importing country.

Barley (*Hordeum distichon*)

This cereal grows in a wider variety of climates than does any other. Its use as a direct food for human beings has diminished considerably during the last 250 years; before that, it was an important ingredient in bread. It is likely that the corn of Egypt mentioned in the Bible was barley, and that the bread of the parable of the loaves and fishes was made of barley; this was probably the species *Hordeum vulgare*. Now it is used almost exclusively for animal fodder or for the production of alcoholic beverages such as beer and Scotch whisky.

See also: Beer; Cereals

Basal metabolism

The metabolism at complete rest, sometimes called 'resting metabolism', is more usually called basal metabolism. Since it is affected by food, by the temperature of the environment, and by movement, the basal metabolic rate (BMR) is measured when the individual has not eaten for some time, usually before breakfast, and when lying down comfortably in a quiet room kept at an equable temperature.

Even these conditions are likely not to represent absolute inactivity; it would therefore perhaps be more correct to speak of 'resting metabolic rate', except that 'BMR' is now so well established.

The BMR is usually assessed by measuring the amount of oxygen that the body is using over a given period; the faster the rate of metabolism, the more rapidly it is using the oxygen it is taking into the lungs. The subject breathes in from a cylinder containing oxygen, and breathes out into the cylinder through a series of vessels where the carbon dioxide of the expired air is absorbed. The reduction in the volume of the oxygen is recorded while this is happening. From the rate of disappearance of oxygen, one can calculate the rate of energy utilization in terms of calories or joules.

The BMR depends, among other things, on the size of the body – more specifically, its surface area. A 'normal' value of BMR can be calculated from the individual's height and weight. Because of this, the BMR is sometimes expressed as a percentage above or below this normal value, so that −10% would mean that the BMR is 90% of normal, and +20% that it is 120% of normal.

The basal metabolic rate is affected by sex, age and climate, as well as by hormonal activity. Men have a higher BMR than women, but this is because women have a greater proportion of body fat, and this has a much lower metabolic rate than has the rest of the body. If allowance is made for this difference in fat, the metabolic rate of the 'fat-free' body, the so-called lean body mass, is the same for men and women.

As age increases, the BMR falls; the fall is somewhat greater for men than for women.

Food increases the metabolic rate by a phenomenon known as thermogenesis, or dietary induced thermogenesis. The older term for this is specific dynamic action. Very cold and very hot climates tend to decrease BMR by some 5% or 10%. The hormones that most affect BMR are those of the thyroid gland; diminished or increased activity of this gland significantly reduces or increases BMR.

In the average moderately active woman, the BMR accounts for about 1,500 kcal a day out of a total daily energy expenditure of about 2,300 kcal. For an average man, both figures will be higher, perhaps 1,600 and 2,500 kcal; the proportion of energy expended by the basal metabolism would be the same, about two thirds of the total.

See also: Benedict; Energy; Metabolism; Thermogenesis

Beer

The fermentation of cereals to produce alcoholic drinks has been carried out for at least 5,000 years. Barley is the cereal most commonly used in the UK to produce beer; in the United States a mixture of barley and maize is often used.

The characteristic feature of modern beer is the addition of hops, nowadays partially or wholly replaced by the relevant pure chemical substances present in natural hops. Traditionally, English ale was brewed without hops until the early fifteenth century. At that time hops were introduced from Flanders; this was resented by the English brewers, who protested to King Henry VI. Even as late as 1542, Andrew Boorde wrote in his *Dyetary of Helth* that beer was 'the naturall drynke for a Dutch man'. He added, 'Now of late days it is moche used in Englande to the detryment of many Englysshe men.'

Hops, however, not only give beer its bitterness and some of its other characteristic flavours, but also help to preserve it; the traditional ale without hops used to deteriorate very rapidly.

The making of beer begins with the malting of the barley. This is a process in which the barley is moistened and allowed to germinate. Some of the starch in the grains is thus digested by the enzyme diastase (amylase), and converted to the sugar maltose. This is an essential preliminary, since the yeast that is added later cannot ferment starch but can ferment maltose. After a few days, 'malting' is carried out, which consists of stopping the activity of the diastase by heating the germinated grain. If the temperature is high enough, some caramelization occurs, and this will ultimately result in a darker beer. The malt is dried, ground and mixed with water to produce the mash. The fluid part, known as the wort, is run off and boiled to destroy any unwanted micro-organisms. Hops are now added, or the chemically produced materials that hops contain. The sterile wort is finally inoculated with yeasts that are kept and grown in the brewery; the character of the beer is very much influenced by the particular strain of yeast used.

What are now called ales tend to contain rather less alcohol and less hops than beers. Stout is stronger and is usually dark because it is made from barley that has been well roasted and perhaps with added caramelized sugar. Like beer, these drinks are made with strains of the yeast *Saccharomyces cerevisiae*, which tends to float to the top of the fermenting vat. Fermentation is carried out at 15°–20° Centigrade for about 7 days. Lager contains less alcohol and is made with strains of the bottom yeast, *Saccharomyces carlsbergiensis*; fermentation continues for 12 days or so at 4°–9°C, and the product is then stored for 3–6 months. The word 'lager' is German for storehouse. Since people do not like their beer to look cloudy, the last stage is the fining of the beer, in which gelatin is added to carry down small floating particles.

Most beers contain about 3g alcohol in 100ml, but strong ale may contain 7g/100ml or even more. A pint of beer will provide some 500–600 kcal, small amounts of riboflavin and nicotinic acid, and insignificant amounts of other nutrients.

See also: **Alcohol; Barley; Maize; Fermentation; Yeast**

Beet

There are three main varieties of the common beet that are used as foods, or for the production of foods. One is the sugar beet, from which about 40% of the world's sugar (sucrose) is made. This is almost white in colour, and was cultivated mostly as an animal feed in the same way as the mangelwurzel is cultivated; incidentally, this too is a variety of the common beet.

A second variety is grown for its leaves; this is known in the US as chard. The third variety, the beetroot, is red; the root of this is eaten raw, or cooked, or pickled. Its pigment may be excreted in the urine, the red colour of which is then liable to cause quite unwarranted alarm.

See also: Sucrose

Behaviour therapy

It has been suggested that, since overweight is the outcome of un-desirable eating behaviour, a change in such behaviour should be encouraged as a means of treating the condition. To this end, some doctors have treated overweight patients by behaviour therapy or behaviour modification. To begin with, the individual has to keep a meticulous diary of all the events that concern eating and drinking: times of eating, what circumstances initiated the eating, what was eaten, where and in what circumstances the eating took place, for how long, and whether they were hungry before or after eating. The therapist then points out aspects of behaviour that require change, for example that food should be eaten slowly, and none taken while walking about or as snacks, but only at the table, with the food on a plate and eaten with a knife and fork or spoon. Sometimes this therapy is combined with an increase in exercise, the use of anorectic drugs, or enlisting co-operation from the spouse or the whole family.

Several studies have shown that for the first few weeks or months the treatment is often effective. However, as in most other treatments of obesity, the majority of individuals are found to have regained much or all of their excessive weight after a year or two.

See also: Anorectic agents; Obesity

Benedict, Francis Gano (1870–1957)

The major contributions that Benedict made to nutrition were in the field of energy metabolism. Born in Milwaukee, Wisconsin, his initial training at Harvard University and in Heidelberg in Germany was in chemistry. He was appointed in 1895 as research assistant at Wesleyan University in Middletown, Connecticut, under W. O. Atwater. Here they both worked on energy metabolism, using a newly constructed calorimeter.

In 1907 Benedict moved to Boston as director of the nutrition laboratories newly established by the Carnegie Corporation. Here he developed several pieces of apparatus for determining oxygen consumption. They were for use both for general research and, with his colleague Roth, for measuring metabolism in individual patients. The apparatus was not very different from the Benedict–Roth spirometer still in use in hospitals.

In 1919, Benedict published *Standards of Basal Metabolism*, which depended on height, weight, age and sex: these standards were thereafter used widely by doctors as an aid in the diagnosis of disease. Benedict believed that basal metabolism was related chiefly to body weight; he thus disagreed with the view of Rubner that it was surface area that determined basal metabolism. It was Rubner's view that ultimately prevailed.

As well as his scientific work, Benedict was very keen on magic and was a member of the Society of American Magicians. He retired from the laboratory in 1937. He died in 1957, in the country home at Machiasport, Marine, which he had long used for summer vacations.

See also: Atwater; Basal metabolism; Energy; Rubner

Beri-beri

During the past thirty years or so, there has been a considerable reduction in the high prevalence of beri-beri that was a feature of many countries of south-east Asia. The disease is associated with diets consisting largely of polished rice; it was much less common in areas in which the rice was lightly milled, or parboiled, that is, milled after boiling for a short time. In India, for example, beri-beri was common in Madras and along the coastal strip 300 or 400 miles northwards, but uncommon in the rest of India, Sri Lanka and Pakistan, where parboiled rice is more often used.

Beri-beri exists in three forms: as infantile beri-beri, or as wet beri-beri or dry beri-beri in children or adults. Infantile beri-beri occurs between the ages of 2 and 5 months in breastfed infants of malnourished mothers, who do not, however, themselves necessarily show the signs of beri-beri. The baby is restless and may have a characterized high-pitched whine – the beri-beri cry. It usually has some degree of oedema and may suddenly develop heart failure and die within a few hours.

In adults, the onset of beri-beri is usually insidious, although it may be exacerbated by sudden physical activity. The patient complains of weakness and loss of appetite. There may be mild oedema, and numbness and pins and needles in the legs. Unless treated, manifest wet beri-beri or dry beri-beri may develop.

Wet beri-beri is characterized by severe general oedema, involving not only the legs but also the face and body, and including accumulation of fluid in the chest and in the abdomen. The heart rate is raised and there are signs of heart failure, which occasionally increase suddenly and lead to rapid death.

Dry beri-beri may occur with little or no oedema. The chief feature is weakness and loss of sensation in the legs. Soon the patient can walk only with the aid of a stick, and ultimately becomes bed-ridden. Some infectious disease often supervenes, from which the patient may die.

Infantile beri-beri and wet beri-beri respond rapidly to treatment with thiamin, so that a patient who appears to be moribund may within a few hours have improved beyond recognition. The neurological changes in dry beri-beri, on the other hand, respond much more slowly, if at all, and much less completely.

The reduction of the prevalence of beri-beri in some countries, such as Japan, has come about by a general improvement in living standards, which as always has been accompanied by a reduced proportion of cereal in the diet, and an increased proportion of other foods. In addition, some governments have introduced legislation requiring a lesser degree of milling of the rice, but this is not always enforced, and the people still prefer the whiter highly polished rice they have been used to. Nor has there been much success in persuading people to parboil rice if they have not traditionally used it in this form. The addition of thiamin to rice has also been attempted by some authorities, but this too is difficult to enforce in the poorer countries.

Although beri-beri is usually found in people whose staple food is polished rice, it does occur, although rarely, in other circumstances. It has been seen, for example, in areas where there has been a high dependence on bread made with highly-milled and unfortified wheat flour.

There are also conditions in which deficiency of thiamin is precipitated by chronic alcoholism.

See also: Alcoholism; Eijkman; Grijns; Rice; Vitamin B_1

Bernard, Claude (1813–78)

The acknowledged founder of modern physiology, Claude Bernard was born in St Julien in France. He left school to become assistant to a druggist, but in his spare time became something of a playwright. His first play was successful enough for him to move to Paris in the hope of pursuing this career, but a well-known critic advised him that he would do better to study medicine. Bernard therefore entered the medical school in Paris and took his MD degree in 1843. In 1854 he was appointed to the first Chair of Experimental Physiology at the Sorbonne. There was no laboratory there, but Napoleon III arranged for one to be built for him at the Jardin des Plantes. A professorship of General Physiology for Claude Bernard was created there in 1868, and he gave up his Chair at the Sorbonne. He died ten years later, and was the first scientist in France to be given a state funeral.

Bernard's thesis for his MD was on the gastric juice, and later he also investigated the digestive function of the pancreatic juice. In 1853 he published his most famous work, on the function of the liver, demonstrating that it forms and stores glycogen, and that glycogen like starch could be hydrolysed to glucose. He discovered that the sympathetic nerves had an effect on the blood vessels, by studying what happened when the nerves were either cut or stimulated. He was also interested in toxicology, making studies with curare and carbon monoxide. It was Claude Bernard who pointed out that the body's chemical and physiological activities were integrated in a way that tended to keep constant the internal environment of the body's tissues, introducing the concept of 'the constancy of the internal environment'.

See also: Glycogen; Liver function

NOUVELLE FONCTION

DU FOIE

CONSIDÉRÉ

COMME ORGANE PRODUCTEUR DE MATIÈRE SUCRÉE

CHEZ L'HOMME ET LES ANIMAUX,

PAR

M. Claude BERNARD,

Docteur en médecine et Docteur ès-sciences;
Professeur de physiologie expérimentale, suppléant de M. Magendie
au Collège de France, Lauréat de l'Institut (Académie des sciences); Membre
des Sociétés de biologie, philomatique de Paris; Correspondant de l'Académie de médecine
de Turin; des Sociétés médicales et des sciences naturelles de Lyon,
de Suisse, de Vienne, etc.

———◦———

A PARIS,

CHEZ J.-B. BAILLIÈRE,

LIBRAIRE DE L'ACADÉMIE IMPÉRIALE DE MÉDECINE,
RUE HAUTEFEUILLE, 19.

A LONDRES, CHEZ H. BAILLIÈRE, 219, REGENT STREET.
A NEW-YORK, CHEZ H. BAILLIÈRE, 290, BROADWAY.
A MADRID, CHEZ C. BAILLY-BAILLIÈRE, CALLE DEL PRINCIPE, 11.

1853.

Bile

The manufacture of bile is one among the many functions of the liver. The bile is produced constantly, and passes to the gall-bladder where it is stored and concentrated. It is released into the intestine after food is eaten, especially if the food contains fat. The gall-bladder then contracts, forcing some bile along the bile duct, where it mixes with the digestive juices from the pancreas before entering the small intestine.

Bile contains two characteristic constituents: the bile salts and the bile pigments. The bile salts are made from cholesterol, and they assist in the digestion of fats in the food by emulsifying them; the resulting minute droplets of fat are then much more readily attacked by the fat-splitting enzyme, lipase, in the intestine. The bile pigments are produced when the red blood cells break down; the haemoglobin releases its iron, which is retained, while the rest of the haemoglobin is converted into the bile pigments. These are then mostly excreted in the faeces, but a part is absorbed from the intestine and appears as one of the colouring substances in the urine.

A third constituent of bile is cholesterol itself. Sometimes the amount of cholesterol is more than can be held in solution in the gall-bladder, where the bile is being concentrated. In that case, it can be a major part of the gallstones that may form.

See also: **Absorption of fat; Digestive juices; Gall-bladder; Liver function**

Biological value of proteins

The nutritional quality of the different proteins in food depends on the sorts and amounts of amino-acids that make up the proteins. There are various ways in which this quality can be determined and can be expressed. The simplest is called the Net Protein Utilization (NPU), which is the percentage of the amount fed retained in the body, expressed in terms of nitrogen, N.

$$NPU = \frac{\text{retained N}}{\text{dietary N}} \times 100$$

That proportion of the protein not retained within the body includes both the part that is not absorbed and the part that, after absorption, is not used by the body. The unabsorbed part appears in the faeces, and the absorbed but unretained part appears in the urine.

If allowance is made for the fact that not all the protein is absorbed, the value so obtained is the Biological Value of the protein, BV rather than NPU. Thus

$$BV = \frac{\text{retained N}}{\text{absorbed N}} \times 100$$

See also: Amino-acids; Protein

Biotin

Biotin is a vitamin for yeast and several species of bacteria, which need quite minute quantities in order to grow and multiply. Human beings also require the vitamin in their bodies, where it acts as a co-enzyme in a variety of metabolic processes involving fats and carbohydrates. It is, however, constantly being produced by the action of some of the micro-organisms residing in the gut, from which some at least is absorbed into the blood; as a result, very little if any needs to be present in the diet. Many foods contain at least some biotin; the richest sources are yeast and kidney, while reasonable sources are pulses, nuts and some vegetables. The average British and US diet provides some 250μg of biotin a day; this is very much more than is needed.

Deficiency occurs in man only when the absorption of the vitamin in the blood is prevented by the consumption of raw egg white, which contains the antivitamin avidin. The effects of the deficiency have been studied in an experiment in 4 volunteers, who took a diet containing the whites of 80 raw eggs a day, which provided 30% of the dietary energy. After about 10 weeks, the volunteers complained of poor appetite and muscular pain, nausea and an excessive tiredness. They developed a dry skin with fine powdery scaling like dandruff; their limbs were sensitive to touch. These effects disappeared with the injection of small amounts of biotin. Apart from this experimental production of biotin deficiency, there have been only three reports of 'spontaneous' dietary deficiency of the vitamin, each of one individual. All had taken a diet containing several raw eggs each day, and all developed one or more of the effects of deficiency as seen in the experiment with the volunteers.

See also: Avidin; Eggs

Blood pressure

The term 'blood pressure' refers to the pressure of blood in the arteries. This is the pressure the contracting heart achieves in forcing the blood through the circulatory system of vessels to the organs and tissues. The blood leaves the heart in a wide artery, the aorta; this divides and sub-divides into smaller and smaller arteries, each of which again divides further into arterioles. Finally, these divide into the tiny capillaries (from the Latin *capillus*, a hair) that carry the blood in between the cells, and 'leak' the dissolved oxygen and other components into the spaces between the cells. Further on, the capillaries join together to form venules, then veins, and ultimately the large subclavian veins that return the blood to the heart.

The narrow diameter of the arterioles offers great resistance to the flow, so that considerable pressure has to be built up in the arteries in order to push the blood through this resistance. Each contraction of the heart is felt as the pulse at the wrist and at other places where the arteries are not too deep. At each contraction of the heart, the pressure rises rapidly and reaches a maximum, which then falls in the half-second or so while the heart rests before the next beat. The maximum pressure at the beat is called the systolic pressure, and the minimum pressure during rest is the diastolic pressure. The pressure is measured, like the barometric pressure, in terms of the height of mercury in millimetres which the pressure can sustain. A typical blood pressure (BP) for a young person is then given as 110/80; this is a systolic pressure of 110mm mercury and a diastolic of 80mm mercury.

The resistance of the arterioles is much affected by their elasticity. Healthy arterioles are elastic enough to expand with each heartbeat. With increasing age, and in some diseases, the elasticity of the arterioles decreases, so that the resistance increases, and with this the blood pressure. The effect is usually first seen in the systolic pressure and later in the diastolic pressure. The result might be, say, 140/90. More serious would be a reading of 160/110; still higher readings would be even more serious, and experience shows that a high diastolic pressure is more worrying than a high systolic.

An increase in BP with increasing age does not occur in every individual; moreover, there are some countries where there is little or no increase. Examples are some of the Pacific Islands. On the other hand, Japan has a greater prevalence of high BP than has any other country.

The causes of high BP (hypertension) are not entirely understood. There are genetic factors, but also environmental factors. Stress and anxiety can cause a transitory increase in BP; it is possible that continual exposure to stress and anxiety might produce permanent hypertension, although this has not yet been established.

As to diet, the most clear association is with obesity, but there is also an increasing amount of evidence that at least in some people a high BP may be the result of a high intake of salt.

Hypertension can also be caused by a variety of diseases, especially of the heart or kidneys. Occasionally, a very high BP develops rapidly without obvious cause and causes disease of the heart and kidneys and many other organs. This is called malignant hypertension. In most cases of hypertension without obvious cause, there are no immediate symptoms. The high blood pressure may be discovered only during a routine examination, for example for life insurance. This condition is given the name of essential hypertension.

It is usual not to treat symptomless mild essential hypertension when the diastolic pressure is no more than 105 and when it is discovered, as it were, inadvertently. However, it is worthwhile to measure the BP again at intervals to see whether it has progressed. If the diastolic pressure is between 105 and 120, it is usually associated with headache and perhaps shortness of breath. The appropriate advice then is to reduce excessive weight, and also to restrict salt intake. If this does not produce a fall in BP, drugs may be prescribed, including diuretic drugs. More severe hypertension, where diastolic pressures are above 120, is usually treated at once with the administration of drugs and with dietary measures.

Hypertension is one of the factors involved in causing two important diseases, coronary heart disease and stroke.

See also: Atherosclerosis; Coronary heart disease; Sodium; Stroke

Body fat

The fat in the body serves several purposes. Firstly, it cushions some of the internal organs such as the kidneys; secondly, the fat that is mostly situated under the skin serves as a store of energy; thirdly, this subcutaneous fat determines to a large extent body contours and hence sexual attraction, and fourthly, it acts as an insulator and so conserves body heat.

The fat is present inside living cells, the adipocytes, which constitute the adipose tissue. This is a metabolically active organ. After a meal, the glucose and fatty acids arising from the food enter these cells and are built up into fat. When no food is taken and energy is required, the fat is broken down into fatty acids and released into the blood for oxidation. Both the synthesis of fat and its breakdown are under the control of hormones, mostly insulin and adrenaline.

The fat that is stored in the adipose tissue tends to be character-istic of the species in whose body it is found; pork fat is different from beef fat. However, a diet rich in fat may influence the nature of what is stored. The fat in a person who habitually takes a high proportion of dietary fat as vegetable oils, for example, will tend to be rather softer than that of a person whose dietary fat is largely the solid fats of animal origin.

It follows from this that the fat does not exist simply as if it were an inert piece of lard or dripping. It is present inside living cells that are continually metabolizing, that is, carrying out innumerable complex reactions common to all the cells of the body, as well as the special reactions involved in the storage and release of the fat. It is important to bear all this in mind when considering some of the ways popularly believed to be effective in the treatment of obesity.

The total fat in the normal individual amounts to about 12% of the body's weight in men, and about 25% in women. A substantially greater proportion than this is considered to denote obesity, where it can amount to 100kg; a substantially lower proportion indicates a degree of starvation or the existence of some wasting disease, where it can be as low as 1kg. A rough assessment of the amount of fat is given by the weight of the body, but this can be deceptive if an unusually higher weight than expected is due to the well-developed musculature of an athlete.

Because much of the surplus store of fat is found just beneath the skin, an assessment of this can be used to estimate the total amount of fat in the body somewhat more accurately than by weighing the body.

It can be done by measuring the thickness of a skin-fold; by doing this at three or four sites on the body, one can get a value that can be judged against standards used by research workers who have calibrated skin-fold thickness against the percentage of body fat. For the same skin-fold thickness, there is rather more fat in the body in older people than in younger. In addition, the same skin-fold thickness indicates more fat in women than in men.

There are two other methods that can be used to measure body fat, but they are elaborate and time-consuming, more suited for research than as a routine.

One such method depends on the fact that the density (specific gravity) of fat is less than that of the rest of the body. Fat weighs rather less than does the same volume of water, and the rest of the body weighs rather more than water. The values for specific gravity are, roughly, 0.90 for fat and 1.10 for the fat-free body. By weighing a person in the ordinary way, that is, in air, and then when he is totally immersed in water, the density of the whole body can readily be determined. From this, the proportion of fat can be calculated; for example, if the density of the body is 1.05, then the proportion of fat can be calculated to be 21% from the formula

$$\% \text{ fat} = \frac{495}{\text{density}} - 450$$

Probably the most accurate way of determining body fat is also the most expensive. It depends on measuring the radioactivity of the body which is a measure of the amount of potassium in the body. Since the potassium is almost entirely in the body's cells, the 'cell mass' can be calculated; the smaller this is in relation to the total weight (mass) of the body, the more fat the body contains. This is because the fat itself, inside the adipose tissue cells in which the fat is stored, contains no cellular material. This method is rarely used because it requires a very expensive piece of equipment called a whole body counter.

See also: Brown adipose tissue; Obesity

Bone

It is wrong to imagine that the bones of a living person are composed of nothing but dry, brittle mineral matter, like the skeletons that can be seen in a museum. Only one half of their substance is mineral matter; the remainder is made up of fat and cellular material, with blood vessels and nerve cells and a great deal of protein fibres.

The outer part of the bones is the densest part; the cavity within this is filled with marrow. In long bones, the marrow consists mostly of fat and is called yellow marrow. In the flat bones of the skull, sternum and pelvis, the marrow is the site of the formation of the red and white blood cells and constitutes the red marrow.

The bones of an adult weigh about 6kg or 14lb. Blacks tend to have somewhat heavier skeletons than whites do, and men somewhat heavier than women. But their weight does not differ much from person to person. Having 'heavy bones' is an unrealistic excuse for someone whose weight is perhaps 20kg or 30kg more than it should be. In chemical terms, bone is composed of about 50% mineral matter, 25% water, 20% protein and 5% fat. Without the cellular and fibrous material the bones would be brittle; without the mineral matter they would be soft, as begins to happen in osteoporosis.

In the child, the growth of the bones is under the control of hormones, especially those of the pituitary gland and the sex glands. The sex hormones, however, which are secreted in greatest quantities from puberty onwards, then stop the growth of the bones at about the age of 18 years. After that, they may still have more mineral added to them for a few years, but from about 40 years of age the hardness of the bones begins to diminish. In women, this takes place quite rapidly after the menopause, which accounts for women having the higher prevalence of osteoporosis.

If a limb is immobilized, for example in a plaster, or if the whole body is immobilized, for example during a prolonged space flight, a gradual demineralization of bone occurs.

There is a constant turnover of mineral matter in the bones, so that in a young child the whole of the mineral is renewed in 1 or 2 years, and in an adult in some 10–12 years. The chemical control of this deposition and removal of the mineral content of the bone is largely influenced directly by the parathyroid hormone and indirectly by vitamin D. The vitamin is the chief factor affecting the absorption of calcium from the intestine.

See also: Calcium; Osteomalacia; Vitamin D

Brain

The average adult brain weighs $1\frac{1}{4}$–$1\frac{1}{2}$kg. In view of its importance, it is not surprising that the brain receives half of its own weight of blood each minute. Moreover, neither this considerable circulation nor the brain's use of energy is significantly affected by the amount of mental work it undertakes, or the amount of physical work that the body undertakes. The brain is very sensitive to oxygen lack. Its activity ceases within a few seconds if the blood supply is cut off for any reason, and permanent damage ensues after a few minutes, then death. Unlike the cells of other tissues, when cells of the brain and other parts of the nervous system die, they cannot be replaced by division of neighbouring cells; brain damage involving the death of cells is therefore irreversible.

Ordinarily, the brain uses glucose in its metabolism. During starvation, however, it adapts to the scarcity of glucose and it then uses the keto acids derived from the body's diminishing stores of fat.

See also: Ketosis; Starvation

Bread

The first bread made was in flat unleavened cakes, produced by roughly pounding wheat or barley or rye grains, moistening with water and cooking over a fire or on a hot stove. It is possible that the discovery of leavened bread followed the discovery of brewing, taking from it some of the scum (barm) from the surface of the beer or wine and adding it to the moistened flour. The yeast in the barm resulted in the risen dough, although this would not occur with barley flour since this grain contains no gluten. Alternatively, leavening might have been discovered by the accidental contamination of the dough with some yeast spores from the air; subsequent loaves of bread were made by mixing a newly-made dough with a small piece of dough kept from a batch made a day or two earlier. This practice is still occasionally used in the making of sourdough bread.

In Europe, North America and Australasia, bread is typically made with flour from wheat, sometimes with varying proportions of rye. In times of shortage of cereals, small amounts of potato flour or soya flour or flour from dried pulses may be added. Other materials, such as milk powder, malt or dried fruits, are occasionally added to make special breads. The common wheaten breads in the UK are white, made with flour of 72% extraction, and brown, with mixed white and wholemeal flour, ending with the equivalent of something like 85% extraction; wholemeal bread is made with flour of 100% extraction.

The spongy consistency of the inner part of the loaf, technically known as the crumb, is produced by carbon dioxide or air. The commonest method of doing this is by the use of yeast, which produces carbon dioxide (CO_2) and alcohol by fermentation. The gluten in the flour, when mixed with water to produce the dough, becomes sticky and viscid, so that small bubbles of the gas are trapped in the dough. Kneading of the dough stretches the gluten into longer fibres, thus helping the entrapment of carbon dioxide. This is seen in the expansion or rising of the dough to about $1\frac{1}{2}$ times its original size. Further expansion occurs when the dough is heated by baking. This also produces the crust, which becomes brown through slight caramelization and by the so-called browning reaction which occurs when carbohydrates and protein are heated together.

Alternative methods of producing gas in the dough are either by using baking powder, a mixture of substances that release CO_2 when moistened, or by using water in which carbon dioxide has been dissolved. The former yields so-called soda bread, and the latter so-called aerated bread.

There are three major processes for the making of dough. The traditional one is the long fermentation process, in which the yeast is allowed to ferment at a warm temperature for an initial 3 hours or so. The partly risen dough is then divided into loaves and allowed to rise ('prove') for a further $1\frac{1}{2}$ hours. About 15% of bread in the UK is made in this way.

The short fermentation process (Chorleywood Bread Process or CBP) eliminates the initial stage by adding ascorbic acid and potassium bromate, sometimes together with azodicarbonamide, and then mixing for 3 minutes at high speed with special machinery. This process uses more yeast than does the long fermentation process; somewhat more water is added too, because the shorter time converts less flour into carbon dioxide and water. The major advantage of the Chorleywood Process is that it produces a good bread with a flour containing less protein than is needed for the long fermentation process. Because of this, more of the soft home-grown wheat can be used and less of the imported harder wheats. Some 75% of bread in the UK is now made using the CBP.

This change, and the increase in duty for the imported wheat, has resulted in the past twenty-five years in an increase from about 40% to about 65% in the proportion of home-grown wheat used for bread-making.

A third process is available to small bakers who do not have the special machinery needed for the Chorleywood Process. For this, cysteine is added to the flour as well as ascorbic acid and potassium bromate; the addition of these substances enables the initial 3-hour fermentation to be considerably reduced, or even eliminated. This process, known as activated dough development, accounts for the remaining 10% of bread production in the UK.

In the United Kingdom and the United States, most of the bread that is eaten is white bread, but the proportion of brown has been increasing, no doubt because of the growing interest in increasing the intake of dietary fibre. In the UK, the fall in consumption of bread which occurred up to 1975 has continued; the average weekly consumption fell from about 50oz to about 30oz between 1956 and 1982. But because there has been a rise in the consumption of brown bread, the proportion of brown has increased appreciably, from about 9% of the total in 1975 to about 18% in 1981.

Home-baked bread often has a more attractive smell and, some maintain, a more attractive taste than does factory-made bread. This is largely because substantially more yeast is used in home bread baking.

In the UK, white bread has by law to be made with flour to which has been added thiamin, nicotinic acid, iron and calcium carbonate. It has been suggested that nicotinic acid and calcium carbonate should no longer be added, because it is no longer considered that they serve any nutritional need. Some authorities also doubt whether there is any purpose in adding iron, because it appears that it is not absorbed by the body.

The argument about whether brown bread is better than white has continued for more than 2,000 years. Most of the early Romans and Greeks ate white bread if they could afford it; it was significantly more expensive, yet some of the best-known figures of those times extolled the virtues of wholemeal bread. Whether it does matter to nutritional wellbeing if white or wholemeal bread is eaten becomes less and less likely as the quantity consumed decreases, and the nutritional value of the remainder of the diet is high. Nevertheless, it is interesting that in the UK it is the wealthier people who eat least bread but take the highest proportion of what they do eat as wholemeal.

Whatever the virtues of wholemeal bread, it is wrong to minimize the values of white bread. With the average daily intake at about 125g, white bread would provide about 10g protein and wholemeal bread about 11g; the practical difference is somewhat less than the apparent 1g, since the protein of wholemeal bread is less well absorbed than that of white bread.

Perhaps the best assessment of the nutritional value of white bread was given by the results of the classic experiment in Germany of McCance and Widdowson in the 1950s. They fed three groups of children in orphanages on a diet of which 75% consisted of bread, 20% of vegetables, and 5% of foods of animal origin; the bread in one group was wholemeal, in another brown bread made from 85% extraction flour, and in the third group it was white bread. The children in all three groups grew equally well.

Staling: When a loaf of bread becomes stale, two processes have occurred. Firstly, moisture passes from the spongy interior (the crumb) to the outside crust, making the inside of the loaf drier, and the crust moister and softer. Secondly, a slow physical change occurs in the structure of the starch granules, making the crumb rather harder. The movement of moisture is to some extent reversible when the bread is warmed, but the change in the nature of the starch is not reversible; warming a stale loaf can therefore 'refresh' the loaf only in the early stages of staling.

See also: Baking; Browning reaction; Cereals; Yeast

Breast-feeding

The composition of human milk is significantly different from that of cows' milk, which is the commonest alternative to human milk. The Table on page 241 gives the content of the major constituents of various milks, including ewes' milk and goats' milk, which are sometimes used either because they are more easily available or because there is a belief that they are more suitable for babies than is cows' milk.

There are also differences in the values for the vitamins; for example, human milk contains more nicotinic acid and much more vitamin D than cows' milk does. It also contains much more vitamin C, especially after pasteurization of cows' milk.

Breast-feeding is commoner in the poorer countries than in the more affluent countries. In the former, however, there has been a tendency among wealthier mothers to adopt artificial feeds based on cows' milk. On the other hand, this trend has recently been reversed in the affluent countries, in that there has been an increase in breast-feeding, especially in the wealthier classes. In 1972, 10% of British mothers were breast-feeding their babies at 6 weeks; by 1982, the proportion had increased to 50%.

Most of the available artificial milk preparations have been formulated from cows' milk, modified so as to minimize the differences between cows' milk and breast milk. For example, dilution and the addition of lactose bring the concentrations of protein and of carbohydrate close to those in human milk.

The promotion of breast milk rather than of cows' milk nowadays is based less on nutrient than on other considerations. In poor countries, the cost of the manufactured powdered infant foods is a temptation to dilute them excessively so that the baby is underfed. Secondly, inadequate facilities for hygiene can readily lead to gastro-intestinal infection, which is a major cause of infant mortality in poorer countries.

Three other disadvantages are claimed for artificial feeds. One is that they lack immune bodies which may contribute to the resistance to infection of the very young infant fed at the breast. Another disadvantage is that the bottle does not give the close contact between mother and child that is of psychological importance. Thirdly, some infants are allergic to cows' milk, in which case they need specially formulated preparations if they are not breast-fed. It remains true, however, that in the developed countries it is possible to feed babies equally well with breast milk or with manufactured preparations of cows' milk.

See also: Lactose intolerance; Milk

Brown adipose tissue (brown fat)

In some animals, especially those that hibernate, there are localized deposits of brown fat under the skin, mainly between the shoulder blades. They have the ability alternately to break the triglycerides down to fatty acids and glycerol, and then rebuild them from these products; the effect is not to change the amount of brown fat, but to produce heat through the metabolic processes that take place. This happens especially when the animals awaken from hibernating, and when they are exposed to cold. Human babies also have a high proportion of brown fat; it is this that may be the heat-producing site when the baby is cold, because it cannot produce heat by shivering. The adult, on the other hand, responds to cold chiefly by shivering; the small amount of brown fat in the adult may, however, be the main site for thermogenesis after food.

See also: Body fat; Thermogenesis

Browning

There are two quite different ways in which food may undergo brown discoloration. One way is the enzymatic browning of the cut surface of foods such as apples or potatoes. It occurs because of the presence of enzymes in the food that oxidize particular substances, phenolic compounds, to other substances that happen to be brown. This phenomenon can be prevented by covering the cut surface to prevent oxidation, for example with lemon juice or a solution of vitamin C or a little sulphur dioxide gas, or a solution of sodium sulphite. The reaction is also prevented if the food is cooked, because this destroys the enzymes.

The other sort of browning occurs when a food containing protein and sugars is stored for a long time, or is heated. A good example is dried milk, produced by roller drying. The browning is sometimes called the Maillard reaction, or non-enzymic browning, or simply the browning reaction. It depends on a chemical reaction between the sugars and the essential amino-acid lysine of the protein. Lysine contains two amino groups, so that there is a free amino group after the lysine has joined with one of the other amino-acids in forming a peptide link of the protein molecule. The effect of the browning reaction is that the lysine is no longer available to the body when the food is eaten, and so the biological value of the protein is reduced.

See also: Amino-acids; Antioxidants; Biological value of proteins

Buckwheat

The cereal buckwheat (*Fagopyrum esculentum*) came originally from Central Asia, which gives it the alternative name of Tartar corn. A more common alternative is Saracen corn, which is said to be derived from the belief that it was the Crusaders who brought it to Europe.

Buckwheat grows in damp, cold climates, and thrives on soils that would not be suitable for other cereals. It is not suitable for making bread, but is used in the US in pancakes, and in Russia as kasha, eaten as a sort of porridge or as an accompaniment to a main dish as an alternative to rice or potatoes. Most of what is grown is fed to animals and especially birds; pheasants in particular are thought to be appreciative of buckwheat.

Buffer

In chemistry and in physiology, the word is used to denote substances that help to prevent a solution from undergoing a change in pH when acid or alkali are added. It can also be used as a verb, so that one may talk of adding something to a solution in order to buffer it. In the body, the buffers are chiefly bicarbonate, phosphate and protein.

See also: Acidosis; pH

Bulimia nervosa

Bulimia is the phenomenon of eating large quantities of food at one time. It is known colloquially as 'binge-eating' or even more colloquially as 'stuffing'. The condition occurs occasionally in people who are overweight, or in people with anorexia nervosa, who are therefore underweight. It also occurs in people of more or less normal weight; mostly, such people are suffering from bulimia nervosa.

As in anorexia nervosa, bulimia nervosa occurs chiefly in women from the better-off families; on the whole, however, they tend to be older. The pattern of eating in bulimia nervosa is the rapid consumption of large quantities of food and drink, mostly items that the individual has been told, or believes, need to be restricted in order to control body weight. She may do this several times a day, almost as a routine, although when other people are present she will eat normally. She ends this stuffing each time either because of abdominal discomfort, or because there is no more food available, or because she has been interrupted. The full stomach is then emptied by vomiting, although purgation is sometimes added to reduce the absorption of food from the gut. Vomiting is induced by putting the fingers into the back of the mouth, but an experienced practitioner may be able to induce vomiting simply at will. The vomiting is followed by a strong feeling of guilt, self-disgust and depression.

The true prevalence of the condition is not known, since the over-eating is usually done secretly and may not be known even to members of the family. For this reason, most doctors have been virtually un-aware of this condition until recently, although it is now suggested that it is in fact quite common.

Bulimia nervosa, then, occurs in people with a great fear of becom-ing fat, who are, however, of normal weight. Like women with an-orexia nervosa, they are industrious and ambitious. Some workers have reported that many of those with bulimia nervosa were previous sufferers from anorexia nervosa.

The effects of bulimia nervosa depend on what the individuals have been eating, the frequency of vomiting, and whether or not there is also purgation. When vomiting is frequent, the teeth may be eroded because of the acidity of the ejected gastric contents. Another conse-quence is that a deficiency of potassium may be induced, which may lead to irregularities of the heart-beat (cardiac arrhythmias) and kidney damage. Epileptic seizures may occur, and also paresthesia, that is, a sensation of pricking and tingling, especially in the limbs. Perhaps unexpectedly, the sufferers frequently have an irregular men-strual pattern, even though their weight is normal.

Occasionally, there is enlargement of the parotid salivary glands, so that the face is puffed up in a way that resembles mumps. This exaggerates the already misjudged body image, and reinforces the belief that the subject needs to control her believed tendency to obesity.

Treatment is usually through psychotherapy. But there are few satisfactory reports about well-controlled treatment or the extent to which it is successful, probably because there is still a great deal of ignorance about the condition and because only a small proportion of sufferers seem to seek treatment.

See also: Anorexia nervosa; Behaviour therapy

Butter

The cream from which butter is made consists of an emulsion of tiny droplets of fat suspended in water; technically, it is an emulsion in which water is the continuous phase and fat is the discontinuous phase. Dissolved in the fat are a few items such as fat-soluble vitamins; dissolved in the water are the milk proteins, lactose, calcium and other mineral salts, and water-soluble vitamins. When the cream is beaten (churned), there is a change in the distribution of the fatty and watery parts; the fat droplets run together, trapping some droplets of water. The emulsion now has a fatty continuous phase and a watery discontinuous phase. Since only a small amount of water can be held in droplets by the fat, much of the water is expressed from the fat. The fat, with its 15% or so of remaining water and its dissolved materials, constitutes butter; the expressed watery material is buttermilk. The amount of water in butter allowed in the UK is a maximum of 16%.

If the butter is made from fresh cream, then the buttermilk is identical in all respects to ordinary fully skimmed milk. More commonly, butter is made from 'ripened' cream, that is, cream that has been allowed to go sour, either by lactic acid organisms ordinarily present in the cream, or more commonly by fermentation produced by the addition of a specially prepared culture of lactic acid bacteria.

Butter contains about 1,300μg vitamin A/100g in the summer, and about 500μg in the winter. There is only about 1μg/100g vitamin D, and this does not differ very much in summer or winter.

See also: Anatto; Margarine; Milk; Oils

C

Caffeine

Caffeine is an alkaloid found not only in coffee but in tea, in maté, and in the cola nut (cola bean). The alkaloid in tea used to be called theine, before it was shown to be identical with caffeine. Maté is made with leaves of a South American plant grown in Paraguay and Brazil; the cola bean comes from tropical Africa. Cola drinks were originally made with extracts of the bean; they are now largely put together from separate ingredients, including pure caffeine.

The amount of caffeine in a cup of beverage can obviously vary greatly, but an average cup of coffee, or of tea as used in the UK, contains about 80–100mg. A cup of instant coffee contains rather less, perhaps 60mg; a 12-oz can of cola drink contains about 35mg. It is quite easy to extract the caffeine from coffee. The caffeine is especially soluble in methylene dichloride or ethylene dichloride, leaving behind almost all the other constituents, which then constitute decaffeinated coffee.

Caffeine is a diuretic; drinking tea or coffee therefore produces a greater volume of urine than would be produced by the same volume of water. It is also a mild stimulant, producing a 'lift' in that it lessens tiredness and sleepiness. In the UK, the average person takes about 6 cups of tea or coffee in a day. Some people take 15 or 20 cups a day, and they sometimes complain of irritability and sleeplessness. On the other hand, these heavy drinkers, and sometimes people taking little more than the average, suffer withdrawal symptoms such as headaches and sleepiness when they suddenly stop taking ordinary tea or coffee.

CAFFEINE IN BEVERAGES

Tea, 5-oz cup (in UK)	80mg
Tea, 5-oz cup (in US)	35mg
Coffee, 5-oz cup (percolated)	100mg
Coffee, 5-oz cup (instant)	60mg
Coca-cola, 12oz	35mg
Tab, 12oz	45mg
Pepsi-cola, 12oz	35mg

Caffeine is sometimes put into pills that are claimed to be an aid to slimming; the rationale for this is that it produces a slight increase in thermogenesis.

See also: Addiction; Coffee; Soft drinks; Tea

Calcium

The body of an adult contains about 1,250g of calcium, more by far than the amount of any other mineral element. Over 99% is in the skeleton, and not more than 10g is in the blood and soft tissues of the body. The amount that is lost and therefore has to be replaced – the so-called turnover – is small, so that it would take about a year in a baby for the whole of the calcium to be replaced, and about 10 years in an adult.

Although the amount of calcium in the soft tissues is so small, calcium is involved in several important functions. These include the clotting of blood and the excitability of nerves and of the muscles, including the heart muscle.

Most of these functions require a constant concentration of calcium in the blood, of about 10mg/100ml blood. When it rises to 13mg or 14mg, the complications of hypercalcaemia are seen; when it falls to 8mg or 7mg, tetany may occur.

The constancy of the concentration of calcium in the blood is achieved by regulation of the amount absorbed from the gut, and regulation of the amount deposited within the bones or withdrawn from the bones. The absorption of calcium does not depend upon the amount in the diet, so long as it is more than enough to allow adequate absorption through the regulatory factors. The most important item controlling absorption is vitamin D, either that contained in the diet or that which is synthesized in the skin.

The vitamin D in its active form 1,25-dihydroxy vitamin D $(1,25-(OH)_2D)$ acts as a hormone, together with two other hormones, calcitonin and parathyroid hormone, in the precise regulation of the calcium concentration in the blood. Since the store of calcium in the bones is so vast in comparison with the amount in the blood, a significant increase in blood concentration from 10mg/100ml to 11mg, or a significant fall to 9mg, would be achieved by as little a change as 0.5g in the 1,250g of calcium in the skeleton. Thus, the function of the bones as a store of calcium is achieved with no discernible change in their function as the supporting framework of the body.

There are not many foods that are rich in calcium. The outstanding exceptions are milk and cheese. Tap water varies in the amount of calcium it contains; some hard waters can supply one-third or more of the adult needs of 500mg a day. In some countries, including the United Kingdom, bread is an important source of calcium, since it is a legal requirement that calcium carbonate (chalk, in the form of creta praeparata) be added to the flour from which all bread except wholemeal is made. The amount is about 0.36%. This legislation was introduced during the Second World War for two reasons. One was the introduction of bread made from flour of higher extraction; the second reason was the decreased production of milk and cheese. By increasing the rate of extraction of flour from the usual 72% for making white bread to the 80–85% for making the National Loaf, less wheat needed to be imported and so shipping space could be saved. But the higher extraction flour contained more phytate, which presumably reduced the absorption of calcium. The amount of calcium added to the flour was more than enough to combine with the phytate of the bread of higher extraction, so that a greater amount could be physiologically available.

Wholemeal flour, surprisingly, does not legally have to have calcium carbonate added, even though it has the greatest amount of phytate. The reason is that many of those who choose to eat wholemeal bread prefer it to be made in the traditional fashion and do not like unusual materials added.

With the increase in consumption of milk and cheese since the end of food rationing, and the return to the white loaf, there is now little reason for the continuation of this measure to ensure an adequate intake of calcium. Moreover, it seems that the body is able to adapt to an increase in dietary phytate. It has been suggested that the legal requirement for the addition of calcium carbonate to bread be rescinded.

It is appropriate here to point out two common fallacies about calcium. One is that additional dietary calcium, in the form of bone-ash, or in the form of salts such as calcium lactate or calcium gluconate, will help to strengthen the nails and thus prevent them from splitting. This is quite untrue, if only for the fact that, although they are hard, nails contain almost no calcium. They consist of keratin, the same protein that is the major constituent of the hair.

The second fallacy concerns the teeth. Although it is possible for severe deficiency of calcium in the diet to produce bones inadequately calcified, the degree of calcification of the teeth is unaffected. Rickets, resulting from deficiency of vitamin D, with or without deficiency of calcium, may delay the eruption of the teeth, but it does not affect their degree of calcification. It is also not true that pregnancy may lead to a reduction of calcium in the teeth, and result in what is often believed to be the almost inevitable loss of 'one tooth for each child'. Whatever calcium the unborn child needs comes either from the diet of the mother or, if this is inadequate, from her skeleton.

In the UK, the recommended allowance of calcium used to be assessed as being around 800mg a day for an adult man, and more for a pregnant woman, a nursing mother, or a growing child. It is now put at 500mg a day, and reduced also for the other categories, although some countries still have the higher figures. The chief reason for these differences and changes is that there are two major observations on which the estimates are made. One is derived from balance experiments, almost all of which have been carried out on individuals in Western countries, whose customary diets have contained a fairly high amount of calcium. The second observation is that, in many of the poorer countries, calcium intake may be 400mg a day or even less, and although their diets may be insufficient in other ways, their bones show no signs of inadequate calcification; the only exception seems to be the occurrence of osteomalacia in women who have had several children and are very deficient in both calcium and vitamin D.

The suggestion then is that the body can adapt to substantially lower amounts of dietary calcium than we had previously supposed. Certainly, a sudden reduction from, say, the 1,000mg a day which is commonly seen in the West, to perhaps 500mg, is likely to result in a loss of calcium from the body, but the loss will probably cease after a few weeks. There is, however, a wide range of individual variation, so that some people would rapidly adapt to the 50% reduction in calcium intake, others adapt slowly, and a few probably not have adapted even after several weeks.

We may wonder how pre-Neolithic man managed to supply his needs of calcium, when he had not yet begun to domesticate animals and use their milk in his diet. Even if he could survive with 400mg of calcium or so a day, he could not have obtained this amount from the food we often imagine constituted his total diet – green vegetables, berries, fruits, meat and fish. The probable answer is that the meat he consumed was not simply the attractive cuts we find in our butchers' shops, but included the soft bones of the animals he obtained by hunting and scavenging.

CALCIUM IN FOODS

Recommended daily intake (RDI) for moderately active man – 500mg

FOOD	PORTION	CALCIUM
		mg
Milk	100ml	120
Cheese, Cheddar	25g	200
cottage	100g	60
Cabbage, boiled	100g	40
Pulses, boiled	100g	15
Bread, wholemeal	30g	8
white, fortified	30g	35
Beef	100g	10

The availability of the calcium in different foods varies considerably, as explained in the text.

See also: Bone; Nutrient balance tests; Vitamin D

Calorie

This measure of energy is defined as the amount of heat required to raise the temperature of 1g of water through 1°C (more strictly, from 15°C to 16°C). Since energy exists in several interchangeable forms, this definition could have been made in terms of solar or chemical or electrical or mechanical energy, rather than thermal energy. Indeed, international convention has agreed that the unit for all sorts of energy should be the joule (J) which is defined in terms of mechanical work. But because the unit of heat, the calorie, has been used for a long time and is more widely known, 'calories' is still much more commonly seen than 'joules' in nutritional writings. It is nevertheless easy to convert one into the other, as one calorie equals 4.2 joules (more exactly, 4.184 joules).

These units are very small in relation to the amount of energy used by the body. For example, an adult might need something like 2,500,000 calories a day. For this reason, it is usual to use units 1,000 times as large, either the kilojoule (kJ) or the kilocalorie (kcal), sometimes confusingly written as Calorie. It is, however, understood in popular speech and writing that 'calories' means 'kilocalories'; a 1,000 calorie diet is a shorthand way of referring to a diet that provides 1,000 kcals a day.

See also: Energy; Joule

Cancer

Apart from the cells of the nervous tissue and usually muscle, cells of all other tissues can divide so as to replace cells that are lost by wear and tear, or by trauma. This cell division, however, is limited to the extent required by replacement. Nevertheless, the cells of a tissue sometimes begin spontaneously to divide in uncontrolled fashion, thus creating a lump or tumour. The tumour may be benign, and grow only locally, often within a defined capsule. The effect is to produce pressure on the adjoining organs, which usually does no harm except in such sites as the thyroid gland, where it may grow enough to interfere with breathing, or in the brain, where it can even cause death by pressure on the normal brain tissues.

Malignant tumours, or cancers, not only grow locally, but they invade adjoining tissues and organs; they also spread through the transmission of some of the cells from the original growth along the blood vessels or lymph vessels and so reach distant organs where new tumours are so to speak seeded. These secondary cancers are known as metastases.

There are considerable differences in the prevalence of some cancers in different countries. Primary cancer of the liver is very rare in most countries, but is not uncommon in some parts of Africa. Cancer of the oesphagus is rare in Western countries, but common in some African countries, around the Caspian Sea, and in China. Cancer of the stomach is common among the Japanese living in Japan, but less common among those living in the US, and also less common among American whites than among American blacks.

These differences indicate that there are likely to be factors in the environment that play a part in the causation of some cancers. Among such environmental causes, diet may well play a part. It has been particularly suspected as a cause of cancer of the colon; the dietary items to which most attention has been drawn are fat, meat, sugar and lack of fibre. However, convincing evidence for any of these items is not available.

Some food additives used in the past have been banned since they were known to cause cancer in experimental animals, or were suspected of doing so. The dye, butter yellow, and the artificial sweetener, cyclamate, are two such substances, although the evidence that cyclamate is carcinogenic, i.e. cancer-producing, is not accepted in some countries, including Germany and Switzerland.

Nitrosamines are chemical substances formed in foods to which nitrates or nitrites are added as preservatives, and are found for example in processed cheese and in meats. There are many different nitrosamines, and some have been found to be carcinogenic in animals when given in amounts at least 1,000 times greater than those likely to be found in foods for human consumption. At present, nitrates and nitrites are deemed to be safe.

The governments of many countries have advisory groups or committees which from time to time check the evidence that a particular substance or contaminant is possibly carcinogenic. The evidence is mostly sought by adding it to the feed of experimental animals, in quantities far greater than are likely to occur in a normal diet. If cancer is produced, the substance is likely to be banned.

In the United Kingdom, any substance proposed as an additive to food has to be approved by the Food Additives and Contaminants Committee, and this includes evidence about its possibly being carcinogenic. In the US, a special law called the Delaney Clause has been in existence since 1958. It says: 'No additive shall be deemed safe if it is found to induce cancer when ingested by man or animal.' This has been interpreted as meaning that a substance is not permitted for human consumption if it produces cancer when fed to any animal species in any quantity for any length of time.

As well as possibly causing cancer, it has been suggested that some dietary constituents may be protective. One such is carotene; another is vitamin B_{17} (Laetrile), which however is neither a normal dietary constituent nor of demonstrable efficacy.

Although it is unlikely that any particular diet can cure cancer or retard its progress, it is important that the morale and comfort of the patient be supported and sustained by careful attention to the diet. It should of course be of a high nutritional standard, so as to reduce as far as possible the loss of weight that is a common effect of cancer. But care must also be taken to ensure that the diet is not only available but is consumed by the patient, whose appetite is likely to be impaired.

It should therefore be as attractive as possible and well presented, and should include favourite foods and some alcoholic beverage if that is desired. On the other hand, foods the patient is known not to like should be avoided, however nutritious they may be. If there is difficulty in taking meals of normal size, frequent small meals may overcome the problem. It may, however, be necessary to give food by naso-gastric tube or by intravenous feeding.

See also: Carotene; Food additives; Laetrile; Nitrates/Nitrites

Carbohydrates

The name implies substances with a chemical structure made up of carbon and water; however, carbohydrates do not have water as such in their composition, but they have hydrogen and oxygen in the proportions in which they occur in water, that is, two hydrogen atoms for each oxygen atom (H_2O). For example, the carbohydrate glucose has the simple chemical formula $C_6H_{12}O_6$.

However, the trouble is that there are several chemical substances that have formulae fitting this description, but not all are carbohy-drates. This is seen when one looks at the formula set out in a more extended way, so as to show better how the atoms are connected with one another. Here are two substances that both have the simple for-mula $C_6H_{12}O_6$, but only one is a carbohydrate:

```
        CHOH                  CHO
        / \                    |
   HOHC   CHOH               CHOH
     |     |                   |
   HOHC   CHOH               CHOH
        \ /                    |
        CHOH                  CHOH
                               |
                             CHOH
                               |
                             CH₂OH
```

INOSITOL   GLUCOSE OR GALACTOSE OR FRUCTOSE
(not a carbohydrate)   (a carbohydrate)

It is possible to write even more elaborate formulae for the chemical structure of these compounds, which give still more information about them:

```
        CHO                    CHO                    CH₂OH
         |                      |                      |
     H · C · OH            H · C · OH                 CO
         |                      |                      |
    HO · C · H            HO · C · H            HO · C · H
         |                      |                      |
     H · C · OH           HO · C · H             H · C · OH
         |                      |                      |
     H · C · OH            H · C · OH            H · C · OH
         |                      |                      |
        CH₂OH                  CH₂OH                  CH₂OH

     GLUCOSE               GALACTOSE              FRUCTOSE
```

—CHO is an aldehyde group

   |
   CO is a keto group
   |

—CH₂OH is a primary alcohol group

   |
   CHOH (or H · C · OH, or HO · C · H) is a secondary alcohol group
   |

From this you can see that the technical characteristics of a carbohydrate, in addition to the simple description with which we began, are that one of the carbon atoms is part of an aldehyde or a keto group, another is part of a primary alcohol group, and the remaining carbon atom or atoms are part of secondary alcohol groups.

A great deal of the carbohydrate in living organisms is formed by green plants and retained by them. These plants synthesize glucose from water and carbon dioxide, with energy provided by sunlight; this is the process of photosynthesis. Part of the glucose is built into the complex carbohydrate cellulose, which forms most of the solid supporting structure of the plant; part is used by the plant for producing the energy it requires for its own metabolism, such as building its protein; part is stored in seeds, fruits and roots, mostly as starch, so as to provide a store of energy for itself and for the embryo when it begins to germinate and before it begins its own photosynthesis.

From the point of view of human nutrition, the carbohydrates can fairly be divided into unavailable and available. The unavailable carbohydrates are virtually indigestible, and so pass through the body without being absorbed, except for extremely small quantities of absorbable material that may be released by microbial action in the gut. These unavailable carbohydrates comprise almost the whole of what is now called dietary fibre and used to be called roughage.

The available carbohydrates can be absorbed by the intestine either directly or after digestion. Carbohydrate forms a large part of man's diet; in the wealthiest countries, it provides about 50% of the total energy, and in the poorer countries it may provide 85% or more.

Chemically, carbohydrates consist of units called monosaccharides, which can exist either by themselves or joined together. Two monosaccharides can join together to form a disaccharide, or many monosaccharides can join to form a polysaccharide, and these polysaccharides sometimes have many hundreds of monosaccharide units. The commonest monosaccharides have 6 carbon atoms; they are glucose, fructose and galactose. There are also less common monosaccharides, with 3, 4, 5 or 7 carbon atoms; the 5-carbon monosaccharide ribose is of particular interest as it is a component of the genetic material DNA.

The commonest sugars are all monosaccharides or disaccharides. The three best-known disaccharides are sucrose (table sugar), which is composed of glucose joined to fructose; lactose (found in milk), which is composed of glucose joined to galactose; and maltose (found in malted barley), which consists of two glucose units joined together.

Polysaccharides may be available or unavailable, depending on whether the particular way in which the monosaccharide units are joined together makes them susceptible to digestion or not. The most important available polysaccharide is starch, found principally in cereals and some vegetables, especially potatoes.

The unavailable carbohydrates consist of cellulose, hemicelluloses, pectin and gums. It is usual to include lignin in this classification, although it is not chemically a carbohydrate; nevertheless, it can form a significant fraction of the dietary fibre.

See also: Fibre; Fructose; Galactose; Glucose; Glycogen; Maltose; Starch; Sucrose

Carnitine

A very few species of animals, notably the mealworm, require in their diet a substance called carnitine, which, as its name implies, is found in meat. It has also been called vitamin BT.

For a long time, it was believed that carnitine was not a vitamin for human beings, since it can readily be produced in the body. However, recent evidence suggests that very rarely a disease of the muscles occurs that responds to the administration of carnitine. There is also some evidence that babies occasionally are unable to produce it in sufficient quantities, so that it is necessary for the deficit to be made up from the carnitine in the diet.

See also: Vitamins

Carotene

There are several carotenes, of somewhat different composition. They are all orange in colour, but of varying nutritional importance because of their varying ability to be converted into vitamin A; this ability accounts for their being given the name provitamin A. The most important is beta-carotene.

The carotenes account for much or all of the colour of some vegetables such as carrots. They also account for part of the colour of green vegetables, where the green colour of the chlorophyll is added to the orange colour of the carotene. Other plants, such as tomatoes, contain carotene together with anthocyanins, which do not have vitamin A activity. Red palm oil contains alpha-carotene, which is only about half as active as beta-carotene. Red palm oil added to some margarines is the source of both their colour and their vitamin A activity; vegetarian margarines in particular could not contain vitamin A from fish or whale oils.

The beautiful pink colour of the flamingo's plumage is derived from the pigments in the shrimps upon which it feeds; these pigments include a high proportion of carotene.

Some of the colour in milk, and thus in cream and butter, is derived from carotenes that have not been entirely converted to vitamin A by the cow; the colour of egg yolk is mostly *not* carotene but other substances that have no vitamin A activity.

On average, about one-sixth of the carotene in fruit and vegetables is converted into vitamin A, and about one-half of the carotene from dairy products and margarine. Tables of food composition usually give carotene in terms of vitamin A equivalent, allowing for the likely proportion of the carotene that will be converted into the vitamin.

For many years, it was thought that the conversion of carotene to vitamin A took place in the liver, a plausible assumption in view of the vast array of chemical activities for which that organ is responsible. It is now known that the conversion takes place within the wall of the intestine as the carotene is being absorbed.

Unlike vitamin A, carotene is not harmful when taken in large quantities. It may accumulate in the blood to an extent that produces a visible orange colour in the palate, but unlike the accumulation of bile pigments in jaundice, it does not colour the conjunctivae of the eyes.

It has been suggested that diets rich in carotene protect the body against some forms of cancer. Whether this is so still remains to be demonstrated.

See also: Vitamin A

Casal, Gaspar (c.1691–1759)

Casal was the first person to give a thorough description of pellagra, in a book published posthumously in 1762.

It is not quite certain when he was born, or even where; some believe he was born in Italy rather than in Spain, where he certainly spent most of his life.

He practised medicine in Madrid and many other cities, but eventually settled in Oviedo in the Asturias. He began his studies on pellagra in 1735, and some fifteen years later moved to Madrid, where his fame as the 'Asturian Hippocrates' was recognized: he received many honours, and was appointed chief court physician to Philip V.

Casal did not publish his observations on pellagra. After his death, they were collected and edited by his friend, Dr Juan Garcia Sevillano, and published in Latin as a chapter entitled 'De Affectione quae Vulgo in hac Regione mal de la Rosa nuncupatur' ('Concerning the affection which in this region is popularly called "mal de la Rosa" ').

Casal clearly described all but one of the classic features of pellagra: the seasonal nature of the disease, the appearance and sites of the skin lesions, the sore mouth, the lassitude, and the mania and melancholia. Curiously, he did not mention diarrhoea. From his excellent description of the dermatitis as it appears around the neck, together with the somewhat unrealistic woodcut illustration in the frontispiece, it is not surprising that we now use the term 'Casal's Collar'.

Casal did not agree with the common belief that pellagra was a contagious disease, a concept that was still being hotly debated as late as the 1920s. He wrote: 'If it were possible to apply to these poverty-

HISTORIA
NATURAL, Y MEDICA
DE EL PRINCIPADO DE ASTURIAS.

OBRA POSTHUMA,

QUE ESCRIBIO EL DOCT. D. GASPAR
Casál, Medico de su Magestad, y su Proto-
Medico de Castilla, Academico de la
Real Academia Medica
Matritense,&c.

LA SACA A LUZ

EL DOCT. JUAN JOSEPH GARCIA
Sevillano, Medico de Familia del Rey
nuestro Señor, Ex-Examinador de su Real
Proto-Medicato, Medico que ha sido de los
Reales Hospitales, y actual de el Real Sitio
de Buen Retiro, Academico de la Real
Academia Medica Matritense, y de
la Real de Oporto, &c.

CON LICENCIA: En Madrid, en la Oficina de Manuel Mar-
tin, Calle de la Cruz. Año de 1762.
*Se hallará en la Librería de Don Francisco Manuel de Mena,
Calle de las Carretas.*

stricken sick the same remedies as to the rich, I would prescribe for them ... above all good and nutritious food.'

Before Casal's book appeared, an account of the disease, with due acknowledgement to Casal, was given by the celebrated French physician, Thierry (1718–92). This precedes the publication of Casal's own observations by seven years.

See also: Pellagra

Cassava

This plant originated in tropical South America, where it is known as manioca or yucca. It is now grown extensively in tropical Africa and Asia. It grows as shrubs or small trees, and is easily propagated by cuttings, producing much food for relatively little effort. The tubers or roots are dug up like potatoes and dried in the sun before being cooked. The outer part of the root contains a goitrogen, and a substance called linamarin, which yields cyanide by the action of an enzyme in the root. Drying destroys the enzyme and thus prevents the release of cyanide. It seems, though, that some cyanide may nevertheless be released from cassava after ingestion, because those for whom this root is an important article of diet have a raised urinary excretion of thiocyanate, a substance formed in the body when it detoxifies cyanide.

The major disadvantage of cassava is that it provides very little protein, less than 2% of its dry weight, and thus much less than potato or yams. It is understandable then that kwashiorkor is commonly found in countries where cassava is the staple food. When dried and powdered cassava is washed well, so that the protein is almost entirely removed, the resulting product is tapioca, which is virtually pure starch.

See also: Poisons in food; Protein-energy malnutrition

Cellulite

Articles on beauty in magazines or newspapers frequently refer to a condition called cellulite. It was described first in France, and is still pronounced 'celluleet'.

It is described as a special deposit of fatty material occurring especially in women, most commonly on the thighs, buttocks and hips.

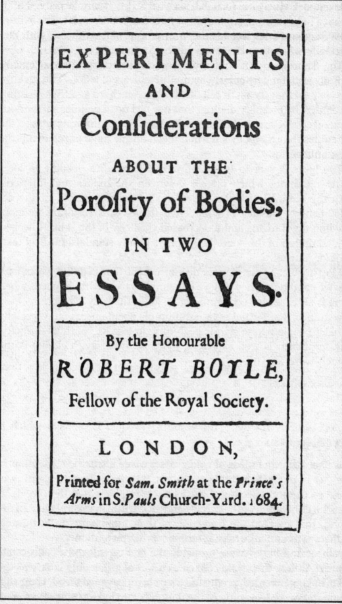

EXPERIMENTS
AND
Confiderations
ABOUT THE
Porofity of Bodies,
IN TWO
ESSAYS.

By the Honourable
ROBERT BOYLE,
Fellow of the Royal Society.

LONDON,

Printed for *Sam. Smith* at the *Prince's Arms* in S. *Pauls* Church-Yard. 1684.

See Osmotic pressure

It is almost always associated with straightforward obesity, but is claimed to be different from ordinary accumulations of fat. The feature most frequently described is the 'orange peel' appearance of the skin, especially when the skin is pinched.

The description of the supposed special structure of the offending deposits is given particularly by manufacturers of lotions and creams. It is claimed that the fat in cellulite has become hard and thus resistant to removal by ordinary dieting; that it is tied up in nodules surrounded by an excessive amount of connective tissue, and that this adds to the difficulties that the body's normal mechanisms have in removing the accumulated fat.

The basis is said to be an hormonal imbalance, leading to local water retention, which presses down on the tissues and interferes with the removal of toxins. These toxins are responsible for the development of threads of connective tissue, thus resulting in more building up of toxins and a decreased elasticity of the skin. However, no description of the condition appears in any standard medical textbook or journal.

Most medical practitioners do not accept that cellulite exists as a specific condition. They believe it is simply part of what happens when there is an excessive accumulation of fat in the body. The orange-peel appearance is a normal manifestation of subcutaneous fat, especially in older people whose skin is beginning to lose its youthful elasticity. The scepticism is well expressed by those who say, 'Cellulite is the French word for fat.'

See also: Obesity

Cereals

It is likely that the seeds of wild grasses made a small contribution to the diet of our pre-neolithic ancestors, but the deliberate planting of these seeds, and selecting them for their yield, created the cereals. It was the cultivation of the cereals, independently in several parts of the world, that marked the transition of their inhabitants from hunter-gatherers to agriculturalists – the neolithic revolution.

Wheat and barley were probably the first cereals to be deliberately grown. At first, they were cooked as a sort of gruel; only later was the art of baking invented, producing a sort of unleavened bread. Later still, fermentation or leavening of the dough before baking was discovered.

There are currently seven major cereals, which tend to be grown in different regions of the world, depending largely on their climates. They are wheat, maize, rice, barley, millet, oats and rye. The Table gives approximate figures for amounts produced annually throughout the world. The proportion used for human food, for animal feed, and for the production of alcohol, varies widely with the different cereals. Much of the maize is produced in the United States, and is used for feeding cattle and pigs; much of the barley is produced in northern climates, and is used for brewing, and for feeding cattle.

The major cereal used in a country is known as 'corn', so that it would imply wheat in the UK and Western Europe, and maize in the United States and parts of Africa. However, the spreading consumption of 'cornflakes' for breakfast is increasing the American usage of corn to mean maize.

Cereals form a large proportion of the diet in some poorer countries, and provide as much as 80% of the total energy intake. The proportion falls as countries become less poor, but even in the UK bread and flour contribute about 20% of the energy in the average diet.

Cereals also supply an appreciable amount of protein, as well as several of the B vitamins, thus belying the belief that they consist of little but starch and so contribute little except calories.

The protein of wheat and of rye is the complex gluten, which is a mixture of gliadin and glutelin. When mixed with water it can be stretched, and being viscid it holds together when distended by gas. Because of this, the production of carbon dioxide in a dough by yeast or by baking powder gives bubbles in a way that makes the dough rise. Bread cannot be made properly from cereals other than wheat and rye, because they have little or no gluten.

Gluten is also the protein to which those suffering from coeliac disease are sensitive, so that they are not allowed to eat products of wheat or rye, but are allowed to eat products of maize or rice.

In considering the nutritional value of a food, that is, what it can contribute to a diet for human beings, it is useful to consider its role in providing for the nutrition of the species from which the food is derived. For example, milk plays an important role in the growth of young organisms of the new generation of mammals, just as eggs and seeds do in the growth of young birds and plants. These items would be expected to provide them with all they need by way of energy or nutrients until they have made themselves partially or wholly independent by being able to obtain for themselves the nourishment they need.

Cereals are the commonest seeds used as food for man. Unlike milk and eggs, they contain little water, thus enabling them to survive from season to season; indeed, the seeds may still be viable after many years. As food for human beings, therefore, they have the great advantage that they can be stored for many months or even, as the Bible story of Joseph tells us, for several years. When they germinate, they provide the energy and nutrients for the initial growth of the root and shoot. The energy is provided mostly from a store of starch. The nutrients exist in the form of the protein, vitamins and mineral elements that the plant requires for early growth. Thus, the vitamins are chiefly those of the B group required especially in the metabolism of carbohydrate, fat and protein for energy release and for tissue building. The mineral elements are mostly potassium, magnesium and phosphorus, with relatively small amounts of a range of other elements. In terms of animal nutrition, the cereals are low in calcium; the plant does not need much calcium because it does not need to produce bone.

Breakfast cereals: Breakfast cereals were introduced in the United States in the 1850s by a Dr John Harvey Kellogg, who was the director of a 'sanitarium' at Battle Creek, Michigan. To a large extent, this was influenced by the demand of vegetarian groups such as the Seventh Day Adventists. The first product was given the brand name 'Granola', and was made of wheat, oatmeal and maize. The first flaked product appeared in 1896, and was called 'Granose'; cornflakes, made from maize, arrived in 1899. Since that time, a health food of limited appeal has become a food of general appeal in many countries.

Breakfast cereals, in themselves, contribute little directly to the nutritional value of the total diet, except those that have been fortified with vitamins and perhaps iron and protein. But in two other ways breakfast cereals make what can be called a vicarious contribution to the diet. It may be a negative contribution, in that they almost always contain sugar and it is usual to add more sugar at the table; on the

WORLD CEREAL PRODUCTION

Approximate annual production, 1979–81, in million tonnes (FAO statistics)

Wheat	240	Barley	80
Rice	145	Millet	43
Maize	130	Oats	26
		Rye	15

other hand, there is a positive contribution from the milk that is usually taken with the cereal.

See also: Individual cereals

Chapati

Traditionally, this is made in India and Pakistan with only water and wheat flour of 95% extraction. The mixture is baked without leaven as a flat cake. Variations in the recipe include the adding of milk, or fat, or egg, or sugar, and occasionally yeast.

Cheese

Cheese has been known for many centuries, and was no doubt discovered as a means of preserving milk, which is easily perishable. When made deliberately, there is a wide choice of starting materials. Firstly, although most of the available cheese is made from cows' milk, some is made from the milk of sheep, goats, or even reindeer or buffalo. Secondly, the cheese may be made from whole milk, or from partly or wholly skimmed milk. There are also variations in the method of manufacture. The first essential step, the production of curd from the milk, may be carried out either by souring the milk with the aid of a bacterial culture, or by the addition of the enzyme rennet, or both.

The final cheese may contain as much as 75% of water (cottage cheese), or less than 30% (Parmesan, Stilton). Some cheeses are deliberately infected with moulds, either within the cheese (so-called blue cheeses, such as Stilton, Roquefort, Gorgonzola), or simply on the surface (Camembert, Brie). It is not surprising that there are said to be more than 900 commercially available varieties of cheese.

The essential early step in making cheese is the production of the curd by clotting. The clot is formed from the chief protein in milk, casein. As it forms, it carries with it most of the fat, much of the vitamins, especially riboflavin, and many of the mineral elements of the milk, especially calcium. The whey is now drained off; this contains 1% protein (lactalbumin and lactoglobulin), lactose and the remaining water-soluble vitamins and salts.

If the curds are simply drained off from the whey, and a little salt added, the result is cottage cheese. Variants of this are cream cheese, which has cream added, and quark, which is made from fully skimmed milk and thus has no fat at all.

The commonest cheese in the UK is Cheddar cheese. In making this, the curds are allowed to settle at the bottom of the trough in which the milk is curdled, first by the addition of bacteria and after a time, during which the milk is warmed, by the addition of rennet. As the curds drain, they tend to form a solid mass; this is cut into slabs in the trough, which are turned from time to time and gradually 'Cheddared', that is, piled on top of one another so that more whey is pressed out. Eventually, the mass is milled, salt added, and the product put into a press to expel more whey and to shape the cheese. It is then allowed to mature in a room in which a cool temperature is maintained. It is at this point that moulds, or perhaps further strains of bacteria, may be encouraged to develop, to produce different varieties of cheese.

Processed cheese is made by the addition of a variety of materials, such as dried milk powder, emulsifiers, and flavours; a preservative such as nitrite may also be added.

Because there are only small quantities of lactose remaining in the curd, cheese does not produce symptoms in individuals with lactose intolerance.

Cheeses contain varying amounts of a substance called tyramine. This can cause a rise in blood pressure. Normally, it is destroyed by an enzyme called monoamine oxidase. There is a group of drugs, however, that act as monoamine oxidase inhibitors, and are sometimes used in the treatment of depression; examples are 'Nardil' and 'Marplan'. People taking such a drug will tend to accumulate tyramine if they eat cheese, and this can have very serious consequences. As well as severe headache and dizziness, they may suffer from a considerable rise in blood pressure, and this may even lead to cerebral haemorrhage, that is, a stroke.

See also: Lactose intolerance; Milk

Chestnuts

Mostly grown in southern Europe, the chestnut tree is valued both for its fruit and for its beautifully grained wood. The fruit is extensively used in some countries, especially Japan, Italy and France, and particularly in Corsica. It can be ground into flour for stews, soups, porridge and stuffing, boiled or roasted and eaten whole, or preserved in sugar to make the delicious French sweet, marrons glacés. It contains 50% or so of water, much more than do other nuts; it also has less protein and fat, and the carbohydrate contains a high proportion of sugar. It was very much a food for the poor, particularly before the widespread use of the potato.

Chestnut trees were abundant in the US until the accidental introduction of a parasitic fungus in the early part of the twentieth century; by the beginning of the Second World War, they had virtually disappeared.

Cholesterol

Although cholesterol itself is found only in animal tissues, it is one of a large number of sterols that are widely distributed in the plant and animal kingdom. Cholesterol is a white waxy material, with a complex structure that includes alcohol groups; it thus exists in the body mostly in the form of esters with fatty acids.

The adult body contains some 140g of cholesterol. Much of it is in the membranes of all the body's cells, especially the nerve cells. In addition, it is the raw material from which the body makes a range of other important substances, including the sex hormones, the hormone cortisol from the adrenal gland, vitamin D_3, and the bile salts.

Some cholesterol is held in a complex form in solution in the blood, a compound in which the cholesterol is combined with lipoprotein. The body is able to make cholesterol, and also obtains some from the diet. The richest sources are eggs and brain, followed by liver and kidney, and then butter and hard cheese.

The amount of cholesterol in the blood is only slightly increased when more is taken in the diet. This is because the increased intake is partly offset by a reduction in the amount that the body synthesizes. Much more effective in changing the concentration of cholesterol in the blood is the amount and type of fat. An increase in blood cholesterol occurs with diets containing much fat, especially saturated fat; a decrease occurs with diets containing little fat, especially if this is mostly polyunsaturated. Some increase in cholesterol also occurs in diets with much sucrose.

The gain in cholesterol from the diet and from bodily synthesis is normally compensated by the excretion of cholesterol. This occurs chiefly in the stools. Some cholesterol is present in the bile, and so finds its way into the small intestine, where it is partially re-absorbed and the rest excreted. In addition, the bile salts themselves are manufactured by the liver from cholesterol and these too pass into the intestine; again, these are partially re-absorbed and the rest excreted in the stools.

The deposits of atheroma in the arteries that occur in atherosclerosis contain cholesterol, as well as several other constituents.

CHOLESTEROL IN SOME FOODS

Average values, mg in 100g food

Brain	2,200	Shrimps	200
Fish roe	600	Meat	100
Kidney	500	Fish	80
Egg	450	Oysters	50
Liver	400	Vegetable foods	0

See also: Atherosclerosis; Bile; Coronary heart disease; Gall-bladder; Lipoprotein

Choline

Choline is often thought to be a vitamin, but although it is an essential component of the body, it is easily produced by the body, so it is not necessary to include it in the diet. Most of the choline in the body is present as lecithin.

See also: Lecithin

Chromium

The evidence from animal experiments indicates that chromium is an essential element. Deficiency causes a diminution in glucose tolerance, and it has been claimed that some diabetics who do not respond very well to conventional treatment are improved when they are given chromium. It is, however, still not certain whether it is a dietary essential for human beings.

See also: Glucose tolerance

Chronic

Lasting a long time, and usually of gradual onset; the opposite of acute.

Cider vinegar

Like the alcohol from any other source, that in cider, which is fermented apple juice, can be oxidized to acetic acid by bacteria; this product is known as cider vinegar.

Cider vinegar has a reputation for curing a range of diseases including, as quoted in one book, 'arthritis and rheumatism, hay fever, asthma, digestive disturbances, heart troubles, and 'flu, colds and catarrh. Above all, it is popular as an aid to weight reduction.'

If any of the claims could be substantiated, which they certainly have not been, it would be extraordinarily difficult to understand by what mechanism these outstanding cures had been achieved by a product of fermented apple juice. Its mineral content, for example, which some writers have suggested is the basis for the cures effected by cider vinegar, is no different from the mineral content of the apple from which the product originated.

See also: Health foods

Citrus fruits

There is now a very wide range of fruits belonging to the citrus family, many of them deliberately cultivated hybrids. The family originated in China, although it is possible that the lime came from India. Surprisingly though, the grapefruit appeared spontaneously less than 200 years ago as an entirely new species in the New World, probably in Jamaica.

Citrus fruits are characterized by containing a juice in which the dissolved constituents are mostly sugars and acids, together with an unusually high quantity of vitamin C. The commonest citrus fruits are oranges and grapefruit, containing much sugar and relatively little acid, and lemons with less sugar and more acid. Tangerines and mandarins are less common, as are a range of hybrids including uglis, tangelos and temples. Even less commonly seen are citrons and kum-quats. The lime, traditionally the fruit associated with the treatment and prevention of scurvy, has less vitamin C than do most of the other citrus fruits: it is, however, not at all certain that it was limes rather than lemons that were used by Dr James Lind, who conducted the first convincing experiments in the search for a cure for scurvy.

The habit of beginning the day with a drink of orange juice, almost universal in the United States, but also popular with the more pros-perous citizens of Western Europe, is one way of ensuring an adequate intake of vitamin C. Whether it is the best way, however, is doubtful, since it is accompanied by a high intake of sugars which, on an empty stomach, may excessively increase the blood concentration of glucose and of the insulin it provokes.

See also: Lind; Scurvy; Vitamin C

Climate

Man is able to live in a wide range of climates because of his ability to provide himself with shelter and with food in very different conditions. The former depends on his skill in the use of tools and in the manufac-ture of materials such as cloth, leather and bricks; the latter depends on his skills in hunting and fishing, on his skills in food production, and on his omnivorous habit.

It is often assumed that the different diets he eats in hot or cold climates indicate differences in physiological needs. There is, however, no evidence for this assumption, and it is much more likely that what determines the climatic variations of diets is climatic variation in the sorts of foods that are available.

One reason why physiological requirements do not depend very much on the general environmental conditions is that the body is exposed more to the micro-environment created by dwelling and clothing. The effect is to reduce considerably the range of temperature and other conditions surrounding the body. This applies more to living in cold climates than in hot; except in the rare situations in which air conditioning is available, it is easier to keep the body warm in a cold climate than cool in a hot climate.

Indirectly, however, the clothes that would be worn to keep a body warm might impede movement sufficiently to increase the effort needed for carrying out physical tasks, and so increase energy expenditure. On the other hand, heat and cold are likely to reduce activity and so reduce energy expenditure. This reduction, however, will only be small.

The need for protein and vitamins is influenced little if at all by climate. Of the minerals, there is a small increase in iron loss through sweating.

It is usually said that an essential requirement in a hot climate is an increase in salt intake. There is now a strong body of opinion that the ability of the body to conserve salt intake by reducing urinary excretion makes it unnecessary for more salt to be taken than is likely to be found in most ordinary diets.

Finally, for persons who have come to either a cold or a hot climate from a temperate one, the psychological effects of their diet are likely to be more important than the physical effects. In their new and unusual surroundings, probably subjected to unusual strains and pressures socially and in their work, the comforting and enjoyable experience of eating good food well prepared, and especially, if possible, the availability of at least some foods to which they are accustomed, will help to maintain their health and reduce possible anxiety and boredom.

See also: Basal metabolism; Sodium

Cobalt

Cobalt is part of vitamin B_{12} and thus an essential dietary constituent for man. Whereas man and many other animals need the vitamin itself in their diet, many ruminants such as sheep and cattle are able to manage with the cobalt salts present in herbage because the vitamin can be synthesized by the micro-organisms in the rumen. Deficiency of cobalt sometimes occurs in cattle, and leads to 'pining disease'.

The amount in the average Western diet is between 0.25mg and 0.5mg a day. In the United States and Canada, cobalt salts were for a time added to beer. It was found to increase the 'head' of beer, that is, the amount of foam, which had been reduced by residues of detergent left on the glass. Since sometimes as much as 1.5mg/litre of cobalt was added, which is 3–6 times the average daily intake, and since some beer drinkers take 10 or more litres a day, the result was cobalt toxicity. This showed itself as a form of heart failure, which in some instances was fatal.

See also: Vitamin B$_{12}$

Cocoa and chocolate

Cocoa is grown on small trees, which produce gourds containing a large number of cacao beans. Its native habitat was originally the Amazon and other parts of South America and Mexico. It is now grown mostly in Ghana and Nigeria. It was consumed as a drink called 'chocolate', from the Aztec word *xocolatl*. This was made by drying the beans in the sun, roasting them, breaking them into 'nibs' and then grinding these. Spices, vanilla and water were added, and the resulting thick drink was drunk cold. Cocoa was brought to Europe by the Spaniards, and then spread to France; it reached England around 1650, and a few years later began to be taken with sugar. It became a popular drink among the gentry, especially the young men about town, who frequented the rapidly-growing number of chocolate houses in the cities.

The cocoa used at that time was excessively fatty because of its high content of cocoa butter, and was made palatable by the admixture of flour and other starchy products. In 1828, Dutch cocoa was produced by Van Houten, who developed a process by which some of the fat was removed under pressure and the cocoa treated with alkali; this is known as 'dutching'. Nevertheless, it was not until 1866 that Cadbury produced a fine cocoa powder similar to that produced by the Dutch, and called it cocoa essence; this had nothing added to it, and made cocoa much more popular.

Drinking chocolate has sugar added to the cocoa powder, and is usually made with milk, or with milk powder and hot water. It is not known when chocolate for eating was first introduced, but it seems to have been around 1830. It was made by grinding the cocoa nibs very finely, and adding cocoa butter that had been expressed in the manufacture of cocoa, together with sugar. The grinding of the mixture is continued with machinery called a melangeur, and then transferred to another type of grinder called a conche. Dried milk powder may be added to produce milk chocolate, an invention of the Swiss firm Peter in 1876. The quality of eating chocolate depends very much on the fineness to which the grinding reduces the mixed ingredients.

Cocoa powder contains roughly 25% fat, 35% carbohydrate and 20% protein. In view of the small quantities consumed, neither the energy nor the nutrients makes a significant contribution to the diet.

Chocolate confectionery, on the other hand, which may be consumed in appreciably larger amounts, may make a measurable contribution to the diet. Although there is great variation in different samples, plain chocolate typically contains about 30% fat, 5% protein and the remainder carbohydrate, and 100g will provide around 500 kcal. The amount of vitamins and mineral elements, however, is small and may be ignored, except for the calcium in milk chocolate; 100g provides 200mg or more of this element.

There are small quantities of alkaloids in cocoa and thus in chocolate. The most important is theobromine, which has a similar action to that of caffeine. There is also some caffeine in the cocoa. Nevertheless, the amounts of caffeine and theobromine are not enough to produce any noticeable effect.

See also: Alkaloid

Coconut

Originating in Malaysia, coconut palms often grow on the shore and are tolerant of salty, sandy soil; they can, however, be cultivated in tropical and sub-tropical regions in other locations, provided the soil is well drained: In West Africa, the coconut provides a most important food. The palms grow rapidly and begin to bear fruit in the sixth year; however, they do not produce their maximum yield until they are about 20 years old, then continue to do so for another 60 years.

The fruit grows at the top of the tree among the leaves. Since it falls only when it is over-ripe, it has to be picked, sometimes by trained monkeys. The unripe fruit contains a fluid, coconut milk, which is slightly sweet and pleasant to drink, but has little nutritive value. The husk yields coir, used for making ropes and coconut matting. The white meat inside the shell can be eaten fresh, or as copra when it has been dried. Copra contains up to 50% oil, which is used in confectionery and cakes, and for the making of cooking oils and margarine. Of the fatty acids in coconut oil, as much as 98% can be saturated; this is a good example of the error of assuming that vegetable oils are necessarily rich in polyunsaturated acids.

The sap of the coconut tree may be used as a drink, known as sweet toddy, or dried to make a raw sugar which the Indians call gharri, or it may be fermented to make a drink known simply as toddy. It is said that when the missionaries in parts of Africa found the local villagers doing this, they persuaded them to give up the habit because it was sinful to drink alcohol. The result was that they became short of the thiamin produced by the fermenting yeast, and developed beri-beri.

See also: Fatty acids

Codex Alimentarius

An increasing amount of food and food products is transferred between countries. Many countries, especially those that are industrialized, have strict food laws governing hygiene, the use of additives and the possible adulteration of foods, while the non-industrialized countries that export a great deal of food often do not have these laws or cannot enforce them. Nevertheless, an attempt was begun in 1963 to set up a universal code of practice, to be prepared jointly by the Food and Agriculture Organization and the World Health Organization (FAO and WHO), to be called the Codex Alimentarius. The intention is that it should cover some 200 foods.

Each country has to decide whether it will accept the proposed standards. There has understandably been great difficulty in getting all the countries to agree to do this, even when the appropriate joint FAO/WHO committee has reached agreement as to what the rules should be.

See also: Food additives; Food adulteration

Cod liver oil

For well over 100 years, cod liver oil has been used in the treatment of many diseases, often ineffectively. Nevertheless, it was certainly used effectively for the treatment of rickets by Armand Trousseau (1801–

67), the famous French physician, in the middle of the nineteenth century. Cod liver oil is rich in vitamin A and vitamin D, although the amounts vary considerably from sample to sample. It is used in several countries, often routinely, for preventing rickets in babies and small children, or for curing it when it occurs.

See also: Rickets; Vitamin A; Vitamin D

Coeliac disease

Children who fail to grow may be suffering from coeliac disease, otherwise known as gluten enteropathy, due to a sensitivity to gluten. This is a mixture of proteins found in wheat and rye, but only in small quantities, if at all, in barley, oats, maize and rice. A similar condition may be seen in adults as one form of 'ideopathic steatorrhoea', and it is now thought that in these instances the disease has been present from childhood but in a mild or symptomless form.

The sensitivity to gluten leads to a destruction of the villi, the tiny threadlike papillae in the mucosa of the small intestine, responsible for the absorption of foods. As a result, part of the food is not digested and is lost in the stools, which are copious and fatty. In addition to diminished growth, there is anaemia and perhaps rickets or osteomalacia. There is a slight tendency for the disease to be familial. It may vary in intensity and sometimes improves spontaneously; on the other hand, the child with coeliac disease may be severely undernourished and stunted, and may die young.

The disease improves remarkably when a gluten-free diet is adopted. This entails the avoidance not only of bread, pasta and other obvious sources of gluten, but also of manufactured foods such as sausages and sauces, to which flour is often added. Many manufacturers of baby foods have omitted gluten from at least some of their products, and this is now indicated by the presence of a recognized symbol on the label. In the UK, extensive information about appropriate foods is available from the Coeliac Society.

See also: Absorption of fat; Cereals

Coffee

An infusion of ground coffee beans was for centuries drunk in Arabia and Ethiopia, where the coffee tree originally grew wild. These are now cultivated in large plantations in Brazil, and in many other countries including India, Africa and Indonesia. The trees grow to 10 or 15 feet. When ripe, the beans are picked, and are then roasted and ground before being infused. The aroma gradually diminishes after roasting and especially after grinding, so that the connoisseur carries out these treatments as near as possible to the time when he intends to brew coffee.

Instant coffee is a powder produced by making the infusion and then either spray-drying it or – for better retention of flavour – freeze-drying it. French coffee contains up to 49% added chicory, and Viennese coffee up to 15% added dried figs; there is no caffeine in either of these materials – coffee connoisseurs might call them adulterants.

Coffee was brought to Europe in the early seventeenth century. The first coffee houses were opened in London in 1659, and rapidly became meeting places for literary and business groups. One of the coffee houses was Lloyds, and the men meeting there formed the nucleus of what later became the world-famous insurance institution.

An average cup of coffee made from ground coffee contains about 100mg of caffeine; a cup of instant coffee usually contains somewhat less caffeine, about 60mg. Coffee also contains nicotinic acid, so that a cup may provide 0.5mg–1mg.

See also: Caffeine

Constipation

Many people believe that it is necessary to pass faeces once a day, and that anything less frequent is constipation. The fact is that, like much else in the way of bodily functions, there is a wide range of normality, from two or even three times a day to twice or even once a week. It is only when defaecation is accompanied by difficulty or discomfort that true constipation exists.

This misconception is itself a main cause of the condition. People who, perhaps from childhood, have been led to believe that daily evacuation of the bowels is important, are inclined to depend heavily on the use of laxatives to achieve that objective. This accounts for the vast sale of laxatives, involving the spending of some £10 million a year by the British public. By the use of laxatives, the normal bowel reflexes are gradually diminished, and they come to be increasingly dependent on the stimulus provided by the laxative.

Constipation often occurs during pregnancy and in the elderly. Relief is best sought from an increase in the amount of dietary fibre. The sudden development of constipation in middle age or later, in persons who have not previously been constipated, warrants early medical examination to discover the cause, which may require attention.

Laxatives have no place in the treatment of obesity. On the one hand, restricted diets taken for weight reduction may result in less frequent defaecation, but do not produce true constipation. On the other hand, laxatives do not help in the treatment of obesity; only when they are taken in vastly excessive quantities, as by some people suffering from bulimia nervosa, does the resulting diarrhoea reduce the absorption of nutrients, and then to a harmful extent.

See also: Fibre

Cooking

The first use of fire, including its use for cooking food, occurred some millions of years ago when men's ancestors learned how to maintain fire that occurred naturally from lightning, earthquake or volcano, and perhaps even from its spontaneous production from the rubbing together of wind-blown dried branches. It was not until perhaps half a million years ago that they gained the ability to make fire, rather than simply to use it when it was accidentally available.

Fire serves many important functions. The heat and light of fire gave protection from wild animals and perhaps from enemies, and extended the period when man could be active after sunset. Much later, the heat of the fire made possible the preparation of bronze and iron, and their use in the production of more efficient tools and weapons.

Fire enables food to be cooked, and this had many important consequences on the sorts of foods that could be included in the diet, and in the proportions of different foods. Some of these effects are more obvious than others.

Starch-rich foods, such as cereals, root vegetables and dried pulses, are difficult to digest, because the plant cells are surrounded by walls composed mostly of cellulose. Cooking makes the starch within them swell, so that cell walls burst. The starch is then available for digestion by the amylase in the saliva and pancreatic juice, and the products of digestion, together with other nutrients from the cells, are available for absorption into the blood.

The cooking of meat and fish makes them more tender and tasty. It results in the breakdown of the collagen that makes up the greater part of the connective tissue. From being a tissue composed chiefly of tough collagen fibres, it is changed to a soft tissue composed largely of gelatin. As a result the food becomes tender, a property that makes it easier to chew. This enhances the time-saving quality of meat in supplying a more concentrated source of nutrition than is supplied by vegetables. In addition, the contraction of the fibres of the meat or the fish expels some of their contents, especially the small molecules of amino-acids and salts that provide the succulent flavour of these cooked foods and the gravy to which they give rise.

Fruits and green vegetables are more readily eaten raw than is meat. On the other hand, the amounts that can easily be eaten of the cooked foods, especially vegetables, are much greater than can be eaten of the raw; the greater concentration of some nutrients in raw vegetables than in cooked is often outweighed by this fact.

The making of jams and jellies from the fruit depends on the heat that releases pectin and acid from the fruit, so that it can react with the sugar and produce a gel.

The effects of cooking on nutritional value are both general and specific. The general effect is that some foods would either not be eaten at all if they were not cooked, or would be eaten in only small quantities. In this connection, it is necessary only to quote the maxim, 'Food that is not eaten has a nutritional value of zero.'

The specific effects on nutritional value are several. Many raw legumes, including groundnuts and soy beans, are not well digested because they contain inhibitors of the protein-digesting enzyme trypsin in the intestine. The inhibitors are destroyed by the heat of cooking. Foods such as bread, which contain both carbohydrate and protein, may lose some of the value of the protein because of the browning reaction. Fatty foods such as meat may lose part of their fat when it melts if it is not incorporated into a gravy or used later. Heating tends to reduce the quantity of linoleic acid and vitamin E that may be present in the fat. Similarly, some of the mineral salts and water-soluble vitamins may be leached out of the food, and will be lost if the gravy is not used. Moreover, some vitamins, especially thiamin and vitamin C, are not very stable, particularly if the food has a neutral pH or if it is alkaline or made alkaline by cooking, for example, with soda. On the other hand, heating increases the availability of the nicotinic acid in cereals.

Perhaps the most important effect of cooking is that it destroys most pathogenic organisms, both microbial and non-microbial, such as the cysts or larvae of some worms. It also destroys many of the organisms that promote spoilage of food, so that cooking extends the period during which food remains wholesome.

Finally, the cooking of various foods and food extracts in combination produces dishes in which novel tastes and textures are created. Even the simplest of these can give great pleasure to people, and make palatable food items which on their own soon become monotonous and so may conduce to inadequate nutrition. On the other hand, such highly palatable 'combination' foods as cakes, confectionery, ice cream and desserts may lead to the over-consumption of nutritionally undesirable food components.

See also: **Appetite; Browning reaction; Neolithic revolution; Nicotinic acid**

Cooking fats

Like margarine, cooking fats are made from a mixture of oils and soft fats, hardened by the process of hydrogenation. Unlike margarine, colouring is not added, since this is not demanded by the consumer. Vitamins are not added either, presumably because lard and similar fats, for which cooking fats are manufactured as a substitute, do not contain them, and their addition is not required by law.

See also: **Margarine; Oils**

Copper

Copper is an essential component of several enzymes in the body, including cytochrome oxidase, one of the enzymes concerned with the oxidative processes that take place in all the cells. Deficiency of copper sometimes occurs in cattle, where it produces a severe anaemia, and in sheep, where it leads to an ataxia called swayback. Deficiency has not been reported in adult human beings, but it does occur, though rarely, in infants. Here it produces chronic diarrhoea and, later, anaemia. Occasionally, some of the symptoms of kwashiorkor have been found to improve when copper was administered, together with the necessary diet.

The total amount of copper in the human body is usually between 100mg and 150mg; the amount in the average Western diet is about 2mg a day.

Since excessive copper is toxic, many countries have legislation that limits the amount permitted in processed foods.

See also: Mineral elements

Coronary heart disease

This is often referred to as CHD, and is sometimes called ischaemic heart disease (IHD), or coronary thrombosis, or myocardial infarction. IHD is a precise synonym for coronary heart disease, but the other two are not exactly the same, as we shall see.

The basis of CHD is a reduction of the blood flow along one or both of the coronary arteries, which are the first branches of the aorta, the main artery carrying blood from the heart. They carry blood to the heart muscle, or myocardium. Obstruction occurs when these arteries are affected by atherosclerosis. This narrows the channel and slows the flow of blood, so reducing the amount of oxygen that can get to the heart muscle that the artery is supplying. Another effect is that the slowly-flowing blood in the coronary artery is more likely to clot.

This can affect an individual in one of three ways. It can produce angina pectoris, which literally means a pain in the chest. It occurs during exercise or under emotional stress, when the heart rate increases. The flow of blood may be just about adequate for a heart beating normally, but is now inadequate, so that the heart becomes ischaemic, or short of blood. This causes the pain in the chest, which normally passes in a short time when the individual rests or calms down.

Secondly, if a clot (thrombus) develops in one of the branches of a coronary artery, the blood supply to a part of the heart muscle may be entirely cut off. Occasionally, this is at once corrected by blood reaching the affected part through some alternative route, from one of the other branches of the artery. If this does not happen, the affected part of the myocardium dies; this phenomenon is called myocardial infarction.

The effect may be a severe pain, like an attack of angina pectoris, but one that does not rapidly disappear with rest. The heart may then stop beating, with a loss of consciousness, until the contractions return, either spontaneously or under appropriate electrical or drug treatment. If the beating of the heart does not resume, clearly the patient dies.

Thirdly, even if there is no clot, the flow of blood through a coronary artery may cease. The effects are just the same; the only difference – and one that is of no interest to the victim – is that no clot can be found if the patient dies and a post mortem examination is carried out. It is believed that this condition occurs in an artery that is atherosclerotic, which for some reason goes into spasm, with the consequent interference in blood flow to an essential part of the conducting tissue in the myocardium that regulates the sequence of events in the contraction of the heart.

Coronary thrombosis as a cause of death seems to have been first described in 1661. It was nevertheless diagnosed infrequently until well into the twentieth century. During the past 60 years or so, however, it has rapidly become a common cause of death in Western countries. It remained rare in the poorer countries of the world, in South America, Africa and most of Asia, but is now beginning to appear increasingly in these countries. The recorded mortality due to CHD, as given in the Table, is likely to be of dubious reliability, especially in the poorer countries, where there are limited facilities for the accurate determination of the cause of death. It is claimed, too, that in Western countries part if not all of the increase in mortality due to CHD recorded in the last half century or so is an artefact, because of under-recording in the earlier period, more accurate recording after the electrocardiograph was introduced in 1903, and possibly over-recording recently, because it is now a more 'fashionable' diagnosis. There is nevertheless broad agreement that the disease is associated with prosperity, so that there is a clear relationship between average incomes of various populations and their experience of CHD, and also generally between the increasing prevalence in the wealthier countries and their increasing prosperity.

The likelihood of developing CHD increases with age. Men are more prone than women, especially up to the age of about 45. After the menopause, this difference diminishes.

Perhaps the most important non-environmental cause is heredity; people are more prone to develop CHD if there is a history of the disease in their family.

There are therefore three factors associated with CHD that cannot be altered: age, sex and family history. On the other hand, there must be one or more factors it should be possible to alter, since there is an association between CHD and affluence. But affluent populations differ in many ways from poor populations. People in prosperous communities tend to be less active physically, smoke more cigarettes, have more competitive stress in their daily lives, eat more food, take diets with more milk, meat, fat, sugar and several other foods, and are more exposed to food additives and to petrol fumes. It is difficult to determine which of these are involved in causing CHD (see Epidemiology).

Among the aspects of the diet that have been implicated are generally excessive intake of food, leading to obesity; an excessive intake of sugar or of fat, especially saturated fat; an excessive intake of coffee; an insufficient intake of polyunsaturated fat, or an insufficient intake of dietary fibre. In spite of the vast amount of research carried out, especially over the past twenty-five years, there is no universal agreement about any of these. The most widely accepted view is that a major cause of the disease is an excessive intake of saturated fat, perhaps together with too little polyunsaturated fat. But there are many highly competent research workers who do not share this view. It must also be stressed that a faulty diet is not the only environmental cause of the disease; there is a great deal of evidence that at least one other factor, cigarette smoking, is involved.

MALE MORTALITY DUE TO
CORONARY HEART DISEASE IN LATE 1970s

Deaths per 100,000 population

Finland	134	France	30
UK	103	Hong Kong	20
USA	100	Japan	13
Sweden	79	Philippines	11
Italy	47	Thailand	0.5

Recently, there has been a slight fall in coronary mortality in some countries, notably the United States. The reasons for this are not known; the observation has simply added fuel to the discussion of the various hypotheses as to the cause or causes of coronary heart disease.

Finally, the epidemiologists believe that all the known hereditary and suspected environmental causes do not totally account for the mortality statistics due to CHD in different countries. It still remains therefore for continuing research to discover what the remaining causes are.

See also: Atherosclerosis; Blood pressure; Cholesterol

Crawford, Adair (1748–95)

Crawford was a successful medical practitioner. He was appointed physician to St Thomas's Hospital, London, and Professor of Chemistry at the Royal Military Academy at Woolwich. Later, he appears to have spent some years in Glasgow and Edinburgh. He was a close associate of Joseph Black (1728–99), who had measured the specific heat of solid and liquid bodies, and had discovered 'fixed air', i.e. carbon dioxide. Crawford also worked in these two fields, and his most important discovery was that the 'alteration' of a given quantity of oxygen by the respiration of guinea pigs, or by the burning of wax or carbon, was about the same. But his publication 'Experiments and Observations on Animal Heat and the Inflammation of Combustible Bodies' met with a considerable amount of criticism. However, Joseph Priestley (1733–1804), to whom Crawford had sent the manuscript, praised his work. Crawford admitted in the second enlarged and corrected edition of 1788 that there were several errors in his measurements, although he maintained justifiably that these did not affect his conclusions. Criticism of his work nevertheless continued; he retired in 1794 and died the following year.

See also: Energy content of food

Cream

The separation of the cream in unhomogenized milk that takes place through the action of ordinary gravity may be effected more quickly through centrifugation. It is then possible to separate the upper layer that is the cream, from the lower layer that is the skimmed milk. Depending on the degree of separation, the skimmed milk will contain more fat or less fat and the cream correspondingly less fat or more fat. In the UK, the law requires a minimum of 48% fat for double cream, 35% for whipping cream, 18% for single cream. Clotted cream is made by heating double cream over a steam bath (*bain marie*) by itself, or by floating it on a layer of milk and skimming off the clotted upper layer. This should contain at least 55% fat; it also contains about 4% protein.

The various sorts of cream may be used directly, for example for adding to fruits such as strawberries, or they may be whipped, a process that results in tiny air bubbles being trapped in the cream so that an air emulsion results. For this to occur, it is necessary for the cream to contain at least 30% fat. Cream may also be made into butter.

See also: Butter; Milk

D

Dates

The date palm is an exceptionally tall tree, nearly 80 feet. It grows in dry, sub-tropical areas, in a belt from Morocco to India and especially in the Middle East and North Africa. There are separate male and female trees; the latter begin to bear fruit from 4 or 5 years, are full fruiting at 15 years, and continue up to 80 years.

The dates grow on strands, each carrying about 30 fruits, with some 40 strands in a bunch. The palm tree can be expected to bear 100lb of fruit or more each year.

Dates are an important part of the diet in many Arab populations. This is especially true of the dry date, which is pressed, or ground into a flour and used in cooking. The date exported on to the world markets is the sweet variety. Dates provide mostly calories, since some 60–70% of their weight is made up of sugars. They have no more than 2% protein, and their only other nutrients even in small degree are iron and nicotinic acid. Like other palms, the date palm yields a sap that can be fermented for toddy, or dried to make sugar.

Dental decay

The tooth is a living organ, with its own blood supply and, as anyone who has had toothache knows, with its own nerve supply. The blood vessel and the nerve enter the central soft tissue, the pulp, at the root of the tooth. The pulp is surrounded by a layer of dentine, which resembles ordinary bone except that it is rather more dense. The dentine in turn is covered by a thin layer of very hard enamel. The dentine and the enamel contain a high proportion of calcium salts, especially a particular phosphate of calcium known as apatite.

Dental decay, also known as dental caries, occurs through the action of streptococcal bacteria. These produce lactic acid by the fermentation of carbohydrates in the food. When enough acid is produced, it begins to dissolve the calcium phosphate of the enamel. Unlike most other tissues, enamel cannot regenerate, so that once it has been damaged, further decay is likely since the bacteria in the damaged tooth tend to be protected from being washed away by saliva. Moreover, a particular strain of mouth bacteria, *Streptococcus mutans*, has the ability to build up larger and insoluble molecules from food carbohydrate; these stick to the teeth and form a plaque which not only harbours more bacteria, but protects them even more from the cleansing action of saliva.

Dental decay is to a large extent a disease of affluence. It was not common in mediaeval times, but later began to be seen among the wealthy, who could afford to use the increasingly available but still very expensive sugar. The German ambassador to the court of Elizabeth I (1558–1603), among his unflattering comments on Her Majesty's physical appearance, included reference to her bad black teeth and bad breath.

Dental decay has recently become so common that the average 12-year-old child in Britain has about 5 decayed, missing or filled teeth ('DMF Index' = 5). Nearly one-third of the population over the age of 16 has no remaining natural teeth. Most caries occurs before the age of 25.

Many dietary carbohydrates are cariogenic, that is, can produce caries. These include not only ordinary sugar (sucrose) but also fructose, glucose, maltose, lactose and starch. In practice, however, some 80% of the dietary carbohydrate in most countries consists of starch and sucrose, and the latter is far more cariogenic than is starch. This is well illustrated by the fact that caries is almost non-existent among those rare individuals who have to avoid sucrose because they have genetic fructose intolerance.

Several factors affect the initiation and development of dental caries. Firstly, the sugar or other cariogenic constituent of food needs to be in contact with the tooth surface for enough time for it to be attacked by the acid-producing bacteria. For this reason sugar in drinks does little harm to the teeth, while at the other extreme, sticky confectionery such as toffee or cakes or sweet biscuits can be potent in producing decay. The effect can be diminished if sweet items are taken during a meal rather than between meals, and if the teeth are brushed after consuming such items. It is doubtful whether ordinary routine toothbrushing once or twice a day is significantly protective.

There is strong evidence that fluoride increases the resistance of the teeth. Ingestion of fluoride seems to be the most effective way this can be done, whether in drinking water or as daily pills. Topical application, for example by the application of fluoride toothpaste, is probably less effective. Nevertheless, there is now evidence that the prevalence of caries in Britain is diminishing somewhat; in England and Wales, the proportion of 9 to 13-year-old children with decayed teeth fell by 10% between 1973 and 1982. The fall may well be due to the increased use of fluoridized toothpaste.

As with much else in living organisms, individuals have varying genetic susceptibility to dental caries.

Because the initiation of caries is by the action of bacteria, notably *Streptococcus mutans*, it may be possible some time in the future to protect the teeth by immunizing individuals against this organism. Although much research has been done to produce such a vaccine, it is not yet available. It is thus still true to say that the best single safeguard in protecting the teeth against decay is to avoid eating sticky, sugary foods as much as possible, and to take fluoride pills if the fluoride content of the local water supply is low.

See also: Bone; Fluorine

Dextrin

There is a range of dextrins, and these are carbohydrates produced during the initial stages of hydrolysis or digestion of starch. The hydrolysis occurs by the application of moist heat to starch, or in the presence of the enzyme amylase. It is usual to use the word 'dextrin' for the mixture of dextrins produced in these ways.

Dextrin is one of the constituents of the crust of bread, where the dough reaches the highest temperature. When dextrin is moistened, it forms a gum; the gum on the backs of stamps is usually made up largely of dextrin.

See also: Carbohydrates

Diabetes

The word 'diabetes' comes from a Greek word meaning 'a flowing through', and refers to the increased amount of urine excreted in the disease, a phenomenon called polyuria. The commonest form is *diabetes mellitus*, or 'sweet flowing through'. In lay terms this is often called sugar diabetes, because glucose appears in the urine, which comes about because the body is unable to metabolize glucose properly. This in turn increases the amount of urine that has to be excreted because the glucose has increased its osmotic pressure. The disease is diagnosed through the assessment of the body's ability to metabolize glucose by measuring the glucose tolerance.

A much rarer cause of glucose appearing in the urine is a fault in the kidney, so that it allows glucose to be excreted at a concentration below the usual threshold of 180mg/100ml blood.

There is also another cause for passing a large volume of urine. This is *diabetes insipidus*, which as the name implies refers to a large volume of tasteless urine, that is, without sugar. It is due to a deficiency of a hormone secreted by the posterior pituitary gland called the anti-diuretic hormone, because it normally controls the amount of water excreted; when there is not enough of the hormone, excessively large volumes of urine are produced.

Individuals with *diabetes mellitus* fall into two broad groups. One affects young people, commonly around the ages of 10 or 12, although it can occur as early as one year and as late as 40. The disease tends to develop rapidly and is severe, and it has to be treated with insulin. This type is called juvenile diabetes, or insulin dependent diabetes.

The second type is more common and occurs in middle-aged people, especially if they are overweight. The name for this is maturity onset diabetes.

The causes of diabetes have not been clearly identified. Heredity plays a part, in that the disease, especially the insulin dependent type, is more likely to occur in people who have close relatives with diabetes. Maturity onset diabetes is somewhat more common in pregnant women and those who have had several children. It is also more common in men and women who are obese. Apart from the excessive diet that causes obesity, there have been suggestions that particular dietary constituents are involved: those which have been especially discussed are excessive fat, excessive sucrose, and inadequate dietary fibre.

Both types of disease show the characteristic excretion of large quantities of glucose-containing urine, and the low glucose tolerance. The polyuria is understandably accompanied both by frequency of micturition and of thirst. There is an excessive breakdown of fat in the body, and it may be more than can be properly oxidized to carbon dioxide and water; ketone bodies then accumulate and produce the condition of ketosis.

Long-standing diabetes may lead to several conditions. One is the ease with which boils and other skin infections occur. A second complication is diabetic retinopathy, affecting the retina of the eye, and this may extend to complete blindness. Another is diabetic nephropathy, in which the kidneys are affected, even to the extent of being a cause of death. Finally, diabetics are particularly prone to develop coronary heart disease.

There seems to be a difference in the metabolic background in the two types of diabetes. Those with juvenile diabetes tend to have no measurable amount of insulin in the blood, and they show degeneration of the special beta cells of the pancreas where insulin is normally manufactured. It is for this reason that they are insulin dependent, and their condition can therefore be said to be due to insulin deficiency. Patients with maturity onset diabetes, on the other hand, do have insulin circulating in their blood, and sometimes a rather higher amount than normal. Their tissues can, however, be shown to be relatively insensitive to insulin. For example, the amount of glucose oxidized by a normal muscle is increased if insulin is injected, but this happens to a much smaller extent to the muscle of an individual with maturity onset diabetes. Nevertheless, patients with this condition may improve if they receive regular injections of insulin, if enough is given.

Dietary treatment is important for both types of diabetes. Indeed, many patients with maturity onset diabetes, unlike those with insulin dependent diabetes, may not need insulin or the oral drugs sometimes used as an alternative to insulin.

There are many views about the sort of diet that is most effective. All agree that it should aim at reducing the overweight that so often occurs with maturity onset diabetes, and that it should contain little or no sucrose. However, some doctors have abandoned the earlier practice of severely restricting starch and other carbohydrates, and give diets that contain the usual proportion of protein, fat and carbohydrate.

See also: Glucose tolerance; Hormones; Ketosis; Osmotic pressure

Dialysis

Dialysis is the process by which small and large molecules that may be together in a solution may be separated. If a solution is placed in a tube consisting of a semi-permeable membrane, the smaller molecules are able to pass through the pores of the membrane, while the larger molecules remain in the solution. Such membranes are now available with predetermined pore size, so that it is possible to separate large molecules of various sizes.

When the kidneys are diseased, they are unable adequately to eliminate from the body excess water and salt, and the waste products of metabolism. The burden on the kidneys can be reduced if the patient is given a diet that is low in protein and in salt. This reduces the amount of salt and of waste products from protein that need to be excreted, as well as the quantity of water needed to take them through the kidney. However, dietary treatment in itself cannot relieve the burden on severely diseased kidneys, but it is now possible to take over much of their function by the process of dialysis by the use of the so-called artificial kidney.

We can understand this process by first recalling the principle of osmosis. Imagine blood being passed through a tube that, somewhat like the blood capillaries, consists of a semi-permeable membrane. Imagine now that the tube is placed in a vessel containing pure water. Then many of the constituents of the blood would pass through the membrane; these would be the constituents with small molecules such as glucose, salts and waste products such as urea, uric acid and creatinine. The larger molecules, such as the blood protein and of course the much larger red and white cells and platelets, would remain inside the tube. Theoretically, if there were an unlimited quantity of blood in the tube, and a small and limited amount of water outside, the glucose and other constituents would flow through the tube until the concentration in the water was the same as that in the blood. Alternatively, if the amount of blood were limited and the amount of water unlimited – for instance, by changing it frequently for fresh water – the blood would soon be entirely cleared of the small molecules, and only the cells and platelets and protein would remain.

Consider now a patient's blood being taken out of an artery, passing through an apparatus where it comes into contact with a semi-permeable membrane, and then returning to the body through a vein. At the same time, on the other side of the membrane, there flows a solution with an appropriate quantity of glucose, salt and other essential blood constituents. The result is that waste products such as urea flow across the membrane from the blood, to be carried away by the dialysis fluid because there are none of these in the fluid. On the other hand, materials such as glucose, which need to remain in the blood, or which need to be increased, can be made to flow across the membrane into the blood by adjusting their concentration in the dialysis fluid.

In the treatment of patients by dialysis with such a kidney machine, this process is repeated two or three times a week, and lasts about 4 hours each time. Modern machines are now suitable for use at home by the patient, who therefore does not need to go to hospital.

Dialysis does not entirely replace all the functions of the healthy kidney. For example, some of the constituents in the blood that are not in the dialysis fluid, such as the amino-acids and some of the water-soluble vitamins, tend to be lost from the blood. These, however, are readily replaced by ensuring that there is adequate protein in the diet, and if necessary by administering additional vitamins.

See also: Aluminium; Kidney; Osmotic pressure

Diet

The word 'diet' comes from the Greek word *diaita*, which roughly means mode of life. The meaning gradually changed, so that it now refers to the habitual pattern of consumption of food and drink. Especially to lay people, the word diet is taken to mean a prescribed regimen of food and drink, taken for the purpose of correcting an abnormal condition such as overweight or dyspepsia, and it brings with it the concept of some temporary restriction in the normal pattern of food consumption. Those concerned professionally in devising these treatments refer to them as special diets. However, general dietary instruction and advice is increasingly given for the purpose of achieving and maintaining health, and so preventing disease rather than curing it. Such advice is given both by qualified individuals and by lay people. The Table gives some indication of the widely different sources from which an individual may derive dietary information. Because nutritional science is, like all other sciences, continually adding facts from new research, much of the advice being given has to be based on incomplete information, which is amplified by experience. There is thus room for differences between individuals in the advice they give, partly because of differences in personality but also because of extraneous influences such as commercial interest. In addition to this, there are the prejudices of those who receive the advice. Understandably, then, the result may well be confusion and contradiction among those who are looking for useful and effective dietary instruction.

From the earliest times, medical writers such as Hippocrates and

Galen believed that diet played a great part in prophylaxis and therapy, that is in the maintenance of health and the curing of disease. For some 2,000 years the diets were based on the theory of the four humours that determined both the temperament of the individual and the character of different foods and drinks. With the development of the science of nutrition, there was a change in these concepts; nevertheless, until quite recently, most of the dietary advice for both the prevention and the curing of disease had little or no scientific basis. There is now a better understanding of what constitutes a healthy diet, and what sorts of dietary regimes help in the treatment of disease, although much of this is submerged or obscured by the plethora of advice from the various sources.

Many people still believe that some foods have particular properties that promote health. The statement that 'Milk is good for you' implies only that it is an excellent source of a wide range of nutrients; the statement that 'Honey is good for you' implies not only that it too is rich in nutrients, which it is not, but also that it positively increases the level of health in an already healthy person – which no known food or drug can do.

A diet for health is one that is wholesome and nutritious: wholesome in that it contains nothing injurious, and nutritious in that it supplies the body with the energy and nutrients it requires in adequate but not excessive amounts. There is reason to believe that such a diet is best achieved by seeking to avoid the wrong sorts of foods rather than by seeking to consume the right sorts of foods; this proposition is discussed in the article on Dietary instinct.

Diets for the treatment of disease, that is therapeutic diets, are now used for fewer diseases than was the case in the first half of the century. On the other hand, several diseases, mostly quite rare, have been identified in which dietary treatment is essential.

The commonest therapeutic diets are the various low-energy diets designed for the treatment of obesity. There are also the diets for individuals who are hypersensitive to particular dietary constituents, such as diets without milk for those with lactose intolerance, or diets without gluten for patients with coeliac disease, or diets without shell-fish or eggs for individuals allergic to these foods. Rarer conditions are phenylketonuria, which is a sensitivity to one of the common amino-acids in proteins, and galactosaemia, a sensitivity to the sugar galactose, which is a part of milk sugar, lactose.

The common condition of chronic dyspepsia, with or without peptic ulcers (gastric or duodenal ulcers), used to be treated with one of a variety of special diets. These are now rarely recommended, partly because they are mostly ineffective and partly because there are now many useful drugs for the treatment of peptic ulcers. Patients with gout are advised to exclude animal food such as liver and kidneys; these contain a high proportion of cells and thus much nucleic acid, which gives rise to uric acid in the body. For high blood pressure it is usual to recommend a diet low in salt, and for some kidney diseases a diet low in protein. Diabetes was until recently almost always treated with a low carbohydrate diet; there is a tendency nowadays not to limit the amount of starch so much, but still to stress the avoidance of sugar.

For these and other conditions, any dietary recommendation should be part of general treatment, and so under the supervision of the doctor, who will also in appropriate instances seek the advice of a qualified dietitian.

In addition to the diseases in the treatment of which diet can play a useful part, there are others where many people believe dietary treatment is effective; examples are arthritis, migraine, asthma and schizophrenia. Apart from a small proportion of patients with migraine or asthma, dietary treatment is ineffective in these conditions.

Sometimes it is difficult or impossible for a patient to take food by mouth; in these instances, solutions of nutrients can be given by intravenous injection. Much research on this problem has been carried out since the middle 1960s, and it is now possible to feed a patient intravenously for months if appropriate solutions are used, and the injection made into a large, deep vein.

SOURCES OF PUBLIC INFORMATION ABOUT NUTRITION

PROFESSIONAL	NON-PROFESSIONAL
Nutritionists and dietitians	Advertisers
Doctors	Journalists and authors
Dentists	(magazines, newspapers, books,
Home economists	radio, TV)
Para-medical (e.g. nurses)	Health food stores
	Relatives (especially
	grandparents)
	Neighbours and friends

See also: **Dietary instinct; Intravenous feeding; Obesity**

Dietary instinct

It is sometimes asked, 'Why do we need nutritional advice?' Animals in their natural habitat, including our early ancestors, ate the foods that they instinctively chose, and those foods when available must be assumed to have supplied all their nutritional needs; natural selection would otherwise have ensured the disappearance of the species. Why then does modern man need to be told how to obtain a 'balanced' diet, with fruit and vegetables for vitamin C, meat, fish, eggs, milk and cheese for protein, and so on?

It has been proposed that this has arisen because man, with his scientific and technological knowledge and skill, can make extracts from foods, mix them in varying proportions, add synthetic flavours and colours, and so produce new foods, more attractive and sometimes cheaper than many of the foods in their natural state. The qualities of attractiveness do not, however, ensure that the foods contain much, if any, of the necessary nutrients. As a result, these new attractive foods may replace other and more nutritious foods in the diet and thus predispose to deficiency, or be eaten in addition to other foods and so predispose to the development of obesity. A further suggestion is that, because the most attractive new foods are those rich in sugar, they lead to an excessive consumption of this undesirable dietary item.

This approach to the question of what is a balanced diet lays stress more on what foods should be avoided than on what foods should be chosen. If the wrong foods are avoided, instinct will determine the amounts and selection from the correct foods. These are the foods that can be gathered, taken out of the soil, or slaughtered: the sorts of foods our ancestors hunted and gathered. They are meat, fish, eggs, fruit and vegetables; because of the constraints of pressure of population and of urbanization, it is usually necessary to add two of the foods introduced in the early days of the agricultural revolution, namely milk and cereal-based foods such as bread. Without these foods, it would in many countries be difficult for the less wealthy to get enough to eat.

According to this argument, dietary instinct determines that we choose a food because we like it rather than because we need it. Dietary instinct cannot therefore be relied upon as an appropriate guide to a healthy diet when it is possible for the food manufacturer, and to some extent the skilled cook, to make foods that are increasingly attractive without regard to their wholesomeness or nutritional value.

See also: Appetite; Neolithic revolution

Dietary intake

In order to assess the nutritive value of what people are eating, it is necessary to know what foods and drinks they consume, how much of each, and the nutrient content of each. There are many ways in which this information may be obtained. Some are direct, and some indirect; some are relatively simple but not very reliable, and some are complicated and laborious but more reliable.

It is relatively easy to know what people of the poorer countries eat, because they have a much smaller range of foods; care must nevertheless be taken to record the items that may be eaten casually by a worker, for example, out of the home. However, it may not be possible for an observer to determine how much persons of a different culture have eaten unless a great deal of time and trouble is taken to enlist their co-operation, especially since they may have cooking and eating practices they are not willing for strangers to observe.

In the wealthier countries, earlier investigators such as Rowntree in York calculated the cost of a diet that, for the least expenditure, would provide what they believed would meet minimum nutritional standards. Although indirect, this method could show that any person or family whose disposable income was less than that of the cost of the minimal diet must have had a nutritionally inadequate diet.

There are several more direct assessments of actual food consumed. For the population of a whole country, it is possible to calculate the nutritional value of an average diet by estimating the total amount of all the available foods, and dividing this by the population of that country. This assumes that reasonably accurate figures are available for food production, exports, imports, increase or decrease of stores, and losses in distribution; this is certainly not true for many countries. Moreover, this method of global assessment says nothing about which people eat what foods, and how much.

A more elaborate method is that used by the Ministry of Agriculture, Fisheries and Food in the United Kingdom, which since 1940 has carried out continual interviews, each involving thousands of families. The head of the household keeps a record of all food entering the home each week, and the number of people at each meal. Other details recorded include income and size of family. Summaries of the information are published quarterly, and a more detailed report published annually.

For an individual, a method often used is the taking of a dietary history by an investigator. The subject is asked to recall what has been consumed during the past 24 hours, and this may be recorded for 2 or 3 days. But it has been shown repeatedly that this method is likely to give results that diverge widely from the true habitual intake; in spite of this, it is still sometimes used. Better results are achieved if the individual keeps a diary of every item consumed, recorded either as 'homely measures', such as 'thin slices of bread thinly buttered', or, ideally, by measuring or weighing all food and drink. These last methods, however, involve the possibility that the food recorded will be modified from that normally consumed. This could be because some foods are not easy to measure or weigh. Or the diet could be deliberately chosen or recorded as a bad diet so as to exaggerate a low income, or as a good diet to impress the investigator.

When the sorts and amounts of food are known, the nutrient intake is calculated with the aid of tables of food composition. By now, information gained by analysis is available for the majority of foods comprising the diet of people in most countries. But different samples of the same food are unlikely to contain exactly the same amounts of the nutrients, especially if the foods are cooked and the nutrients to be assessed are being depleted during cooking. This objection can to a large extent be overcome if at the time of consumption a duplicate dish or meal is prepared, as nearly as possible of identical foods in identical amounts; this is then taken to the laboratory and analysed. The procedure is clearly enormously laborious and costly, and in most instances prohibitively so. The fact is that there is no way in which the amounts of the various nutrients can be measured in the foods actually being consumed; a food that is eaten cannot be analysed, and a food that is analysed cannot be eaten.

One last question that remains is the length of time for which it is necessary to collect records of food consumption. Since the object is usually to record habitual intake, it is certainly necessary to take a record for more than one day. In the poorer countries, where the choice is small, the variation from day to day is likely not to be great, but the variation from season to season may be considerable; measurements for 2 or 3 consecutive days, 3 or 4 times a year, may then be appropriate. In the wealthier countries, however, modern methods of transport and preservation have minimized seasonal variation, but people themselves tend to change their choice of food from day to day. It has been shown that the nutrient value of their diets may vary significantly, even from week to week. For most people, the smallest variation is in the amounts of calories and protein, and the greatest variation is in the amount of vitamin C, and especially in the amounts of vitamins A and D. It is, however, usually impractical to expect people to keep a record for more than a week, and so a 7-day dietary record is usually accepted as being a reasonable compromise between accuracy and convenience.

See also: Tables of food composition

Dietary requirements

In assessing whether the diet of a person provides the amount of energy and of nutrients needed to assure optimal health, it is necessary to know both what the diet is providing (the dietary intake) and how much the body requires in terms of energy and of each of the nutrients. This information is used in planning food supplies for a population, for example during a war or after a disaster, or for improving food supplies by improved production or imports in a developing country, or for planning meals for institutions or for individuals such as patients in a hospital.

The requirement for energy is that which meets the basal metabolism, together with the amount needed for standing, walking, climbing the stairs, working in the house or in the fields or at a factory, as well as additional voluntary activities. It is usual to say that the energy requirement is the amount needed to maintain an individual's physical activity and his normal weight, together with that needed for growth or pregnancy or lactation. We now know that this is not entirely true, because there can be an adaptation to a slight excess or a slight deficit (see Obesity and Thermogenesis).

The methods used for assessing requirements of nutrients are not the same for all of them. One method is to measure the intake of, say, thiamin or iron in individuals of a population in which beri-beri or iron deficiency anaemia is endemic; examination of the diets of individuals with and without the disease should then give at least a reasonable measure of the amounts of the nutrient that prevent deficiency or that fail to prevent it.

Another method is an experimental modification of this last method. Experiments are conducted in which groups of people are given diets containing different amounts of the nutrient. They are then examined regularly to see which groups develop signs of deficiency and which do not.

A third method is by balance studies. This is suitable for nutrients that are not destroyed, such as the mineral elements, or for protein which can be measured indirectly by measuring the amount of nitrogen. Diets with decreasing amounts of the nutrient are given, each for a few days, and the amount of the nutrient (or the nitrogen) is measured in the urine and faeces. If the individual is not growing, or is not pregnant or lactating, and if the amount of the nutrient is enough or more than enough, the amount excreted is the same as that in the diet, because there is no net gain or loss. When the intake is decreased, excretion also decreases; there comes a time, however, when a further decrease in intake does not cause decreased excretion, an indication that intake has fallen below requirement, because there is a net loss.

Somewhat similar to balance studies are saturation tests. When the habitual diet contains small quantities of vitamin C, it is used up in the body and little appears in the urine. When a very large dose of vitamin C is then consumed, it is also taken up by the 'unsaturated' tissues and again only a little is excreted. On the other hand, a person who is accustomed to a high intake of vitamin C will have tissues 'saturated' with the vitamin, so that a large dose would result in a large increase in the amount excreted in the urine. It is then possible to determine how much vitamin C should be taken in the habitual diet in order to ensure saturation. Groups are given diets with varying amounts of the vitamin for a time, and then they are tested with a large dose of vitamin C to see which group was taking the lowest amount that results in saturation.

These and other methods have been used to determine how much of each nutrient is needed to meet the particular test. But problems still remain. Firstly, is it good enough to have in the diet the minimal amount that will prevent a disease, or are there advantages in having more than this? Secondly, if it is better to take more than the minimal amount, how much should this be? Thirdly, what decision is to be taken if, by measuring requirements by more than one method, different results are obtained? Fourthly, how accurately can one determine what the requirements are for people of different ages, sizes and activities? These and other questions are still being debated, and differences of opinion have resulted in differences evident in the recommendations from the various national and international authorities. For example, the British authorities recommend 30mg of vitamin C a day for an adult; the American authorities recommend 45mg.

For all of these reasons, many authorities no longer speak of requirements for nutrients; in the UK, the term is Recommended Dietary

Intake (RDI); in the US, Recommended Daily Allowance (RDA). These are more than the amounts needed to prevent overt deficiency disease, and allow both for some people having requirements more than the average, and for the possible improvement in some aspect of health not easily measurable. Because of these considerations, it is quite possible for an individual to be taking significantly less of a nutrient than its RDI, and yet having quite enough for optimal health. Thus, it is quite wrong to say that a moderately active man whose diet provides on average 0.8mg of thiamin a day instead of the RDI of 1.1mg, or 6mg of iron instead of the RDI of 10mg, is suffering from beri-beri or anaemia; all one can say is that the extent to which either of these nutrients falls below the RDI increases the *likelihood* that he is deficient in that nutrient.

As the Table shows, it is a convention that RDIs are given on a daily basis. This does not imply that precisely these amounts of energy and nutrients need to be consumed each day. It is possible to eat more or less than one's needs to satisfy energy requirements on one day, or even to fast for a few days, without coming to any harm. Similarly, any person whose habitual diet is adequate will not suffer the effects of

Recommended daily intakes (RDI) for energy and nutrients for UK published in 1979. For men and women.

	Man aged 35–64, moderately active	Woman aged 35–64, moderately active
Energy, kcal	2,750	2,500
Protein, g	69	62
Thiamin, mg	1.1	1.0
Riboflavin, mg	1.6	1.3
Nicotinic acid equivalent, mg	18	15
Folate, μg	300	300
Ascorbic acid, mg	30	30
Vitamin A (Retinol equivalent), μg	750	750
Vitamin D, μg	0*	0*
Calcium, mg	500	500
Iron, mg	10	12

* No dietary sources may be necessary for those sufficiently exposed to sunlight; if not, a supplement of 10μg daily may be needed.

nutrient deficiency if his intake of any one or more of the nutrients is below the RDI for several weeks, even if his diet is entirely lacking in them; this has been demonstrated for example with vitamin C. Much longer periods of low dietary intake of the fat-soluble vitamins can usually be sustained with no ill effects.

See also: **Nutrient balance tests**

Dietitian (alt. sp. Dietician)

A dietitian is someone who has a training in the principles of nutrition, to which is added training in its practical application to the feeding of groups and individuals, including the construction and preparation of special diets for the treatment and prevention of disease. Because the basis of this practical work is the science of nutrition, a well-trained and experienced dietitian may well be doing the work of a nutritionist, so that there is often little to distinguish the practitioners of the two professions.

In the UK, dietitians who work in the National Health Service need to have had a recognized training leading to the diploma of SRD (State Registered Dietitian). However, there is at present nothing to stop anyone from claiming to be a dietitian.

See also: **Nutritionist**

Digestibility

The word digestibility has three different meanings. To the layman, a food is digestible if it is unlikely to cause pain or discomfort after it is eaten. Thus, for some people, lobster and melted cheese are indigestible in this sense.

A second meaning for digestibility is to do with the speed with which a food is broken down by the digestive juices. This can be measured in the laboratory by adding some digestive juice to the food and measuring the rate at which it disappears, or the rate at which the digestion products appear. A food is then considered to be more digestible than another if these events happen faster. A little oil will for a long time remain unchanged when shaken gently with an extract of pancreas; on the other hand, it will rapidly be digested if a small amount of lecithin is added. The digestibility of the oil has been increased by the emulsifying action of the lecithin.

The third meaning is the one used especially by nutritionists. It refers to how much of the food is absorbed into the blood as it goes through the alimentary canal. This is assessed by measuring the composition of the food consumed, and then the composition of the stools, to see how much has not been absorbed. In general terms, something like 90% of the total diet is absorbed, as indicated by the fact that about 10% in terms of energy is found in the stools. As for individual foods, it transpires that about 90% of the protein in white bread is digested on this definition, and about 85% of the protein in wholemeal bread.

It will be seen that it is necessary to take care not to transfer one meaning of the word digestible to another meaning. It is for instance not reasonable to say that wholemeal bread is more indigestible than white bread, giving the impression that it is more likely to lead to abdominal discomfort.

From the average meal, about 90% of the protein, fat and carbohydrate is absorbed. The chief constituent that is not absorbed is what is now described as dietary fibre. Meals with a high proportion of fibre tend slightly to increase the amount of the other constituents that are not absorbed, but this additional loss would not amount to more than the equivalent of 100 kcal or so.

See also: Absorption; Digestive juices; Fibre

Digestive juices

In the mouth, the food is mixed with saliva secreted by the three pairs of salivary glands. This secretion is stimulated by the sight, smell and taste of food, and sometimes even by the thought of food. One function of the saliva is to moisten the food, which helps in the process of swallowing. In addition, saliva contains the enzyme ptyalin, also known as salivary amylase. This converts starch into the sugar maltose; if a piece of bread is chewed for a minute or two without swallowing, one can begin to taste the sweetness of the maltose.

In the stomach, the food comes into contact with the gastric juice, the secretion of which is stimulated by food in the stomach, although like the secretion of saliva its flow is stimulated also by the sight, smell and taste of food. The gastric juice is strongly acid (pH about 1.5), containing as it does hydrochloric acid. The action of saliva ceases when the acid gastric juice penetrates the bolus of swallowed food, but until it does so, the digestion of starch continues. The gastric juice, especially that of infants, contains rennin, which clots milk. More importantly, it contains pepsin, which requires acid for its action. This digests protein as far as polypeptides, chains of a few amino-acids that are appreciably smaller than the complex of amino-acids that form the protein.

The mixture of partly digested food, sometimes called chyme, now passes in small spurts into the duodenum through the pylorus of the stomach. Here it meets the mixture of bile from the gall-bladder and the digestive juice from the pancreas. The mixture is somewhat alkaline, so that it neutralizes the acidity of the chyme. The bile salts emulsify the fat in chyme, so enormously increasing the surface of the fat exposed to the fat-splitting enzyme lipase of the pancreatic juice. This juice also contains another starch-splitting enzyme, pancreatic amylase. Finally, the pancreatic juice contains some enzymes that digest protein, known collectively as trypsin. They are secreted in an inactive form, trypsinogen, which is converted into trypsin by one of the intestinal enzymes called enterokinase.

The small intestine secretes a digestive juice that is sometimes called *succus entericus*, which is Latin for 'intestinal juice'. As well as enterokinase, it has an enzyme polypeptidase that digests the polypeptides to their individual amino-acids. The disaccharide sugars are digested into their constituent monosaccharides: sucrase (invertase) digests sucrose to glucose and fructose, lactase digests lactose to glucose and galactose, and maltase digests maltose to glucose. In addition to these enzymes, intestinal juice contains enzymes that digest a variety of other constituents of food, including lipoproteins and nucleic acids; these give rise to a range of substances including lecithin, phosphates and xanthine, and this last in turn is converted into uric acid in the body.

See also: Enzymes; pH

Dried fruits

The preservation of fruits such as apples, peaches, apricots, plums, grapes and figs by drying has been carried out from the earliest times.

Dried fruits are used in many ways and make an attractive article of food.

It is often believed that dried fruits, particularly the vine fruits such as raisins and sultanas, have a high nutritional value and are especially rich in iron. Neither the general nor the particular claim is valid. The nutrient content of dried fruits cannot be greater than that of the original fresh fruit, unless something is added during the processing.

The misunderstanding arises from comparing a given weight of the fresh and the dried fruit, while forgetting that it is necessary to use perhaps 4–5oz of grapes in order to produce 1oz of raisins. In some instances it is true that there is marginally more iron in dried fruits than can be accounted for by the fact that they are more concentrated; this is because in some areas the drying process is carried out on metal trays, and traces of iron may be picked up by the fruit. This is analogous to the small amounts of iron present in raw sugar, most of which derives from the machinery employed in the several processes that go into preparing the sugar from the cane. Apart from the special case of iron, and allowing for the effect of drying in increasing the concentration but not the amount of nutrients, the true nutritional value of dried fruits is lower than that of fresh fruits. Most of the vitamin C is destroyed, and a good part of the thiamin. The other vitamins of the B group and carotene, together with most of the mineral elements, are unaffected by the process.

See also: Food preservation; Quantities

Drummond, Jack Cecil (1891–1952)

Drummond came to prominence as the Scientific Adviser to the British Ministry of Food during the Second World War. He had graduated in chemistry in 1912, and succeeded Funk in 1918 as biochemist to the Cancer Hospital Research Institute, London.

In 1920 he suggested that 'accessory food factors' should be known by the simpler name of vitamins, dropping the final 'e' in the name originally suggested by Funk in 1912, because it was now clear that not all the newly discovered factors were amines. In 1922 he was appointed to the new Chair of Biochemistry at University College, London. With Ann Wilbraham, who later became his second wife, he published, in 1939, *The Englishman's Food*.

THE
ENGLISHMAN'S FOOD

A History of Five Centuries of
English Diet

by

J. C. DRUMMOND

*Professor of Biochemistry, University
College, London*

and

ANNE WILBRAHAM

*La destinée des nations dépend de la
manière dont elles se nourrissent.*
BRILLAT-SAVARIN
La Physiologie du Gout, 1825

JONATHAN CAPE
THIRTY BEDFORD SQUARE
LONDON

As Scientific Adviser to the Ministry of Food, Drummond suggested that the extraction rate of bread flour should be increased from 72% to 85%. This had the two-fold effect of reducing the volume of imports and improving the nutritional value of the diet.

After the war, the American Public Health Association made an award to the British Ministry of Food, mentioning by name Drummond and three of his colleagues 'for the greatest demonstration in public health administration that the world has ever seen'.

Drummond later became Director of Research at the Boots Drug Company; he nevertheless continued as adviser to the Ministry of Food for one more year. In 1952, Sir Jack Drummond, his wife and 10-year-old daughter were murdered while on a holiday in the south of France.

See also: Food rationing; Vitamins

Du Bois, Eugene Floyd (1882–1959)

The method of measuring metabolic rate, and the relationship of the basal metabolic rate to size, sex and age, were largely the work of E. F. du Bois. It was he who translated the German word *Grundumsatz*, the concept developed by Magnus-Levy, into 'basal metabolism', and with his colleagues established much of what we know about metabolism and its measurement.

Du Bois was born in New Brighton, New York State, in 1882 and took his MD degree at the College of Physicians and Surgeons at Columbia University in 1903. He spent most of his subsequent working life in a succession of posts in the medical school of Cornell University. During the Second World War he was chairman of the Committee of Aviation Medicine of the US Naval Research Council.

His early research on metabolism was carried out in collaboration with Graham Lusk. He confirmed the discovery of Rubner that the basal metabolism was proportional to the surface area of the body and also that, on the basis of surface area, it was on average 7% less in women. With a cousin, D. du Bois, he devised an improved formula for the calculation of surface area. From measurements of metabolism carried out both in healthy individuals and in patients, he demonstrated that the total energy released was that derived from the oxidation of ingested food. He measured his own basal metabolic rate over a period of 14 years and found it constant within ±2.8%.

His best-known book was *Basal Metabolism in Health and Disease*, first published in 1924.

See also: Basal metabolism; Energy; Lusk; Rubner

Dyspepsia

Indigestion or dyspepsia may be defined as discomfort, distension, pain, nausea or heartburn after a meal. The commonest causes are gastritis, peptic ulcer and hiatus hernia. However, dyspepsia may also be a symptom of disease of some other organ, such as the gall-bladder or the pancreas.

Elaborate diets do not seem to be of much use, or at least are unnecessary, in the treatment of simple dyspepsia. With careful observation, it may be possible to recognize particular items of diet that produce symptoms, so that clearly these should be avoided. In addition, many people find relief with diets low in carbohydrate, and especially with diets low in sugar-rich foods such as cakes, sweet biscuits, most desserts and confectionery.

See also: Digestibility; Peptic ulcers

E

Eggs

The following account refers to the hen's egg; the composition of other eggs is much the same, the only noteworthy difference being in the size.

Because the egg has to supply the needs of the chick for the 21 days during which it grows from a single cell to an independent and completely formed young bird, it contains all the essential nutrients in significant amounts. In terms of the human diet, therefore, it is a nutritious food, except that, not surprisingly, it contains no vitamin C, which the chick does not require. The edible part also contains only small amounts of calcium, which the chick embryo obtains from the shell.

In the UK, eggs are graded in size from above 70g (Grade 1) to below 45g (Grade 7). Of the average egg of about 60g, some 20g is yolk, 35g white, and the rest the shell and membranes. The whole egg provides about 100 kcal, and contains 8g protein, 8g fat, 1.5mg iron and significant amounts of vitamins A, D, E and the B group. Most of these items are contained in the yolk; the only important exception is that the white contains about half of the riboflavin and half of the protein. The average of 4 eggs a week eaten in the UK does not therefore contribute very much to the nutritional value of the British diet.

Eggs contain more cholesterol than do most other foods; one egg contains about 250mg. This may be compared with the average daily intake of cholesterol in the Western diet, which is about 500mg. The average consumption of eggs in the UK will thus contribute about 150mg of cholesterol a day.

The proteins include small quantities of avidin and conalbumin, which can interfere with the absorption of biotin and iron. The total proteins of the egg are of high biological value, and are sometimes used as a standard against which the biological value of other proteins is assessed.

White eggs and brown eggs have the same composition. There is, however, a slight difference in the eggs from free-range hens compared with those from battery hens: the former have a greater amount of vitamin B_{12} and of folic acid.

The white of a hard-boiled egg often has a dark ring where it is in contact with the yolk; this is due to the formation of iron sulphide, the iron coming from the yolk and the sulphide from the proteins of the white.

As eggs become older, there is an increase in the amount of air in the air space; this can be used as a test for a stale egg, which will float in water. Meanwhile, there is a slow change in the nature of the proteins; ultimately they break down and release hydrogen sulphide gas, which is responsible for the characteristic foul smell of bad eggs.

See also: Albumin; Avidin; Biological value of proteins

Eijkman, Christiaan (1858–1930)

Eijkman was born in the Netherlands and graduated in medicine in 1883. He worked in the Colonial Service in the Dutch East Indies (now Indonesia) for the next two years, but was invalided home. He went back to the East Indies as a member of the Government Study Commission on beri-beri. Most members agreed that the disease was a bacterial infection, and returned home. Eijkman, however, remained as director of a new research laboratory. He began his research on fowls in the military hospital that were being fed on kitchen scraps. He noticed that the birds developed paralysis, polyneuritis, which resembled (dry) human beri-beri. A new director of the hospital prevented Eijkman from continuing to use kitchen scraps, which consisted largely of polished rice, so he began to feed his fowls on whole rice. With this diet, the paralysis improved and did not recur. Eijkman's suggestion that the polyneuritis of the fowls was related to human beri-beri was rejected by other workers.

Eijkman himself interpreted the results of his experiments as being due to a toxin present in the polished rice, with an anti-toxin in the outer layers of the rice. His colleague, Grijns, however, was not satisfied with this explanation, and suggested that beri-beri was caused by the absence of some essential dietary substance present in the rice polishings. Eijkman's contribution to what turned out to be the discovery of the vitamins was recognized when in 1929 he received the Nobel Prize for Physiology and Medicine jointly with F. G. Hopkins.

In 1898 Eijkman returned to the Netherlands and became Professor of Hygiene at the University of Utrecht.

See also: Beri-beri; Grijns; Hopkins; Vitamin B; Vitamin history

Elasticity

Economists have used this term to denote change in the amount of a commodity bought, or sold, in relation to a change in price, or to a change in income. Nutritionists are mostly concerned with income elasticity and price elasticity of food. They are each expressed as the percentage change in the amount of a food bought when the income, or the price of the food, is increased by 1%.

Butter and margarine provide a good example of both income elasticity and price elasticity. When income increases, people tend to eat more butter and less margarine. Recent figures for the UK show that the figure of income elasticity for butter was 0.15 and that for margarine was −0.28. These figures, derived from families with a wide range of income, mean that an increase in income of 1% resulted in an increase in butter consumption of 0.15%, and a fall (hence the negative figure) in margarine consumption of 0.28%. Again, the figures for price elasticity were −0.40 and +0.65; as the price of butter increased (relative to that of margarine) by 1%, the consumption of butter fell by 0.40%, and that of margarine rose by 0.65%.

Electrolytes

When dissolved in water, some chemical substances split into positive and negative ions. A solution in water (aqueous solution) of sodium chloride or common salt splits into positive sodium ions and negative chloride ions; magnesium sulphate (Epsom salts) splits into positive magnesium ions and negative sulphate ions. The process is called ionization. A mixture of sodium chloride and magnesium sulphate in water exists as ions of sodium, magnesium, chloride and sulphate; when this solution is dried, the solid left is a mixture of four different salts: sodium chloride, sodium sulphate, magnesium chloride and magnesium sulphate.

Other substances, such as glucose and urea, do not ionize, and may therefore be called non-electrolytes.

The membranes of cells, including those that constitute the walls of capillaries, are permeable to all the small molecules, both electrolytes and non-electrolytes. One would then expect the concentrations of sodium ions and potassium ions to be the same inside the cells and outside the cells in the blood plasma, lymph and intercellular fluid.

But in fact, most of the potassium is kept inside the cells, and most of the sodium outside the cells. A great deal of the energy used by the body is expended in maintaining the different concentrations of the body's ions on the right side of the cell membranes.

See also: Basal metabolism

Emulsifiers and stabilizers

The purpose of using an emulsifier or a stabilizer in the preparation of some foods is to prevent the separation of constituents that are in a different physical state (e.g. air and water, or solid and water), or do not ordinarily mix (e.g. oil and water). An instance of each of these three uses are ice cream, which is kept light and foamy by tiny bubbles of air, fruit juices in which the particles of fruit are kept suspended, and mayonnaise in which the oil does not separate from the other ingredients. In ice cream, for example, the emulsifier helps mostly in the formation of the tiny bubbles of air or droplets of fat, and the stabilizer helps to keep them apart by surrounding the air or fat with a layer that makes it difficult for them to join together again. Many of the substances used act in both ways.

Commonly used emulsifiers and stabilizers are egg yolk, lecithin, agar, alginates, carageenin, egg albumin and glyceryl monostearate.

See also: Food additives

Endemic

This is an adjective describing a disease constantly present in a particular population. Thus, malaria is endemic in Central Africa; pneumoconiosis is still endemic among miners in Britain, although less common than it used to be.

See also: Epidemic

Energy

The body requires a constant source of energy for carrying out mechanical work, for growth and for maintaining and repairing the tissues so that they remain in good working condition. The energy comes from the precisely controlled oxidation of the components of food, all but a tiny fraction being the energy released from oxidizing its protein, fat, carbohydrate and perhaps alcohol.

As in all other instances where energy is used – motor engines, electric light bulbs, a falling pile-driver – the energy is ultimately dissipated as heat. Thus, one can measure the energy utilized by a person by measuring the amount of heat produced, either directly or indirectly. Directly, it is done with a calorimeter, in which the person is placed; this is a chamber constructed in such a way that all the heat he emits can be measured. Indirectly, it can be done by measuring the amount of oxygen he consumes, since we know how much energy is produced when a given amount of oxygen is used to oxidize the body's fuel.

The former method requires a room big enough to hold a person comfortably. Preferably it should be big enough to allow him also to do different sorts of work or movement, so that the energy required for these activities can be measured; there will, however, clearly be a limit to the sorts of activity that can be done in a confined space. The most difficult practical aspect is to build a room rigorously insulated, and with a sensitive method of measuring heat output.

The method of measuring oxygen consumption requires that the subject wear a mask, and this too imposes a limit on the sort of activity that can be undertaken, even though there now exist some quite light machines that can be strapped to the back.

See also: Basal metabolism; Benedict; Lavoisier; Liebig; Oxidation

Energy content of food

It is the oxidation of the major constituents of food that releases the energy required by the body. The amount of energy in a food can be measured by burning a measured quantity of it in a bomb calorimeter. This consists of a chamber which, for ease of combustion, is filled with oxygen. It carries a small sample of the food in a vessel that can be heated by an electric current so that it ignites the food. The vessel is surrounded by a water jacket, and the rise in temperature of the water is a measure of the heat released.

With this method, we now know that on combustion 1g of carbohydrate releases about 4 kcal, 1g of fat releases about 9 kcal, and 1g of alcohol about 7 kcal. These figures were first determined by the German physiologist, Max Rubner (1858–1932). Protein burned in the calorimeter releases about 5.25 kcal, but as protein in the body is not so completely oxidized as it is in the calorimeter, it is necessary to correct for the incompletely oxidized products which are excreted in the urine. These have a caloric value of about 1.25 kcal for each gram of protein metabolized, so that the energy released to the body by 1g of protein is 4 kcal.

One other correction may need to be made to the caloric value obtained by burning the food in the calorimeter, and that is for its fibre, since this is not oxidized in the body. It can be ignored if it is about 5% or less; if it is greater than this, an appropriate reduction must be made to the figure given by the calorimeter in converting it to the amount of energy available to the body.

If the content in grams of protein, fat and carbohydrate (and alcohol) in a given sample of food is known, it is of course quite easy to calculate its caloric value by multiplying these quantities by the factors 4, 9 and 4 (and 7); the sum of these will then be the number of kcal in the sample of food.

See also: Atwater; Calorie; Crawford; Joule; Rubner

Enzymes

An enzyme is a protein made by living cells, which acts as a catalyst in promoting one or more of the very large numbers of reactions in the body. Consider one of the digestive enzymes, ptyalin, also called diastase or salivary amylase. A solution of starch left to itself would not perceptibly undergo change even over a long time. If it is boiled with a small amount of acid, starch will quite rapidly be changed into the sugar maltose. The same reaction will occur if the starch is moistened with saliva; for example, if one chews without swallowing a starchy food such as bread, it gradually begins to taste sweet as maltose is released by the catalytic activity of ptyalin.

The enzymes in the digestive juices in the alimentary canal break down the large molecules of food components, such as protein, starch

MAJOR DIGESTIVE ENZYMES

SECRETED BY	SECRETION	MAIN ENZYMES	MAIN ACTIONS
Mouth	Saliva	Salivary amylase (ptyalin)	Starch and dextrins $\longrightarrow$ maltose
Stomach	Gastric juice	Pepsin	Proteins $\longrightarrow$ polypeptides
		Rennin	Caseinogen $\longrightarrow$ casein
Pancreas	Pancreatic juice	Trypsin (from trypsinogen)	Proteins $\longrightarrow$ polypeptides $\longrightarrow$ amino-acids
		Pancreatic amylase	Starch $\longrightarrow$ maltose
		Lipase	Fat $\longrightarrow$ fatty acids + glycerol
Duodenum	Duodenal juice	Enterokinase	Trypsinogen $\longrightarrow$ trypsin
Small intestine	Succus entericus	Sucrase (invertase)	Sucrose $\longrightarrow$ glucose + fructose
		Lactase	Lactose $\longrightarrow$ glucose + galactose
		Maltase	Maltose $\longrightarrow$ glucose
		Erepsin	Polypeptides $\longrightarrow$ amino-acids
		Lipase	Fats $\longrightarrow$ fatty acids + glycerol

and fat, so that the smaller molecules that are released can be absorbed through the alimentary canal wall into the bloodstream. Other enzymes remain inside the cells of the body and carry out a vast range of metabolic reactions in which these smaller molecules are oxidized to release energy, or are built up into other molecules so as to preserve the overall integrity of the body's tissues. Most of the enzymes act specifically on particular substances, or on a range of substances of similar chemical composition. The substance on which an enzyme acts is called its substrate, and the substrate often determines the name of the enzyme. The enzyme that digests maltose is maltase; the enzyme that oxidizes amino-acids is amino-acid oxidase.

Some of the enzymes can work only in the presence of other substances; these are called co-enzymes. They are not proteins, but are much simpler substances; several are members of the B group of vitamins, including thiamin, nicotinic acid, riboflavin, pyridoxine and pantothenic acid.

All living processes are dependent on the action of enzymes, but many enzymes can continue to be active after they are separated from the living cells that produce them. Examples are the enzymes in the digestive juices, or the enzymes that can be extracted from yeast but are still available to ferment sugar. Incidentally, since much of the early work on enzymes was carried out with yeast juice, enzymes are still sometimes called 'ferments'.

Enzymes act faster as the temperature rises up to 40°C or so, but most begin to be destroyed at higher temperatures. Saliva heated to 50°C will not digest starch, nor will boiled yeast ferment sugar. Finally, each enzyme acts best at a particular pH. Pepsin is most active at the pH of around 1.5 or 2, which is the degree of acidity in the stomach; trypsin is most active at the slightly alkaline pH of about 8.

See also: Fischer; Hydrolysis; pH

Epidemic

An epidemic describes an outbreak of a disease affecting many people in a population. There was an epidemic of influenza in Europe in 1918 and 1919, in which about 200,000 people died in England and Wales alone. An epidemic that spreads to many countries, or even becomes worldwide, is sometimes called a pandemic; such an outbreak of influenza occurred in 1889–90.

More recently, the term epidemic has been used in relation to the widespread occurrence of coronary heart disease in the developed world.

See also: Endemic

Epidemiology

One important way in which the cause or causes of a disease may be established is by the use of epidemiology. This is done by seeking to identify differences between, on the one hand, individuals who develop the disease or populations in which the disease occurs, and on the other hand, individuals or populations without the disease. One of the earliest examples was the observation by Dr John Snow that all those who developed cholera in an epidemic in London in 1854 had been drinking water from the same pump. That the disease was caused by the water was confirmed by the removal of the pump handle, whereupon the epidemic stopped.

Epidemiology has been used a great deal in searching for the causes of disease; examples in nutrition are the recognition that pellagra occurred largely where maize was an important item of diet; beri-beri where it was polished rice, and scurvy where no fresh food was eaten. However, these discoveries did not in themselves identify the specific cause of these conditions, namely the deficiency of the essential dietary constituents later called vitamins.

For epidemiological studies to be effective in helping to identify the cause of a disease, it is necessary to know what information is needed, how it is to be obtained, and how it is to be interpreted. For populations, the required information is the incidence or prevalence of the disease, and the prevalence of the suspected cause in the populations to be compared. The information can be collected in one of three different ways – by prospective studies, by retrospective studies, and by cross-sectional studies. Prospective studies identify the cases as they occur from the beginning of the investigation, and at the same time record how many have the characteristics that have been suggested as possible causes of the disease. They then examine a number of individuals who have not developed the disease, and again count the number who have those same characteristics. Retrospective studies ideally study current cases of the disease and then seek to discover past characteristics or events that may have caused the disease. A retrospective study would find a number of patients with lung cancer, a similar number without the disease matched for age, sex and, if possible, class and nationality, and question them all about their smoking habits.

The third possible method is by cross-sectional studies or surveys. This is a relatively simple method of seeking associations, such as the prevalence of measles in children in relation to the income of their parents.

More recently, epidemiological studies have been used extensively in attempts to discover the causes of coronary heart disease, cancer of specific sites, diabetes, and other diseases generally believed to be more common now than they used to be, and more common in the wealthier countries than in the poorer countries.

Epidemiological studies have indeed identified some characteristics of populations or people more likely than others to develop coronary disease; for example, they have higher than average cholesterol in the blood. It has also been shown that an increase in cholesterol can be produced experimentally by changes in the diet: by increasing consumption of fat, or the proportion of saturated to unsaturated fat, or the consumption of sucrose. However, the assumption that this observation in itself proves that fat or sugar is a cause of coronary disease is unwarranted.

It must also be borne in mind that an association may simply be an indirect association. An example is the observation that in Britain the rise in the number of people dying of coronary disease closely follows the rise in the number of households with radio and television. This is simply a measure of rising income, which in turn is associated with increasing leisure, cigarette smoking, dietary fat, dietary sugar – all of which have been suggested as real causes of the disease.

In the language of the epidemiologist, a characteristic that is associated with an increased chance or likelihood or risk of a disease is called a risk factor. This expression has probably strengthened the belief that anything that increases the cholesterol in the blood, such as a diet rich in saturated fat, can actually cause coronary heart disease, and anything that lowers it, such as a diet rich in poly-unsaturated fat, will prevent it. But 'risk factor' is a statistical concept, and means no more than that the presence of the factor is an indicator of an increased risk, and not that it is a cause.

See also: Coronary heart disease; Diabetes

Essential

Most commonly, a constituent of a food is referred to as being essential if, in its absence, the body does not function properly or indeed is not able to survive. Thus, the vitamins and many of the mineral elements are essential. Essential too are some though not all of the amino-acids and some of the fatty acids, and they are differentiated from those the body does not need in its vital processes, or can make for itself, by being known as essential amino-acids or essential fatty acids (EFA).

A second use of 'essential' conveys the meaning of 'essence' rather than 'vital importance'. Spices and herbs owe their flavour, and flowers their smell, to constituents that are called essential oils. Unscrupulous distributors of these oils have been known to word their advertisements in such a way as to imply that the health of anyone not using their products is in some way in jeopardy.

Expeditions

The experience of many explorers, some of it calamitous, has gradually provided considerable knowledge of what foods are appropriate on expeditions, and how best they can be packaged. To begin with, the explorers must, before they begin their journey, be healthy and active, and adequately trained in general as well as in the specific tasks they are likely to undertake. The assessment of their dietary needs has to take into account how active they will have to be on the expedition. Apart from this, their needs are no different from those at home. Particular care must be taken, however, to ensure adequate supplies of water, something that is often given insufficient attention. If the supplies are likely to be short in the terrain to be explored, it will be necessary to carry water on the expedition, even though this will aggravate the problem of weight.

The weight of the foods themselves can be reduced by having them prepared beforehand, so that inedible parts are removed. If local water supplies are known to be adequate, it may be further reduced by having dehydrated foods. Modern lightweight packaging is also now available. If any of the methods of preparing the foods is likely to reduce their nutrient content, appropriate precautions should be taken. It has been said that the deaths of Scott and some of his colleagues at the South Pole in 1912 were at least partly caused by the development of scurvy from the lack of vitamin C in their diet.

See also: Survival rations; Water

Eye

The ordinary defects of refraction, that is, short or long sight or astigmatism, are probably not affected by nutritional factors, although from time to time it has been suggested that such defects might be caused by a generally poor diet, or by excess or deficiency of items such as sugar or protein.

There are, however, several conditions that affect the integrity or functioning of the eye. Deficiency of riboflavin can produce a conjunctivitis and corneal vascularization. The symptoms are itching of the eyes, together with dislike of the light (photophobia) and excessive production of tears (lacrymation). Deficiency of vitamin A results in night blindness; later, xerophthalmia may occur, in which the conjunctiva become thickened and dry; Bitot's spots may also be present on the conjunctiva as small, whitish plaques. If the condition is severe, the cornea becomes soft, and may break down and become infected, so that blindness ensues. Blindness due to deficiency of vitamin A is said to occur in large numbers of children in south and east Asia; in India, as many as 20,000 new cases are added to the total each year. It is disturbing to realize that this is entirely preventable by simple dietary change.

During the Second World War, it became evident that people who had been taking a grossly deficient diet for prolonged periods gradually lost their vision. The initial impairment was of central vision, so that they had difficulty in reading or in recognizing people. When treated early with yeast or yeast extract, they usually recovered rapidly and completely; if the condition had progressed considerably, it often turned out to be irreversible. The precise nutritional component involved has not been identified.

See also: Riboflavin; Vitamin A; Yeast

F

Factory farming

In Western countries, the production of meat, eggs and milk is increasingly carried out by intensive methods that are less costly than the conventional methods of farming in free range or pasture. It is because of the efficiency of such production that the consumer is able to buy so cheaply such foods as chicken, which up to the 1950s was an expensive item of the diet. Repeated investigations can show no difference in the nutrient content of food produced by factory farming, except that eggs from battery hens contain rather less vitamin B_{12} and folic acid than those from free-range hens.

Many people claim that foods produced intensively have less flavour than those produced conventionally. This is no doubt true for chicken. It occurs because the carefully controlled feeding programme allows them to reach slaughter weight faster, and young animals have less flavour than do older ones. It is arguable, however, whether anyone can really tell the difference in taste in eggs or pork.

See also: Health foods

Famine

This article deals with fasting, famine and starvation. Fasting is a condition imposed voluntarily, in which an individual deliberately refrains from taking food, and sometimes also drink. This may be done for religious reasons, at particular times of the year or on particular occasions, or it may be done for political reasons, such as a hunger strike.

Starvation refers to a similar abstention from food, perhaps from drink too, but through imposed causes rather than voluntary. Famine is a situation in which a large number of people are deprived of food, again involuntarily.

So long as water is taken, an adult can live for many weeks without food. The length of time depends on several factors, one being the amount of reserve energy in the body; a fat person is likely to survive longer than a thin person, an adult will survive longer than a child, and an inactive person longer than one who is physically active. The expected survival time without any food whatsoever is about 8 or 10 weeks.

The first energy store to be used is the glycogen in the liver and muscle. During the first 5 days without food, 200g or so of the total glycogen store of about 500g is converted to glucose and then oxidized. During this time, amino-acids from muscle protein begin to be broken down, yielding more glucose from some 65g of protein each day. This release of glucose is especially important, because normally it is the only material that can be used by the brain. Later, however, protein breakdown is reduced; by 5 weeks, it has fallen to around 20g a day. At this time, fat oxidation is the main source of energy and the brain is able to use the products of ketosis, which come from the incomplete oxidation of some of the fat.

A person can survive a loss of about 25% of body weight, so that an average man of 70kg (about 155lb) could lose about 17kg in weight. Of this, about 3kg are protein, 7kg fat, 6kg water, and the remaining 0.5–1kg carbohydrates and salts. The different organs lose very different proportions of their original weight, according to how important their function is in preserving life. Death by starvation is accompanied by a loss of only 3% of the weight of the brain and heart, 30% of the weight of the muscles, 70% of the weight of the spleen, and 95% or more of the weight of the adipose tissue.

From the experiences in Nazi concentration camps, and the continuing famines in different countries, we now know a great deal about the physical and mental changes that occur in starvation. The skin becomes loose, dry and pigmented, and the sunken face gives a false impression of protruding eyes. In the later stages, oedema occurs, including the characteristic swollen abdomen associated with famine oedema. The pulse rate and the blood pressure are low. A starving person becomes physically listless and mentally irritable. His thoughts are concerned mostly with food, and interest in other matters is minimal. In the late stages, there is complete breakdown of moral standards, so that food may be stolen from one's own family. Resistance to infection is low, so that death commonly occurs because of tuberculosis, malaria, or some other disease.

Cancrum oris is an horrific complication of starvation, usually in children but sometimes in adults. It consists of gangrene of the lips and cheeks. The effect is the spreading destruction of parts of the face; the only treatment is surgical removal of the affected parts, although death is the most likely outcome when this condition arises.

Almost as serious is the occurrence of diarrhoea, especially in famine, where people are likely to be taking quite unsuitable objects as food, such as roots and grass. The intestine by this time will have degenerated and wasted to a thin wall with very little of its mucous membrane lining. It therefore reacts to the irritation of these foreign items with excessive contractions. When diarrhoea occurs, the chances are that death will soon supervene.

The treatment of starvation depends on whether there are, on the one hand, one or a few individuals with access to modern hospital facilities, or, on the other hand, large numbers of people, as in a famine, and few facilities. In the former instance, it is possible to feed small quantities of bland foods, or to institute intravenous injections containing glucose, amino-acids and mineral salts, together perhaps with vitamins.

In famine conditions, the problems are largely those of logistics, in bringing appropriate foods, cooking vessels and shelter to the afflicted areas. The major need is to supply sources of energy, first in small quantities of food. It is usually quite inappropriate to organize supplies of vitamin pills for people whose wasted bodies demand a supply of energy. Reconstituted skim milk in frequent small feeds is a good way of beginning rehabilitation. Later, a slow increase in the quantity of food, and a widening of the range, is indicated; in a week or two, as much as 500 kcal a day may be demanded. Some individuals, however, do not respond satisfactorily to the initial stage of feeding; even after several weeks they may die because of the permanent damage sustained by the organs, especially the heart.

See also: Ketosis; Oedema; Water

Fat

The word 'fat' is used to indicate a number of chemical substances not soluble in water, but soluble in solvents such as benzene and chloroform. There is no essential difference between the terms 'fat' and 'oil', which are used simply to indicate whether the fat is solid or liquid.

This entry deals with the fat in food; body fat is dealt with under that heading.

Most of the fat in food is chemically known as triglyceride. This is a compound of glycerol (glycerine) and fatty acids. Since there are many fatty acids, there are also many triglycerides. When these are heated with an alkali such as caustic soda, the glycerol and the fatty acids are separated, and the acids combine with the soda to form soap.

A fatty acid contains a chain of carbon atoms, most commonly about 16 or 18 atoms long. On to these carbon atoms are attached hydrogen atoms. If the fatty acids in the fat have the maximum number of hydrogen atoms they can possibly have, the fat is called saturated. If they have fewer than the maximum, it is called unsaturated, and if they hold several fewer than the maximum, it is called polyunsaturated. Nutritionists have their own name for polyunsaturated fatty acid; they call it PUFA.

Fats rich in unsaturated fatty acids, and especially in polyunsaturated fatty acids, are liquid at ordinary temperatures, and are therefore oils. They oxidize quite readily unless they are treated, either by refining them or by adding small quantities of antioxidants. When they do become oxidized, they become solid. This is the basis of 'drying' in oil paints, which often contain linseed oil. They do not dry in the ordinary sense by the evaporation of liquid, but by the conversion of the liquid oil into solid oxidized oil.

The fats in animal foods, such as milk, meat and butter, are mostly saturated fats and the unsaturated fat that contains oleic acid. The fats in vegetable foods, mostly from seeds such as maize or soya or sunflower, are usually oils and tend to be rich in polyunsaturated fat; an important exception is coconut oil.

Average fat intake in different countries is to a large extent dependent on average incomes. In the poorest countries, fat may contribute 10% or so of the energy content of the diet; in the wealthiest countries, it amounts to about 40% and contains a large proportion of animal fat.

Fats serve four purposes in the diet. The most important is the supply of energy. Fat is the most concentrated form of energy in the diet: 1g releases 9 kcal, compared with 7 kcal for alcohol, 4 kcal for protein and 4 kcal for carbohydrate.

The second function of fats is that they help to make the diet palatable; diets with little or no fat are quite unattractive. The third function is to provide the 'essential fatty acids' (EFA). These are linoleic acid and linolenic acid. Both are polyunsaturated, and derive their names from linseed oil, which contains these fatty acids. If they are lacking in the diet, signs of deficiency occur. Another polyunsaturated acid, arachidonic, is essential in the body, but it can be made from linoleic acid and so need not itself be taken if the diet contains enough linoleic acid.

Finally, the dietary fats are the normal carriers of the fat-soluble vitamins A, D, E and K.

See also: Absorption of fat; Fatty acids; Oils

Fatty acids

Most of the fat in our food, and in our bodies, is made up of triglycerides. These are readily broken down either by heating with acid or alkaline, or by the digestive enzymes in the intestine, into their constituents, which are glycerol (glycerine) and fatty acids.

There are altogether 40 or so different fatty acids in food and in the body. Most of the time they are present as part of the triglycerides (neutral fat), but in the body there is constantly a small amount of triglyceride being broken down into its constituent glycerol and fatty acids, or conversely some triglyceride being built up from the glycerol and fatty acids. In addition, there are some other materials in the body that are composed partly of fatty acids, notably the phospholipids and lipoproteins.

The fatty acids differ from one another in three ways. The following description gives an outline of these differences; the Table amplifies this description with some chemical formulae.

The first difference is that, since they are made up of a sort of backbone in the form of a chain of carbon atoms, they may differ in the number of carbon atoms in this chain. They almost all have an even number of carbon atoms; the commonest ones have 16 or 18, but they can have between 4 and 24. A second difference is in the number of hydrogen atoms that are attached to the carbons of the chain. Apart from the carbon atom at the two ends of the chain, each with a particular chemical group attached, the atoms in the chain can each hold a maximum of two hydrogen atoms. However, it is possible for an adjacent pair of carbon atoms to hold only one each; the carbon atoms would then have what is called a double bond between them, instead of the single bond that exists when each carbon has two hydrogen atoms. If the chain has all the possible hydrogen ions attached to the carbons, the result is a saturated fatty acid. If it has fewer than the maximum, so that it has one or more double bonds, it is an unsaturated fatty acid; it would be monounsaturated if it had one double bond, and polyunsaturated if it had two or more.

The third difference that may exist between different fatty acids

FORMULAE OF FATTY ACIDS

Most naturally occurring fatty acids have an even number of carbon atoms. A simple, short-chain acid such as caproic acid can be written

$CH_3 \cdot CH_2 \cdot CH_2 \cdot CH_2 \cdot CH_2 \cdot COOH$
CAPROIC ACID

More simply, caproic acid can be written

$CH_3 \cdot (CH_2)_4 \cdot COOH$

Most fatty acids have longer chains, with 16, 18 or 20 carbon atoms

$CH_3 \cdot (CH_2)_{14} \cdot COOH$ $CH_3 \cdot (CH_2)_{16} \cdot COOH$ $CH_3 \cdot (CH_2)_{18} \cdot COOH$
PALMITIC ACID   STEARIC ACID   ARACHIDIC ACID

All of these are saturated acids. An unsaturated acid has fewer hydrogen atoms and consequently has one or more 'double bonds'. Oleic acid is an example of a monounsaturated acid, and linoleic acid an example of a polyunsaturated acid.

$CH_3 \cdot (CH_2)_7 \cdot CH = CH \cdot (CH_2)_7 \cdot COOH$
OLEIC ACID

$CH_3 \cdot (CH_2)_7 \cdot CH = CH \cdot CH_2 \cdot CH = CH \cdot (CH_2)_4 \cdot COOH$
LINOLEIC ACID

A fatty acid with one double bond can exist in either of two different forms called stereo-isomers. Oleic acid, strictly speaking, is only one form of the acid with the formula written above, and should be written in the 'cis form

$CH_3 \cdot (CH_2)_7 \cdot CH$
$\|$
$HOOC \cdot (CH_2)_7 \cdot CH$
OLEIC ACID (CIS)

Its isomer is elaidic acid, which is a 'trans' acid

$CH_3 \cdot (CH_2)_7 \cdot CH$
$\|$
$CH \cdot (CH_2)_7 \cdot COOH$
ELAIDIC ACID (TRANS)

A fatty acid with two double bonds can exist in four different forms, since either double bond can be 'cis' or 'trans'. The naturally occurring unsaturated fatty acids all exist in the 'cis' form; however, some of the unsaturated acids are changed into the 'trans' isomers during the process of hydrogenation in the manufacture of cooking fats and margarine.

relates only to the unsaturated ones. At the point of a double bond, a molecule may exist in either of two forms, depending on whether the rest of the chain turns back on itself (cis) or proceeds in the original direction (trans).

The body's enzymes can recognize the difference between cis and trans fatty acids; for example, the naturally occurring essential fatty acid, linoleic acid, is polyunsaturated with two double bonds, and both are in the cis form.

If they are in the trans form, the acid cannot act as an essential fatty acid.

See also: Arachidonic acid; Body fat; Linoleic acid; Lipoproteins; Margarine

Favism

This is a particular sort of anaemia which may occur in people who are born with an inability to manufacture the enzyme glucose-6-phosphate dehydrogenase, an enzyme that helps to maintain the integrity of the red blood cells. The condition is genetically determined, and is found in some Mediterranean people and black Americans. Severe anaemia occurs only when affected persons are treated with one of several drugs, which include anti-malarials, anti-pyretics and analgesics, or when they eat broad beans, *Vicia faba*. When the bean is a common article of the diet of the affected person, the anaemia so developed can be very severe and the condition is then known as favism.

See also: Poisons in food; Pulses

Fermentation

The action of micro-organisms upon carbohydrates, especially when there is little or no oxygen present, is known as fermentation. The effects may be desirable or undesirable. On the one hand, people consider it undesirable to have milk that curdles when added to their coffee or tea because bacteria have produced some lactic acid in the milk by fermentation. On the other hand, continued action of the same bacteria in the milk produces enough lactic acid for the milk to become quite solid and then to be eaten as yoghurt. Again, a fruit salad will be rejected by many people if it has begun to undergo alcoholic fermentation through the growth of yeast, yet this is precisely the process that ultimately produces wines from grapes and other fruit.

Alcoholic and lactic acid fermentations are the best known, and the most used in food production. The former produces carbon dioxide as well as alcohol, and so is used for making not only beer and wine and, indirectly, spirits, but also for making bread. Although the best-known products of fermentation are alcohol, lactic acid and carbon dioxide, other substances are produced by the growing micro-organisms and several of these are made commercially. Examples are riboflavin, citric acid, vinegar, and several antibiotics including penicillin and streptomycin.

See also: Alcohol; Beer; Bread; Wine; Yeast; Yoghurt

Fertility

Demographers differentiate between the actual numbers of babies born – fertility – and the ability to have children – fecundity. Physicians and biologists on the other hand tend to use 'fertility' to mean either of these indices.

Animal experiments have shown that almost any sort or degree of nutritional deficiency results in a reduced ability to produce young. But in human beings the relation between nutrition and the ability to have children is not clear-cut. In poor countries, people tend to have larger families than those in wealthier countries, and some sociologists have suggested that this is caused by a higher reproductive capacity (fecundity) with poor nutrition. They go on to offer a teleological explanation for this, suggesting that the higher birthrate is a compensatory mechanism making up for the higher death rates that are to be found in the impoverished countries.

The few facts that are known, and from which only uncertain deductions can be made, relate to fertility rather than fecundity. It seems that extremely poor families have a birth rate of perhaps 40 per 1,000 of population, and that it is a little higher, between 45 and 50, in marginally less poor countries. The difference may in fact be due to the low fecundity of a very poor woman, who suffers from diseases, including those of the reproductive organs, that reduce her chance of conceiving or of delivering live babies; somewhat better nutrition thus diminishes these disabilities, so that rather more children are born. When a population begins to be less poor, fertility decreases steadily from the high levels of around 45 per 1,000 until it reaches the current low levels in the affluent countries of 15 or less. There is every reason to believe that these low levels have nothing to do with nutritional state, but are the result of deliberate family limitation.

It might also be argued that inadequate nutrition does reduce fecundity and therefore fertility, as shown by the amenorrhoea seen in anorexia nervosa, or seen in Western Europe in the period of severe food shortage towards the end of the Second World War. These acute situations in which sudden nutritional deficiency is imposed on previously well-nourished people may well produce physical and hormonal effects different from those in populations who all their lives have been subject to a low dietary intake.

See also: Population

Fever

Technically, a fever or pyrexia is a condition in which the body's temperature is, for any length of time, above the normal for that individual. Although it is usual to say that the normal temperature as measured in the mouth is 98.6°F or 37°C, it is lowest in the morning and highest in the evening. It also varies during the menstrual cycle, being highest at ovulation.

It is possible to raise the temperature of the body by having a hot bath or by strenuous exercise; this rise lasts for not more than one hour.

Since the introduction of antibiotics and other drugs for diseases such as pneumonia and tuberculosis, it is much rarer for fever to be prolonged. Short-term fevers are best treated with nutritious foods such as milk, perhaps with the addition of beaten eggs, and fruit juices. As the patient improves, the diet can be extended with meat and fish, although not fried. Bread, cereals and milk puddings are often recommended, but it should be remembered that some patients may develop heartburn and other symptoms of indigestion with these foods.

If the fever is prolonged, there is no need to change these principles. It may, however, be necessary to take even more care to make the serving of the meals attractive and varied, and to introduce favoured foods, unless for any reason these would be unsuitable, for example because they cause abdominal discomfort.

The advice is sometimes given to 'feed a cold and starve a fever'. One interpretation of this is that it is good practice to eat when one has a cold, but not to eat when one has a fever; an alternative interpretation is that to eat when one has a cold is liable to produce fever. These contradictory recommendations are clearly of no help as a guide to appropriate dietary treatment for either condition.

Fibre

There are several food constituents that are not digested and absorbed by the human body. Some are partly attacked by micro-organisms when they reach the large intestine, but the products of this 'digestion' are mostly lost in the faeces.

An older name for the indigestible matter in the diet was roughage. It was also called unavailable carbohydrate, although some of the materials in the fibre are not chemically carbohydrates. The new name is dietary fibre, but this too is not strictly accurate because the materials involved include pectin, which does not consist of fibres.

Dietary fibre is made up of several different chemical substances. It is present only in vegetable foods. Most of it is cellulose, which constitutes the major part of cotton and paper. There are also compounds called hemicelluloses, which with cellulose are the chief supporting structure of plant leaves and stems. Lignin is the hard material in wood, and in woody parts of plants. Pectin is found in soft fruits; when boiled with sugar, it produces the jelly that is the characteristic feature of jams. Other indigestible plant constituents are gums such as guar gum, from a leguminous plant grown in India and the southern US, and alginates such as agar from seaweed.

Foods that supply a high proportion of dietary fibre include leafy vegetables, most fruits and bran. Wholemeal bread thus contains significantly more dietary fibre than does white bread.

It has been suggested that the lack of dietary fibre is an important cause of the 'diseases of civilization': e.g. dental decay, overweight, diabetes and coronary thrombosis. The chief evidence for this is that these diseases are rare in poor rural areas of the non-industrialized countries, where the diets contain much more dietary fibre because they include a high proportion of unrefined cereals. It has also been suggested that several diseases of the digestive system are prevented by a high intake of dietary fibre; some of these are constipation, diverticulitis, gall-bladder disease and cancer of the large bowel.

It has to be remembered that the populations of the poorer countries and those in the more affluent countries, with their very different patterns of diseases, have many differences in lifestyle in addition to the quantity of fibre in their diets. It requires therefore not only studies in epidemiology to implicate lack of dietary fibre as a cause of the diseases of affluence, but experimental studies to determine the effects of dietary fibre in the body. Such experiments have shown that an increase in cereal fibre in the diet increases the speed at which food passes through the bowel, decreasing what is called the transit time between eating food and eliminating the undigested residue. Similarly, cereal fibre increases the bulk of the stools and the frequency of defaecation, so there is a consensus that constipation can often be relieved by dietary fibre. Pectin, but not cereal fibre, lowers the concentration of cholesterol in the blood, and so may play a part in preventing heart attacks; this suggestion is not, however, universally accepted. Pectin and guar gum, but again not cereal fibre, slow down the absorption of glucose into the blood, and may be useful in the treatment of diabetes and, some say, also in its prevention; here again, not every nutritionist agrees with this conclusion. Dietary fibre has also been recommended for the prevention or treatment of obesity. This is based on the supposition that the presence of dietary fibre increases the sensation of satiety and so reduces food intake, while at the same time reducing the absorption of food in the intestine. This too is an area where there is no universal agreement.

The effects of an increase in dietary fibre are not all beneficial. In some people, it produces abdominal discomfort, an excessive frequency of defaecation and an unwelcome degree of flatulence. The fibre also combines with some of the mineral elements in the intestine, and so reduces the amounts absorbed from the food. This is particularly important in regard to iron and zinc, where a high-fibre diet can be an important cause of producing anaemia or zinc deficiency.

See also: Cancer; Carbohydrate; Constipation; Coronary heart disease; Diabetes; Epidemiology; Obesity; Zinc

Fischer, Emil (1852–1919)

Emil Fischer was an important German chemist who made fundamental discoveries in the structures of the purines, the sugars and the amino-acids. He was also a pioneer in the use of enzymes, especially those of yeast, in carrying out biological reactions; it was he who first suggested the 'lock and key' analogy of the action of enzymes on particular chemical substances.

Fischer was born in Prussia in 1852, the son of a merchant. In 1871 he became a student with Kekulé, the chemist who suggested the ring formula for benzene and who thus laid the foundations for the understanding of aromatic organic chemistry. Fischer became Professor of Chemistry in Erlangen in 1882, and then moved to Würzburg and finally to the Chemical Institute in Berlin University in 1892. His distinctions included the award of the Nobel Prize in Chemistry in 1902. He died in Berlin.

See also: Enzymes

Fish

The nutrient composition of fish is in some respects comparable to that of meat, except that there are no obvious deposits of fat. Those fish that have a fair amount of fat, such as salmon, mackerel and herrings, contain between 10% and 15%, interspersed invisibly between the muscle fibres. The fat content is somewhat lower in the winter, or in young fish. White fish such as cod, haddock and whiting contain only 0.5%–4% of fat. The amount of protein in both white and fatty fish is about 15%–18%, and so rather less than in many sorts of meat.

Most fish contain fair amounts of the vitamins of the B group, and of iodine. The fatty fish, and the livers of all fish, are good sources of vitamins A and D. In addition, quite appreciable amounts of calcium can be consumed from fish with soft bones, such as canned sardines or salmon, or from other fish cooked in vinegar, such as soused herring.

Roe, including caviare, has a protein content of 20–25%, and is especially rich in vitamin B_{12} and purines; for this reason, it is commonly excluded from the diet of persons with gout.

Shellfish have much the same composition as white fish. They are noteworthy on two counts. Firstly, more people are allergic to shellfish than to other fish or to meat. Secondly, molluscs such as oysters or mussels are often harvested at the seashore near the output of sewage, and thus may convey food poisoning, especially salmonella infection. Proper supervision is necessary of both the disposal of sewage and the sites for harvesting, especially for oysters when these are to be eaten raw. Mussels and whelks must in any case be well cooked.

Fluorine

It is not certain whether fluorine is an essential element in the body. It does play a part in the protection of the teeth from dental decay, but this could be said in any case not to occur to any significant extent in the absence of sucrose (sugar) in the diet, or of 'refined' starchy foods that might readily stick to the teeth. From this point of view, one could say that fluorine is an antidote to the harmful effects of sugar and starch on the teeth. On the other hand, since rats fed diets entirely free from fluorine do not grow to their full potential, it may be that, in addition to its effect on the teeth, the element plays some part in the body that is not yet apparent. Although, as we shall see, the amount in the diet varies considerably, it is impossible to find a human diet quite free from fluorine; by contrast, the diets fed to experimental animals can be made to contain virtually no fluorine.

The amount of fluorine that prevents dental decay is about 1mg a day; German authorities quote this amount as the daily requirement for an adult. The average intake is between 1mg and 3mg a day. Much of this comes from drinking water; with a concentration of 1mg per litre of fluorine (as fluoride), i.e. one part per million (1 ppm), this would provide about 1mg a day. Tea also supplies a significant amount, and may contribute up to a further 1–2mg a day. Water supplies, however, vary in their content of fluorine; in some areas they may contain almost none, and in a few there may be more than 5 ppm. These high concentrations cause mottling of the teeth, which occurs as brown bands separated by chalky white patches on the surface of the enamel. Apart from this, fluorine in water causes no harm to the body until it reaches concentrations of more than 10 ppm. Nevertheless, there are many people who object to the policy of adding fluoride to public water supplies that contain low amounts of fluoride, so that it reaches 1 ppm. Apart from the unwarranted belief that this poses a danger to health, there is also the ethical objection to fluoridation on the ground that it involves the compulsory ingestion of a chemical and does not allow freedom of choice. For this reason, it is suggested that other ways of taking fluoride should be available. One would be to take pills containing fluoride. Another is the use of fluoridized toothpaste, or the application of fluoride-containing materials on to the teeth by the dentist. Since the protective action of fluroide occurs mostly in young children, and hardly at all in adults, it has been proposed that fluoridized milk should be available to children in school.

Toxicity due to high intake of fluoride occurs in areas in Asia, South Africa and South America, where there is a fluoride concentration of more than 10 ppm to the water supply. This fluorosis is also seen in workers who come into frequent contact with fluoride-containing minerals used in smelting aluminium. The symptoms of fluorosis begin with a loss of appetite; later, osteosclerosis may develop. In this condition the bones become denser; more importantly, the ligaments of the spinal vertebrae become calcified, so that a stiff 'poker back' results.

Because of these effects of high fluoride intake, some physicians have administered sodium fluoride to patients with osteoporosis. There is, however, still uncertainty about the efficacy of this treatment.

See also: Bone; Dental decay

Folic acid

Anaemia is very common in tropical countries, especially among pregnant women. In the early 1930s Dr Lucy Wills in India discovered that a similar sort of anaemia could be produced in monkeys given a diet like that of her anaemic patients, and consisting largely of polished rice and white bread. The monkeys were cured when they were given extracts of yeast, and the same extracts also cured the anaemia of her patients.

A few years later, a substance was isolated from leaves and given the name folic acid (also called folacin), and this too was found to cure the experimental anaemia in monkeys. Incidentally, folic acid turned out to be related chemically to the pigment of butterfly wings, a subject of some of the very earliest research carried out in the 1880s by F. G. Hopkins who some 20 years later was one of the discoverers of the vitamins.

Folic acid was shown also to improve the anaemia of pernicious anaemia, but it soon turned out that the accompanying subacute combined degeneration of the cord in pernicious anaemia was if anything made worse. Vitamin B_{12}, which does cure both the anaemia and the nerve degeneration, has some similarities in action to folic acid, but they cannot entirely replace each other.

Anaemia caused by folic acid deficiency is common in Third World countries, especially in pregnant women. It is rarely seen in affluent countries, except during pregnancy. Some doctors give folic acid routinely during pregnancy. Persons with anaemia that has not been fully diagnosed should not be treated with folic acid, because the improvement in the anaemia might hide the fact that the underlying condition was pernicious anaemia, which might not be diagnosed until perhaps irreversible changes have occurred in the nervous system.

Folic acid is a water-soluble vitamin, present in sizeable amounts in liver and in most green vegetables; on the other hand, meat, milk and most fruits do not contain very much. It is present in foods and in the body mostly as the salt, folate, and as several related substances of varying folic acid activity. The RDI for adults is $300\mu g$ of total folate. Canning and cooking, especially if the cooking water is discarded, can lead to considerable loss of the vitamin.

As well as deficiency of the vitamin in the diet, secondary deficiency of folic acid may occur because of gastro-intestinal disease leading to diminished absorption, or in some people because of the prolonged administration of anti-epileptic drugs or oral contraceptives.

The anaemia of folic deficiency is a macrocytic anaemia or megaloblastic anaemia, so that the red blood cells are similar to those found in pernicious anaemia.

See also: Anaemia; Pregnancy; Vitamin B_{12}; Yeast

Food

As with so many words that are universally used and presumably universally understood, it is not easy to produce a necessary and sufficient definition of food. Here are some of the definitions found in different reference books:

Substances taken in by mouth which maintain life and growth, i.e. supply energy, and build and replace tissue.
  – Dictionary of Nutrition and Food Technology, Bender

Any substance containing nutrients, such as carbohydrates, proteins and fats, that can be ingested by a living organism and metabolized into energy and body tissue.
  – Collins English Dictionary

Victuals; provision for the mouth.
  – Dictionary of the English Language, Samuel Johnson

What one takes into the system to maintain life and growth, and to supply waste; aliment, nourishment, victuals.
  – Shorter Oxford Dictionary

What is taken into the system to maintain life and growth, and to supply the waste of tissue; aliment, nourishment, provision, victuals.
  – Oxford Dictionary

Anything which, when taken into the body, serves to nourish or build up the tissues or to supply body heat; aliment; nutriment.
  – Dorland's Illustrated Medical Dictionary

Some of the differences among these definitions are rather subtle; for example, the *Oxford Dictionary*, unlike Bender's *Dictionary*, implies that an intravenous drip containing glucose or vitamins, or even common salt, can be classed as food. The *Shorter Dictionary*'s phrase 'to supply waste' suggests that one of the functions of food is to contribute to the content of the faeces; that must please those who believe that food should contain roughage or dietary fibre.

Food additives

Materials may be added to foods for a variety of reasons. Usually, food additives are thought of in terms of chemical substances used by food manufacturers, but the cook in the kitchen also uses food additives with the same objectives: to enhance flavour, to add colour, to preserve, to change the consistence. These objectives are achieved by such items as nutmeg, cochineal, salt, cornflour. The additives used by food manufacturers are now, in most countries, controlled by legislation in the form of lists of permitted substances. The presence of additives in food has to be indicated in the manner laid down in regulations governing food labelling. These lists of permitted additives are rarely the same for any two countries. The reasons are often political rather than being caused by differences of opinion about safety. For example, if the particular chemical substance long permitted as a safe additive in one country turns out to be different from that permitted in another country, there may be little incentive for either country to make a change. This would require new legislation and, with it, changes both in the enforcement agencies and in the industry.

Preservatives: Some of the substances formerly used as preservatives, including boric acid, are no longer permitted. Those that are permitted are considered in the entry 'Food preservation'.

Colouring agents: Most coloured confectionery, as well as many cakes and drinks, has colour added. Colours are especially important when the food or drink is given a flavour such as that of a fruit which is normally associated with a particular colour. An experiment in which 6 people were given colourless sweets with a blackcurrant flavour showed that only one person identified the flavour. It was, however, immediately recognized by all 6 when they were given similar sweets to which the usual purple colour had been added.

Flavouring agents: The distinctive flavours of different foods are due to the presence, often in minute quantities, of a very large number of chemical substances. With the advances in analytical chemistry, especially the techniques of chromotography since the early 1940s, chemists have been able to identify most of these materials. It is therefore now possible for food manufacturers not only to use extracts made from foods and spices, but also in many instances to have the appropriate chemical substances, or closely related ones, synthesized. In addition, there are sometimes quite different chemical substances available that happen to have a flavour close to that required.

In the EEC, there now exist more than 2,000 flavours on the permitted list. About half of these are synthetic chemical substances. Examples are acetaldehyde with an apple flavour, benzaldehyde (almond), propyl acetate (pear) and diacetyl (butter).

Monosodium glutamate (MSG) occupies a unique position in that it is used not so much because of its own flavour but because it enhances the meaty flavour of stews, soups and savoury sauces. In small quantities, it also improves the flavour of cooked vegetables. MSG is the sodium salt of glutamic acid, one of the amino-acids found in most proteins and thus present in the gravies of cooked meats, in meat and yeast extracts, and in such protein derivatives as hydrolysed vegetable protein (HVP).

MSG is found in many Chinese foods, partly because it is present in soya sauce and partly because the pure substance is now used in Chinese restaurants; it is also found in dried soups and many other prepared foods. Some individuals react to MSG by what is called the Chinese Restaurant Syndrome. This is characterized by pain in the neck, headache and perhaps palpitations. One of the early descriptions of the condition was made by a Dr Kwok in 1967, and it was then given the name 'Kwok's Quease' by one of the British medical journals. This condition is only transitory, however, and individuals sensitive to MSG soon learn to avoid eating foods containing a great deal of it. At one time, it was suggested that MSG could cause brain damage in babies and young children. Although there is no evidence at all that it produces this or any other harm, except the temporary Chinese Restaurant Syndrome in people sensitive to a large intake, most manufacturers of baby foods who used to add MSG now do not do so.

The legislation governing the use of food additives is an extension of the 1955 Food and Drugs Act (see Food Adulteration). Whereas the early legislation gave lists of substances prohibited because they were known to be harmful, there are now lists of substances permitted because they are safe.

No legislation would be effective without means of enforcement. In the UK, there are officials employed by local authorities, who are able to have samples of food analysed in laboratories belonging to the authorities, or in private laboratories. Where a prosecution is undertaken, it is brought before a magistrates' court.

In the United States, satisfactory legislation was delayed by the various attempts by different states to solve their own problems. The first federal act was introduced in 1906. This was superseded in 1938 by the much more effective Food, Drug and Cosmetic Act, and one of its first actions was the creation of the Food and Drug Administration. Twenty years later, the Food Additives Amendment was passed and, like the British 1955 Food and Drugs Act, it changed the governing principle in the use of food additives from forbidding substances known or suspected of being harmful, to allowing named substances accepted as safe. The permitted additives have either been tested for safety or have been in use for many years with no evidence that they are harmful; the latter group of additives are called 'GRAS', that is, generally recognized as safe.

The Food Additives Amendment also includes the so-called 'Delaney Clause', which says 'no additive shall be deemed safe if it is found to induce cancer when ingested by man or animal'. This has been interpreted as forbidding the use of any substance which, in any quantity however great, produces cancer in any species of animal. It was this clause that led to the banning of cyclamates, which experiments had suggested produced cancer of the kidney in some rats after a very long time with enormous doses.

The chief reason why food legislation is non-existent or ineffective in many of the poorer countries is the absence of skilled personnel and properly equipped laboratories for inspection, and inadequate procedures for enforcement.

See also: Appetite; Food adulteration; Food preservation

Food adulteration

Deliberate adulteration of food in the home is rare, apart from the occasional attempt to poison an errant husband or wife. For those who make foods for sale, however, it is always tempting to add materials that extend the food, or that improve its appearance. Flour, bread and beer have for centuries been subject to adulteration by dishonest millers, bakers and brewers. Soon after the introduction of tea into Europe in the seventeenth century, some of the merchants and shopkeepers learned how to add sand or sweepings or dried herbs, especially those that gave an astringency to the infusion. Within this century, school arithmetic books had sums in which children were asked to calculate the profit made by a shopkeeper when he added a particular proportion of sand to his tea leaves. Vinegar has been adulterated with sulphuric acid, and with caramel or oak chippings to colour it; wilted vegetables made to look green with copper salts; chalk added to milk, which readily lent itself also to dilution, sometimes with unsalubrious water from the nearest pond or ditch.

The use of all these adulterants, and more, increased with the increasing migration from the country to the town that led to increasing dependence by people on the buying of food from retailers. By the early nineteenth century, food adulteration was so widespread that a chemist named Frederick Accum (1769–1818) was moved to publish the results of his analyses of a wide range of foods and drinks in a book entitled *Treatise on the adulteration of food and culinary poisons*, which appeared in 1820. It immediately created a storm of indignation. The public was shocked to learn that the addition of alum to bread was a common bakery practice, and that wine was often simply artificially coloured spoiled cider; the manufacturers, many of whom were named by Accum, were incensed, and they abused and persecuted him.

The second indictment of food manufacturers, published some ten years later by an anonymous author, attacked the purveyors of adulterated food even more vehemently, in a book called *Deadly adulteration and slow poisoning; or disease and death in the pot and bottle*. However, this publication was much less accurate than Accum's, and many of its allegations were without foundation.

Nevertheless, the interest in the problem of food adulteration did not subside, and it led to a series of food analyses carried out chiefly by a doctor, A. H. Hassall (1817–94), on behalf of the founder and first editor of the medical weekly, the *Lancet*, Thomas Wakley (1795–1862). Beginning in 1851, and continuing over a period of four years, the *Lancet* carried details of the analysis of several dozen food items, and a list of more than 3,000 tradesmen whose wares had been found to be grossly contaminated. The forecast that there would be innumerable libel suits from infuriated purveyors of these foods and drinks did not materialize; instead, there was considerable support for the reports from much of the press and particularly from the medical profession. The outcome was the first piece of legislation produced in any country designed to combat these malpractices, the 1860 Adulteration of Food and Drink Act. This, however, proved quite ineffective in reducing the activities of the rogues in the food industry, and it was replaced by the Sale of Food and Drugs Act of 1875. A large number of other legislative measures followed, culminating in the 1955 Food and Drugs Act. This introduced two momentous principles in British food legislation: first, that food must be fit for human consumption and free from hazards to health, and second, that it must be of the nature, substance and quality demanded. Most other countries have and enforce similar laws; the exceptions are some of the countries of the Third World, where there are either no laws or there are laws but not enough inspectors and scientists who can monitor them.

There are now in the UK two bodies responsible for advising about legislation, and for monitoring its application; they are the Food Standards Committee and the Food Additives and Contaminants Committee. Some sorts of additives, such as colorants, sweeteners and preservatives, may be used only if they are on a permitted list.

The corresponding agency in the US is the Food and Drug Administration (FDA).

See also: Codex Alimentarius; Food additives

Food fortification

The addition of particular nutrients to improve the nutritional quality of a food is called fortification, or enrichment, or sometimes ennoblement. It was first carried out voluntarily by some British margarine manufacturers, when in 1925 they added vitamins A and D to some of their brands. In 1940, these additions were made compulsory; the reason given by the authorities was that, since it is used as an alternative to butter which contains these vitamins, margarine should have a nutritional value similar to that of butter.

Thus, one reason for adding nutrients to a food is to bring its nutritional value nearer to that which it would be expected to have. This is also the reason for the addition in the UK of iron, thiamin and nicotinic acid to bread flour, other than wholemeal, thus replacing at least part of these vitamins removed during milling.

A second reason for fortification is to add nutrients as a public health measure to foods that ordinarily contain little or none, to reduce the prevalence of specific deficiencies. Calcium carbonate has since 1940 been added to flour in the UK, again except to wholemeal flour; the reason was partly because of the expected shortage of milk and thus possibly a shortage of calcium during the Second World War, and partly because of the use of higher extraction flours for breadmaking, with its higher phytate content.

Other examples are the addition of iodide to salt in several countries to prevent simple goitre, lysine to bread to improve the biological value of its protein, and iron to bread flour to reduce the prevalence of anaemia caused by iron deficiency.

It is debatable whether some of the examples quoted have been necessary or have made any significant impact on the nutritional health in the countries where they have been used. This is true for the addition of calcium and iron to bread in the UK. On the other hand, there is a stronger argument for the fortification of foods in poorer countries, where deficiencies of items such as thiamin, nicotinamide, vitamin A, folic acid and iron are common. But although fortification schemes have been tried in some countries, they are accompanied by considerable problems of enforcement and of distribution that are not easy to overcome.

See also: Bread; Margarine

Food habits

It is common to make personal judgements on what and how people eat, especially if these are very different from what and how we ourselves eat. It is as if we are saying, 'We have food preferences, you have food prejudices, they are food cranks.'

It is useful to distinguish the different attitudes and behaviour of people towards food.

Food preferences: Particular foods an individual likes or dislikes.
Food choice: The foods selected by an individual at a given time.
Food habits: The sum of the food choices of an individual, constituting his total diet.
Food customs: These properly refer to the patterns of consumption of populations or groups, perhaps a family. Nevertheless, such group patterns are often referred to as food habits.

Food preferences are determined mostly by attractiveness, that is, the appearance, colour, smell, texture and flavour. Other determinants are familiarity with the food, the culture in which one lives, and religious injunction.

Food choice can be at several levels. It can be a choice between a Golden Delicious apple or a Granny Smith apple, or between Brand A and Brand B frozen peas. It can be between peas and beans, or between beef and lamb. It can be between meat and cheese. Or it can be between an egg sandwich and a chocolate bar. The nutritional significance of the choice may therefore be negligible, moderate or considerable.

Food choice is determined largely by food preference and by cost. It is, however, also influenced by convenience, especially in relation to ease of purchase, of preparation and of storage. To what extent food choice is determined by advertising is debatable; it is likely that advertising and other methods of marketing can determine choice between Brand A and Brand B, rather than choice of commodity, for example between meat and fish.

One other factor that may determine food choice is the perceived wholesomeness or nutritional value of food, that is, its health qualities. This is rarely an overriding factor, except in a small proportion of the population, usually the professional classes. An example is the consumption of brown bread rather than white, partly because of the supposed benefits of dietary fibre. It is no doubt the recent publicity about the suggested nutritional superiority of brown bread that has been responsible for its increased consumption since 1980 or 1981.

Attempts to change food habits or food customs are made for two reasons. One is an attempt by food producers or food manufacturers to increase the consumption of their product; the second reason is the attempt of some authority to improve people's nutritional health.

It is often said that people are very resistant to change in their food habits, yet one can point to many and rapid changes that have occurred, especially in Western countries, during the past 30 years or so. But the fact that spontaneous change has occurred in the consumption of some sorts of food is not the same as saying that induced change for other foods is easy to achieve. It is tempting to make generalizations about what sorts of foods seem to be rigidly resistant to change – for example, the staple food such as bread or pasta – and what new foods are readily accepted – for example, the very palatable soft drinks and the very convenient hamburgers. But little serious experimental work has been done in identifying and quantifying change or resistance to change. Nor has much been done to distinguish between the acceptance of an unaccustomed food, such as breakfast cereals, and the discarding of an accustomed food, such as jam or fish.

Experience in the last few years has repeatedly shown that the introduction of new foods, such as the single-cell proteins, largely in order to contribute to improved nutrition, will fail if they are not attractive; it is not enough for them to be 'acceptable'. The lesson to be learned from these disappointing examples is that the chief reason why people eat particular foods is because they like them.

See also: Appetite; Novel protein foods

Food labelling

With a few exceptions, all prepacked food sold retail in the UK must provide information as laid down in legislation that came into force in 1983. The label must describe the produce without misleading the customer. It must give a list of ingredients in descending order of weight, and this must include any additives that are present. Because some of the additives have chemical names that would have little meaning for most consumers, the UK uses code numbers agreed by the members of the European Economic Community (EEC). The net quantity of the contents must be shown, and the package must give either the 'Sell by' date or the 'Best before' date. Other information required to be given includes details of special storage that may be needed, and the name and address of the manufacturer, packer or seller of the food.

The label may give other information as well, so long as it is not misleading. There is nothing, however, to prevent its being unconsciously amusing. The label on a can packed in the US and available in the UK tells you that it contains 'Large olives'. However, it also tells you that these are the smallest olives the firm produces by listing a range of sizes, starting with the 'Large' and continuing with 'Extra Large', 'Mammoth', 'Giant', 'Jumbo', 'Colossal' and 'Extra Colossal'.

EXAMPLES OF EEC CODE NUMBERS

E150   Caramel
E210   Benzoic acid
E232   2-(Thiazol-4-yl)benzimidazole
E300   Ascorbic acid (vitamin C)
E320   Butylated hydroxyanisole (BHA)
E321   Butylated hydroxytoluene (BHT)
E330   Citric acid
E412   Guar gum

See also: Codex Alimentarius

Food preservation

The availability of fresh food is rarely continuous; it may vary considerably from season to season, or because of changes in the environment such as drought or flood, or because of disease or war.

Because of the tendency of most foods to undergo spoilage, those that need to be kept for any length of time have to be preserved in some way. Sometimes preservation is not difficult. Cereals keep well so long as they are dry; this is illustrated in the biblical story of Joseph's advice to Pharaoh to store part of the corn harvests from the seven years of plenty so that it would be available for the seven years of famine that followed.

Some methods of preservation have been used since prehistoric times. Examples are the drying of fruits, legumes, meat or fish; the addition of chemical substances such as salt, sugar, vinegar or alcohol; the use of cold by bringing blocks of ice from the mountains into caves.

Methods of food preservation in use at the present time are either chemical or physical. Chemical methods include those that have been used for centuries. Acetic acid produced by acid fermentation, as in the making of sauerkraut from cabbage, reduces the pH to a level at which few micro-organisms can grow. Acid fermentation was also the method by which pickled gherkins and pickled cucumbers were made, but nowadays acetic acid is often used directly. It is also used for making pickled herring. Sugar and salt preserve because they produce a high osmotic pressure in solution and thus deprive micro-organisms of the water necessary for them to be able to grow. More recently, sodium nitrate (saltpetre, or more correctly Chile saltpetre) and sodium nitrite have been used and still are used for pickling meat such as ham and bacon. Other chemical preservatives include sodium sulphite, which releases sulphur dioxide, or sulphur dioxide itself; these are used for preserving wine, beer, fruit, vegetables and some sauces.

Many countries now allow only those chemical preservatives that are on a permitted list. The list also controls the foods to which the preservatives may be added and the maximum amounts that may be used. Different countries do not necessarily have the same lists. This may be due to differences of opinion among the scientists advising the various governments as to the safety of particular additives; sometimes the decision is influenced by political considerations, such as whether a particular chemical is manufactured in the country or has to be imported.

Physical methods of food preservation, by drying, cooling, heating and irradiation, avoid the problem about whether the addition of chemical preservatives is harmful to health.

Drying in the atmosphere, especially in the sunshine, was one of the earliest ways in which food was preserved. Most of the chemical reactions food may undergo, all its enzymatic reactions, and all growth of micro-organisms, cannot take place without sufficient moisture; adequate drying of food will thus prevent these causes of deterioration. One of the reasons why cereals became such an important source of food for neolithic man was because they keep well with their normal content of moisture of around 10%. This is why cereals harvested in wet conditions have to be dried before storage.

Many fruits and vegetables are re-named after drying: examples are prunes from plums; sultanas, raisins and currants from different varieties of grapes; pulses, such as dried beans, peas, lentils and grams. Drying may be carried out simply by spreading the foods out on trays or mats that are then left in the open air. In modern factories the process is accelerated by placing the trays in cabinets or tunnels and passing warm air over them.

A low temperature retards the rate of food spoilage because all the causes of deterioration then proceed more slowly. The routine keeping of foods at low temperatures became possible with the invention of methods of refrigeration in the 1860s. Its first use for food preservation on a large scale was the transport of chilled meat to Britain from New Zealand in 1882. Even better preservation is achieved by freezing. Damage to the food by the development of ice crystals is avoided by freezing very rapidly, so that only tiny crystals are formed. Quick freezing causes little damage: nevertheless, some soft fruits such as strawberries are found to be softer when they are thawed. A major limitation of this method of preservation is that the food has to be stored at $-18°C$ continuously until it is to be used.

A fairly recent method of preservation that causes minimal change in the food is freeze-drying. The food is first quick-frozen and then dried by vacuum, or by a combination of vacuum and heating. The vacuum removes the moisture, now ice, and in doing so lowers the temperature of the food still further. This makes it more difficult for the moisture to be removed by the vacuum. The application of a controlled amount of heat, however, prevents the lowering of the temperature and so the drying process does not slow down. This combined process is called accelerated freeze-drying (AFD). The quality of food dried in this way, and reconstituted, is very high indeed, even when it is applied to soft fruits. However, the process of AFD is expensive and so is used for only a few foods that are worth the additional cost. At present, the most common use is in the production of freeze-dried coffee.

Heating destroys bacteria and fungi; ordinary cooking, that is at temperatures of about 100°C, will help prevent deterioration of food for perhaps a few days, especially if it is covered. However, cooking temperatures do not normally destroy microbial spores that may be present, and these may very well germinate so that further infection with micro-organisms can occur. This can be prevented by the use of higher temperatures, of around 120°. The principle of canning foods, invented by the Frenchman, Appert (1752–1841), in 1810, depends both on the use of such a temperature and the sealing of the can so as to keep out further organisms. If there is no flaw in the can, food will keep for many years. The belief that it will become unfit to eat if it is not removed immediately from an opened can is not justified; it will deteriorate no faster in the can than in any other vessel.

It is also possible to sterilize food in bulk and to put it into sterilized cans and glass vessels with aseptic precautions. The advantage of this technique of aseptic filling is that it is not necessary that foods be heated for as long as would be necessary for canning; the result is less damage to their colour and taste.

Irradiation of food by ultraviolet light will kill micro-organisms on the surface of food, but the rays do not penetrate to any depth. The process is therefore useful for such purposes as the prevention of growth of moulds on cakes and other baked products. On the other hand, irradiation with ionizing radiation does penetrate food quite deeply and is thus potentially of great promise. However, its use is confined to specified foods, and only in some countries; the US allows its use in only three or four foods and the UK does not allow it for any. The suggestion that this method is harmful seems unwarranted, however, for all the evidence points to its being safe.

There is widespread belief that all physical methods of food preservation cause significant or even considerable diminution in the nutritional value of the foods. The only method for which this is true is drying, other than freeze-drying. The major loss then is in vitamin C in fruit and vegetables. Very little of this vitamin remains, for example, in dried pulses.

It is unreasonable to compare, for example, the vitamin C content of canned vegetables with that of fresh vegetables. Canned peas are cooked, and need only to be heated before being served. Fresh peas will need to be cooked, and the amount of vitamin C they contain when served will depend on the way the cooking has been done. In practice, when neither the canned peas nor the fresh peas have been overcooked, the amount of vitamin C is very similar. It should be added that so-called processed peas have lost most of their vitamin C before they are put in the can because they have been dried. Quick-frozen foods in particular can have a high nutritional value, since vegetables for example are frozen within a very short time of picking; so-called fresh vegetables bought in the market or in shops tend to be several days from picking, and may have undergone significant loss, again of vitamin C, before they are bought. There is little loss of most of the other nutrients, including protein, mineral salts and other vitamins.

Finally, the comparison of the nutrient content of preserved and fresh foods is often misleading. Many preserved foods are available when fresh foods are not. Even if the preserved food, such as dried peas, has lost a great deal of one or more of its nutrients, its consumption clearly provides more than does the unavailable fresh food.

See also: Food additives; Nitrates/Nitrites

Food rationing

Food is never universally distributed. Even if season and locality have not imposed a shortage of food, some items will be more expensive than others, and thus more readily available to those with higher incomes. Nutritionally, this is of no great importance, so long as those items that are still able to be bought by the least affluent constitute a diet that is adequate both quantitatively and qualitatively.

This, however, becomes unlikely if food supplies diminish so that prices rise; the more nutritious foods such as milk, meat, eggs, fish and fruit, which tend to be the more expensive foods, will then become available only to the relatively wealthy, and the poor will be able to afford only the less nutritious foods such as bread and root vegetables; they may even be limited in the quantities of these foods that they are able to buy.

A well-organized scheme of rationing can prevent this undesirable maldistribution of important foods, or at least can minimize it. In the UK, some foods were rationed during the Second World War and for a few years after it; the most important were meat, milk, cheese, eggs, sugar and fats. In addition, there was a range of other foods from which a choice could be made on the basis of 'points'. In many instances, there was less of a particular food available for distribution; in one or two instances, such as milk, total consumption increased during the period of rationing. In both instances, however, rationing ensured a more uniform distribution of particular foods than had existed previously.

A scheme of rationing is characterized by two features. Firstly, people are issued with documents that allow them to purchase a given amount of rationed foods each week or month. Secondly, the prices of a range of foods are kept at levels to make them more readily available to those with low incomes. Price control can be achieved in a variety of ways, including subsidizing of fertilizer prices to farmers, paying them more than the prices ordinary market forces would ensure, subsidizing food producers, or allowing 'vulnerable groups' to purchase some foods at especially low prices or even to get them free.

With the important proviso that the administration and enforcement of price control and ration documents can be well implemented, the result is that the more affluent people will take less of the more expensive foods, and the least affluent will have more. This redistribution is not always appreciated by the more affluent, who are aware only that their own consumption has been restricted. The fact is that, during the period of rationing in the United Kingdom, many people realized for the first time that there was a section of the population, usually the poor from the city centres, who had previously rarely eaten an egg and whose consumption of milk had been confined to small quantities from a tin of condensed milk.

See also: Drummond

Food spoilage

The plants and animals that provide our food, like all living organisms, begin to deteriorate as soon as they are harvested or slaughtered. It is only exceptional and refined foods that do not deteriorate. These are items such as sugar and oils made by extracting and separating individual chemical constituents of plants and animals.

There are three main processes that may occur in food as it is kept. These are chemical changes, enzymatic changes, and changes caused by micro-organisms. The reason why separated and purified food items are immune from spoilage is that they contain no substances that undergo spontaneous chemical change, nor enzymes, nor sufficient nourishment to sustain the growth and multiplication of micro-organisms.

As an example of chemical change, we may refer to the rancidity occurring with time in fats and oils. The process is partly a hydrolysis (splitting) of the triglycerides into their constituents, glycerol and fatty acids; it is also partly an oxidation.

Rancidity is promoted by increased temperature and by the presence of light, as well as the existence of impurities such as traces of copper and other metals in the oils or fats. Rancidity is thus less likely if these foods have been carefully refined. Polyunsaturated oils are more likely to undergo rancidity than are saturated fats. On the other hand, rancidity is retarded by the presence of vitamin E, a constituent of many vegetable oils.

The most obvious enzymatic changes are those that occur when meat and fish soften on keeping. This process is often desired for meats, which are hung for a few days, or in the case of game, for many days. It depends on the breakdown and even partial liquefaction of the proteins of the tissues through digestion by its own enzymes. This self-digestion is called autolysis. It is not desirable for fish, since it readily produces unpleasant smells and taste.

Micro-organisms grow readily on most foods, except such refined foods as sugar and oils. The spores of many species of bacteria and fungi present in the air can readily germinate on or in many foods, such as meat, fish and milk, as well as in many made-up dishes.

The effects of such micro-organisms on the food depend both on the nature of the infective organism and on the components of the food. Many of the species of bacteria and yeasts that attack sugary liquids such as fruit syrups will cause fermentation and produce chiefly alcohol and carbon dioxide. The micro-organisms that grow best on meat and fish produce chiefly putrefaction, in which unpleasant smells and taste result from the breakdown of the food protein into nitrogen compounds such as ammonia and a variety of amines.

See also: Aflatoxins; Poisons in food

Fructose

Fructose is also known as laevulose, or, as the name suggests, fruit sugar. It occurs, however, only in some fruits, but as it is a component of sucrose, it is produced when this is digested (hydrolysed). This occurs by the action of the appropriate enzyme in the intestine, or by acid or alkali, so that some hydrolysis occurs even in the acid of the stomach. The products of digestion of sucrose are equal amounts of glucose and fructose, a mixture known as invert sugar.

Fructose is about twice as sweet as sucrose. It can therefore be used as a sweetener for slimmers, so saving half the calories. It is also used for diabetics because, unlike glucose, it does not stimulate the immediate release of insulin or require insulin for its metabolism. Until recently, fructose was expensive to produce, but it is now much cheaper because there are methods of making it from glucose, which in turn can be readily produced from starch. Nevertheless, there is increasing concern about its use by diabetic patients, or indeed for non-diabetic individuals, because it increases the concentration of triglyceride in the blood; it may also increase the uric acid in the blood and so precipitate an attack of gout. In the long term, too, it may increase the concentration of insulin in the blood.

There is a rare congenital disease, hereditary fructose intolerance, in which infants develop serious symptoms when sucrose or fruit containing fructose is introduced into the diet. The condition arises because of the inability properly to metabolize fructose, and the consequent interference with the release of glucose from glycogen in the liver. There follows hypoglycaemia, vomiting and failure to thrive, and death may occur. The symptoms cease when sucrose and fructose are eliminated from the diet; as the affected child grows up, he learns to avoid the offending food and can then remain symptom-free. One effect of not taking sucrose, for example, by people with fructose intolerance, is that they do not develop dental decay.

See also: Carbohydrates; Glucose; Invert sugar; Sucrose

Fungi

Fungi are plants that have no chlorophyll and reproduce by spores. They include mushrooms, mildews, moulds and rusts.

Only a few varieties of mushrooms are not safe to eat; it can certainly be assumed that the species that are commercially available are safe. Although there are very many different edible species, few are eaten in Britain; many more are eaten in most other countries in Europe. Mushrooms provide little energy and little protein, and almost nothing of the fat-soluble vitamins. On analysis, they appear relatively rich in nicotinic acid, riboflavin and pantothenic acid; however, in the quantities usually consumed, their contribution to the diet is far more in terms of taste and texture than in terms of nutrients.

Some fungi are important in that they produce powerful toxins. In this connection, the best known are aflatoxin and ergot. Ergot is an infection of rye; the contaminated cereal is eaten only when other foods are scarce. The result is ergotism, otherwise known as St Anthony's Fire. This is characterized by cramps and spasms, or by gangrene of the extremities.

A few fungi are not only not toxic, but are deliberately used in the making of cheeses, such as Stilton, Danish Blue and Gorgonzola. More recently, particular fungi are being grown and harvested commercially as sources of 'single cell protein' for feeding animals or human subjects.

See also: Aflatoxins; Novel protein foods; Poisons in food

Funk, Casimir (1884–1967)

The name vitamin, spelt at first as vitamine, was coined by Casimir Funk in 1912. He was born in Warsaw, studied biology and chemistry in Switzerland, and then went to Paris to work in the Pasteur Institute. In 1906 he moved to Berlin and worked with Emil Fischer, publishing a number of papers on the chemistry and metabolism of protein. He moved to Wiesbaden in 1907, but continued his research in collaboration with Fischer's assistant, Abderhalden (1877–1950).

The next move, in 1910, was to the Lister Institute in London, where research was being conducted on beri-beri. Funk showed that dietary polyneuritis in pigeons, the equivalent of the polyneuritis in chickens produced in Batavia by Eijkman and Grijns, could be prevented by extracts from rice polishings. In 1912, Funk published the work that introduced the term 'vitamine' in a sentence stating 'the deficient substances which are of the nature of organic bases we will call vitamines, which means a substance preventing a special disease'. He postulated that beri-beri, scurvy and pellagra were caused by a

Die Vitamine

ihre Bedeutung für die Physiologie und Pathologie

mit besonderer Berücksichtigung der

Avitaminosen:

(Beriberi, Skorbut, Pellagra, Rachitis)

Anhang:

Die Wachstumsubstanz und das Krebsproblem

Von

Casimir Funk,

Leiter des physiologisch chemischen Laboratoriums
Cancer Hospital Research Institute, London

Mit 38 Abbildungen im Text und 2 Tafeln.

Wiesbaden

Verlag von J. F. Bergmann

1914

dietary deficiency of the appropriate vitamine. His book *Die Vitamine* was published in 1914.

When the First World War began, Funk moved to New York, where he worked until 1923. From there, he moved first to Warsaw, then to Paris; in 1939 he returned to New York, taking mostly appointments in industry until he retired in 1963 at the age of 79. He died in New York four years later.

See also: Beri-beri; Eijkman; Grijns; Vitamin B₁; Vitamin history

G

Galactose

By far the major natural source of galactose is as one of the monosaccharides that, with glucose, makes up the disaccharide lactose (milk sugar). Since some of the complex chemical substances present in the brain and nerve tissues contain small quantities of galactose, it was suggested that lactose was an essential dietary component for infants, and explained the presence of this unusual sugar in what is primarily a food for young animals. However, this attractive hypothesis has not been substantiated.

Galactosaemia is a rare genetic disease affecting some infants, which is the inability to convert galactose to glucose in the ordinary fashion; this results in an accumulation in the blood of galactose and its first metabolic product, galactose phosphate. The effect is a failure of growth, mental retardation, a large liver, and especially cataract of the eyes and blindness.

The diagnosis can be made by testing for galactose in the urine of infants who are not thriving, or even better by routine testing of blood at the time of screening for phenylketonuria. Once the diagnosis is made, treatment consists simply in avoiding milk or any milk-based food that contains lactose. If treatment begins soon enough, there is no chance of any disability arising, although it must be remembered that the genetic defect persists throughout life.

See also: Carbohydrates; Milk; Phenylketonuria

Gall-bladder

The gall-bladder stores and concentrates bile made by the liver. It contracts from time to time so as to pass the concentrated bile through the bile duct into the duodenum, the first part of the small intestine. The contractions of the gall-bladder that perform this function are caused by the stimulus of a hormone, cholecystokinin, which is released into the blood. This happens when the small intestine is stimulated by food reaching it, especially if the food contains fat.

The gall-bladder is commonly the site of disease. The three most common, in decreasing order of frequency, are gallstones (cholelithiasis), gall-bladder inflammation (cholecystitis) and obstructive jaundice. It is said that about 20% of adults have gallstones, although they often produce no symptoms. They are more frequently found in women, and in both men and women who are obese. Most commonly, there are many stones in the gall-bladder; they usually consist largely of cholesterol, with some bile pigments; occasionally, they also contain calcium salts, in which case they can be visualized by X-rays. Rarely, there is just one large stone, made up almost exclusively of cholesterol.

About 50% of people with gallstones have no symptoms. However, when they cause obstruction of the bile duct, the stones give rise either to inflammation of the gall-bladder or to obstructive jaundice. Either of these conditions may be accompanied by severe pain.

The usual treatment of gallstones is surgical removal. There are some physicians, however, who treat the condition by administering the expensive drug chenodeoxycholic acid, although there is still some debate as to its efficacy.

Cholecystitis is accompanied by periods of mild pain, with occasional bouts of more severe pain. It is accompanied by dyspepsia and nausea, and occasionally mild jaundice. Symptoms often follow the consumption of fatty foods. The symptoms may be diminished by the avoidance of such foods, with the apparently paradoxical administration of an occasional fatty meal to facilitate the emptying of the gall-bladder.

Obstruction of the gall-bladder by a stone or by narrowing of the bile duct by scarring or by the growth of a cancer, usually of the pancreas, causes jaundice. Because the bile continues to be produced by the liver, but is prevented from flowing into the intestine, the bile pigments and the bile salts that it contains pile up in the blood. The pigments are responsible for the yellow colour of the skin in jaundice; the high concentration of the bile salts in the blood results in considerable itching of the skin. Moreover, the lack of bile salts in the intestine prevents the proper absorption of the dietary fats and their accompanying fat-soluble vitamins. As a result, there is an excessive amount of fat excreted in the faeces, and perhaps the development of signs of deficiency of vitamins A, D and K. The last especially is important, since it could result in a reduction of the clotting power of the blood and so in excessive and perhaps uncontrollable bleeding. This excessive tendency to bleed is a hazard especially if an operation is being undertaken to remove the biliary obstruction; this hazard is avoided if the operation is preceded by the administration of adequate vitamin K to the patient by injection.

See also: Absorption of fat; Bile; Vitamin K

Gastritis

Acute gastritis is typified by the nausea, pain and vomiting that occur the morning after a rather exuberantly alcoholic night before, or in the small boy who has climbed into an orchard and over-indulged in unripe apples – the so-called green apple sickness. Aspirin, or arsenic provided by an unsophisticated attempted murderer, are other causes of this acute inflammation of the gastric mucosa. The most important treatment, especially if vomiting is persistent, is to ensure an adequate intake of fluid. This can be achieved by fruit juices or by milk; fluids sweetened excessively with sugar may continue to irritate the already inflamed mucosa. If the gastritis and vomiting are severe, it may be necessary to treat the ensuing dehydration by intravenous saline, perhaps containing glucose.

Chronic gastritis results in atrophy (degeneration) of the chronically inflamed mucosa; there is a great diminution in the thickness of the mucosa, and a complete or almost complete disappearance of its gastric glands. Causes are likely to be irregular meals quickly swallowed, continuing consumption of foods that are irritating, alcohol, and frequent use of aspirin. The first essential treatment is the correction of the cause. This is then followed by a diet that is known to cause no symptoms; if this is not known, the diet can be carefully monitored by the patient until he discovers which foods are for him innocuous, and which cause symptoms.

See also: Dyspepsia; Peptic ulcers

Gelatin

The most notable characteristic of gelatin is that it is soluble in hot water, but in sufficient concentration forms a solid jelly when it cools. The Latin word *gelatus* means frozen, and is recalled in the Italian word for ice cream, *gelati*. When its concentration is 2% or more, solutions of gelatin set at ordinary room temperatures of 15°C to 25°C.

Gelatin is a protein, and is formed from collagen, which is the chief protein in connective tissue. Bones, skin and gristly meat are a major source of gelatin; a good example is calf's foot. By itself, gelatin has a low biological value because it contains no tryptophan and little phenylalanine. Commercial jellies with their sugar and flavour make an attractive dessert, but with their 2% of an inferior protein, together with sugar and flavouring, it is unrealistic to suppose that because they are solid they add significantly to the nourishment of a convalescent.

See also: Agar; Biological value of proteins

Ghee

In India, clarified butter, called ghee, is widely used; in the Middle East, it is called samna. It is made from the milk of the cow or buffalo, or more rarely that of the sheep or goat. The process involves heating the butter so that the fat melts and the watery part evaporates. The milk solids that remain are then skimmed off. Because it has little or no water, ghee keeps better than butter does.

The Indians also make vanaspati, a margarine equivalent of ghee; it is produced by hydrogenation of vegetable oils, but with no water.

Gilbert, Joseph Henry (1817–1901)

Gilbert was born in Hull, England, and studied analytical chemistry in Glasgow. Here he lost an eye through an accidental gunshot wound. His first research was at University College, London, where he met Lawes; he then spent some time in Giessen with Liebig. In 1843 he was invited to join Lawes at Rothamsted, to take charge of his Agricultural Research Institute, which was the first such institute to be created anywhere.

There followed nearly 60 years of close collaboration, during which he and Lawes published some 130 research papers. These were concerned mostly with the use of chemical fertilizers for crops, and the effects of different constituents of feed on the growth of farm animals and on the composition of the carcase.

THE ROTHAMSTED EXPERIMENTS;

BEING AN ACCOUNT OF SOME OF THE

RESULTS OF THE AGRICULTURAL INVESTIGATIONS CONDUCTED AT ROTHAMSTED,

IN THE FIELD, THE FEEDING SHED, AND THE LABORATORY

OVER A PERIOD OF FIFTY YEARS.

BY

SIR JOHN BENNET LAWES, BART.

D.C.L., Sc.D., F.R.S.

AND

SIR J. HENRY GILBERT

LL.D., Sc.D., F.R.S.

From the
'Transactions of the Highland and Agricultural Society of Scotland'
Fifth Series, Vol. VII., 1895

Printed by

WILLIAM BLACKWOOD AND SONS

EDINBURGH AND LONDON

MDCCCXCV

Their partnership was close and cordial, and the death of Lawes in 1900 affected Gilbert greatly; he died in December 1901.

See also: Lawes; Liebig

Glisson, Francis (1597–1677)

Francis Glisson was born in Dorset in England and studied medicine in Cambridge, where he was appointed Regius Professor of Physic in 1636. He took part in the meetings that led to the formation of the Royal Society in 1660, and was one of the founding Fellows. He lived and practised medicine in Colchester and London for much of the time, and died in London having held the Regius Professorship for 41 years.

He had for several years made notes on his observations on rickets, mostly in Dorset children, and discussed them with colleagues at meetings of the Royal College of Physicians. These observations formed the basis of his *De rachitide sive morbo puerili, qui vulgo The Rickets dicitur* ('On rickets or the disease of children colloquially known as The Rickets'). The first edition appeared in 1650 and an English translation in 1651. His anatomical and clinical descriptions of the disease were precise, and have hardly been improved to this day. The book has been called 'one of the glories of British medicine'.

It has been suggested that the material on rickets published by Daniel Whistler in 1645 was based mostly on the observations of Glisson and his colleagues, rather than on original observations by Whistler himself.

Glisson is also known for his work on the normal and the diseased liver. It was he who first described the fibrous sheath still called Glisson's capsule.

See also: Rickets; Whistler

Glucose

Glucose, also known as dextrose, is a sugar – more specifically, a monosaccharide – found in a few foods, grapes and honey being the best known. The word 'glucose' is sometimes used commercially to refer not to the one monosaccharide glucose, but to the mixture of

DE
RACHITIDE
SIVE
MORBO PUERILI,

qui vulgo

The Rickets dicitur,

Tractatus;

Operâ primò ac potissimùm

FRANCISCI GLISSONII

Doctoris & publici Professoris Medi-
cinæ in almâ *Cantabrigiæ* Academiâ,
& Socii Collegii Medicorum
Londinensium, conscriptus :

Adscitis in operis societatem

GEORGIO BATE,
&
AHASUERO REGEMORTERO·

*Medicinæ quoque Doctoribus, & pariter Sociis
Collegii Medicorum* Londinensium.

LONDINI,

Typis *Guil. Du-gardi*; Impensis *Laurentii Sadler*, &
Roberti Beaumont : apud quos veneunt in vico
vulgò-vocato Little Britain 1650.

carbohydrates produced by the digestion of starch by acids or by enzymes. It consists then of the range of substances produced by the breaking down of the large starch molecules; they include dextrins, which are still quite large molecules, through smaller molecules consisting perhaps of three or four glucose units, then maltose with its two glucose units, and finally glucose itself; the glucose constitutes perhaps 25% of the total carbohydrate in the mixture. Often, this commercial glucose is left in the form of a syrup and is not crystallized. It is variously called glucose syrup, or corn syrup, or liquid glucose. Food manufacturers then use the word 'dextrose' when they refer to the sugar itself.

Commercial glucose is not as sweet as when the starch is hydrolysed completely to glucose, because the other components in the mixture are less sweet than glucose.

A major use of glucose syrup is in making sugar confectionery such as boiled sweets, because it prevents crystallization occurring when the sweets are cooled.

Glucose in the body arises chiefly from digested starch, and digested disaccharides such as maltose, lactose and sucrose. Some is also formed from the amino-acids from protein, and a little from fats. The glucose makes up a great part of the material used by the body as a source of energy.

The body has an elaborate system by which it tends to keep constant the concentration of glucose in the blood, which is often referred to as the blood sugar. After a meal, there is a rise in glucose concentration. This leads to an increase in the amount of the hormone insulin put into the blood from the pancreas, which reduces the amount of the glucose in the blood. This it does partly by increasing the amount oxidized, and partly by building the glucose up into a large molecule, glycogen. Glycogen, like starch, is formed by the joining together of many glucose molecules, and it is then stored either in the liver or in the muscles. Between meals, and especially during physical activity, glucose is being used up, but the amount in the blood is then restored by being released from the glycogen stored; this is controlled chiefly by another hormone, glucagon.

Since glucose is the major fuel in the body, it is commonly supposed that the consumption of glucose is a particularly useful way of supplying the body with energy. The only possible advantage of glucose over other foods might be in the assumed rapid absorption of ingested glucose. But many other carbohydrates release glucose quite rapidly during digestion in the alimentary canal, so that the difference in the rate of absorption is small. In severe exercise of long duration, it may nevertheless be worthwhile to take advantage of the somewhat more rapid absorption of glucose.

In starvation, or in conditions such as prolonged unconsciousness, or where ordinary feeding is impossible, intravenous solutions of glucose can provide adequate energy for some days. If more prolonged feeding is necessary, amino-acids, salts and vitamins can be added.

See also: Carbohydrates; Glucose tolerance; Glycogen; Hypoglycaemia

Glucose tolerance

When glucose is taken by mouth, it causes a temporary rise in the concentration of glucose in the blood. If the conditions in which this is done are standardized, so that 50g or 100g are taken before breakfast, and the concentration measured at intervals of 15 minutes or 30 minutes for $2\frac{1}{2}$ or 3 hours, it is possible to measure what is called glucose tolerance. In normal individuals, the concentration of glucose begins at about 80mg/100ml blood, rises to about 150mg, and returns to the 'fasting' concentration of 80mg or so within 2 hours. Abnormal values are seen in diabetes and hypoglycaemia. In diabetes, the initial concentration is likely to be significantly above 80mg/100ml, the maximum higher than 180mg/100ml, and the time when it returns to the fasting level more than 2 hours. When the glucose concentration exceeds about 180mg/100ml, some spills over into the urine (glycosuria).

See also: Diabetes; Hypoglycaemia

Gluten

Gluten is a mixture of two proteins, gliadin and glutenin. It is the presence of gluten in wheat and rye that makes these cereals suitable for the production of bread. When mixed with water and kneaded, the gluten in wheat or rye flour becomes elastic and traps small bubbles of carbon dioxide from yeast fermentation. The flour of other cereals, such as oats or maize, with little or no gluten, can be used only for flat cakes such as oat-cakes or tortillas.

Children with coeliac disease, and some adults with a similar disease known as sprue, have a sensitivity to gluten which causes damage to the intestinal villi so that they are unable properly to digest and absorb some of the food components, especially fat. It has been suggested that several other unrelated diseases, including schizophrenia, may at least in some patients be caused by a sensitivity to gluten, but the evidence for these claims is not conclusive. Again, it has been said that people with multiple sclerosis improve on gluten-free diets if they are also given linoleic acid; this too has not been substantiated.

Nevertheless, it does seem as if some babies without obvious coeliac disease are sensitive to gluten although they lose this sensitivity gradually through their first few months or years. For this reason, many manufacturers of baby foods avoid using gluten-containing items in their products.

See also: Absorption; Absorption of fat; Coeliac disease

Glycogen

Like starch, glycogen is a large molecule made up of glucose units; it is indeed sometimes called animal starch, recalling that its main function is as a store of energy for the organism. Most of it is held in the liver and the muscle cells, the total quantity in the adult body being somewhat less than 1kg. Strenuous or prolonged exercise can considerably deplete the glycogen stores, for example a quick walk for 2–3 hours. Because of this, some diets for athletes attempt to increase the glycogen stores before an event such as long-distance running.

When the body is physically active, the glycogen in the muscles releases energy by being converted first to lactic acid, which occurs without the intervention of oxidation; this is anaerobic metabolism. Later, more energy is produced by oxidizing part of the lactic acid, so that the rest is converted back to glycogen. This uptake of oxygen after exercise has ceased is the so-called oxygen debt, and accounts for the noticeably high rate and depth of breathing that continues after strenuous exertion.

The liver is the main organ that keeps the concentration of the blood glucose constant, by storing glucose as glycogen or releasing glucose from the glycogen. The glucose from which the glycogen is synthesized is derived mostly from the carbohydrate in the diet, but about two-thirds of the dietary protein and 10% of the dietary fat, namely the glycerol of the triglycerides, is also converted to glucose.

See also: Bernard; Energy; Glucose; Insulin

Goats' milk

There seems to have been an increase in the use of goats' milk for infants who are not being breastfed. The reason given by the parents is that cows' milk is more likely than goats' milk to cause allergic reactions; this does not seem to be so.

There is little difference between goats' milk and cows' milk in the amounts of protein and carbohydrate they contain. On the other hand, goats' milk contains about one-third more fat. It also has very little folic acid, so that anaemia may develop in infants fed on nothing but goats' milk. A more important hazard is that of infection if goats' milk is not boiled, because rarely if ever is pasteurization carried out.

See also: Allergy; Milk

Goldberger, Joseph (1881–1929)

More than any other person, Joseph Goldberger was responsible for the demonstration that pellagra is caused by a deficiency of a vitamin. At the age of 7, he was taken by his parents to New York from the small mid-European town where he was born. As a youth, he studied civil engineering and then medicine. Two years later, he joined the US Public Health Service.

Goldberger was involved in the study of several infectious diseases, including two to which he himself fell victim – yellow fever and typhus. In 1914 he was invited to join an expert commission to study pellagra, which at that time was rife, especially in the southern United States. There were then some 100,000 cases a year and some 10,000 deaths. The commission had recently reported that it was 'an intestinal infection, transmitted by contaminated food', supporting the common opinion of the medical profession. In his first report, published after three months, Goldberger wrote that he thought the disease was due to a dietary deficiency rather than an infection. He demonstrated that the disease occurred with diets lacking in meat, milk and eggs, that it was cured when these foods were added, and that pellagra was not transmitted by contagion. The dietary component that prevented pellagra was shown to be present in a watery extract of liver and yeast. Goldberger gave it the name of pellagra-preventing (P-P) factor.

He died in 1929, so that he did not live to see the identification by Elvejhem in 1937 of the P-P factor as nicotinic acid.

See also: Nicotinic acid; Pellagra

Gout

One of the several kinds of arthritis is gout, which affects chiefly the small joints of the fingers and especially the toes. The joints become inflamed and swollen, and the pain may become quite excruciating. There have been many cartoons illustrating the bad-tempered gentleman lying with his big toe bandaged and obviously in considerable pain. Usually the attacks last a few days and then subside; thereafter, they may recur at shorter and shorter intervals. The disease occurs mostly in middle age and is ten times more common in men than in women, who tend to have the disease after the menopause. In this and in its tendency to be commoner in overweight people, gout resembles coronary disease, with which incidentally it is linked in that both diseases tend to occur in the same person. There is a slight but distinct hereditary element in the chances that a person will develop gout. Attacks of gout have for generations been associated with the good life; the victim tends to eat too much, eat too much meat, and partake excessively of alcohol.

The most characteristic feature of gout is that it is usually accompanied by an increase in the amount of uric acid in the blood. The normal concentration of uric acid is about 4mg/100ml. In gout, it is about 7mg/100ml. Urates, i.e. salts of uric acid, are sometimes but not always found in the affected joint; occasionally these deposits can be seen as small raised areas, tophi, under the skin over the finger joints or on the ear. Another result of the excessive uric acid in the blood is that it increases the risk of uric acid stones forming in the urinary tract.

Uric acid is the end product of the body's metabolism of substances called purines. These are compounds that form part of the RNA and DNA of the nuclei of the body's cells. Not all purines, however, are converted into uric acid in the body; the caffeine in tea and coffee, and

DEADLY ADULTERATION

AND

SLOW POISONING;

OR,

DISEASE AND DEATH

In the Pot and the Bottle;

IN WHICH

THE BLOOD-EMPOISONING AND LIFE-DESTROYING ADULTERATIONS

OF

WINES, SPIRITS, BEER, BREAD, FLOUR, TEA, SUGAR, SPICES, CHEESEMONGERY
PASTRY, CONFECTIONARY, MEDICINES, &c. &c. &c.

ARE LAID OPEN TO THE PUBLIC,

WITH

TESTS OR METHODS

FOR ASCERTAINING AND DETECTING THE
FRAUDULENT AND DELETERIOUS ADULTERATIONS
AND THE GOOD AND BAD QUALITIES
OF THOSE ARTICLES:

With an Exposé of Medical Empiricism and Imposture, Quacks and
Quackery, Regular and Irregular, Legitimate and Illegitimate ; and
The Frauds and Mal-practices of Pawnbrokers and Madhouse keepers.

BY AN ENEMY OF FRAUD AND VILLANY.

" The Workshop of the Distillery [and of the Wine and Spirit Compounder] is the Elaboratory of Disease and of Premature Death."—*Manual for Invalids.*

Devoted to disease by baker, butcher, grocer, wine-merchant, spirit-dealer, cheesemonger, pastry-cook, and confectioner; the physician is called to our assistance; but here again the pernicious system of fraud, as it has given the blow, steps in to defeat the remedy :—the unprincipled dealers in drugs and medicines exert the most diabolical ingenuity in sophisticating the most potent and necessary drugs, (viz. peruvian bark, rhubarb, ipecacuanha, magnesia, calomel, castor-oil, spirits of hartshorn, and almost every other medical commodity in general demand;) and chemical preparations used in pharmacy.
Literary Gazette.

LONDON:

PUBLISHED BY SHERWOOD, GILBERT AND PIPER,
23, PATERNOSTER ROW.

See Food Additives

theobromine in cocoa and chocolate, are purines that do not produce uric acid. Since the purines that do produce uric acid are found chiefly in cells, especially animal cells, the purine-rich foods are liver, kidney, sweetbreads and fish roes, because these have an unusually high proportion of cells.

The treatment of gout has traditionally been through diet; however, there are now drugs that either reduce the inflammatory response in the joints, or increase the excretion of uric acid in the urine. Nevertheless, dietary measures are still useful for patients who are sensitive to the drugs, or who have a general reluctance to take drugs if they can be avoided, or for those who believe that the dietary recommendations are likely to be of general benefit. The aims of these recommendations, then, are to reduce overweight if present, to reduce alcohol intake, to avoid purine-rich foods, and to drink freely of non-alcoholic drinks so as to reduce the risk of the formation of kidney stones.

See also: Arthritis

Grijns, Gerrit (1865–1944)

Grijns was born in Leerdam, Netherlands, and studied medicine in Utrecht. His first post was as a military surgeon in Batavia, Dutch East Indies (now Indonesia). Here he met Eijkman, who was at the time with the commission sent by the Netherlands government to study beri-beri. When the commission returned home, Eijkman and Grijns remained to continue their research studies. By then, their work with chickens convinced them that beri-beri was not caused by an infection, which was the view commonly held. Eijkman became convinced that the disease was due to a toxin in polished rice, and that the pericarp of the rice, which was removed in polishing, contained an antidote to this toxin. Grijns did not accept this view, and showed that polyneuritis in chickens did not occur with a meat diet, but did occur if the meat had been heated for a long time.

Grijns's work ended in 1900 and the results were published in Dutch in 1901. After a few years back in Europe, Grijns returned to Batavia and worked as a sub-director and then director of a rather primitive laboratory for bacteriology and pathological anatomy. In 1917 he went back to the Netherlands, where he continued his scientific work until he retired in 1935.

See also: Beri-beri; Eijkman; Vitamin B₁; Vitamin history

Groundnuts

The alternative names for these are monkey-nuts, earthnuts or pea-nuts. The last name helps us to remember that the product is a pulse, that is, it is related to peas, beans and lentils. Thus, as a member of the Leguminosae, it does not properly fall into the botanists' classification of nuts. The names groundnut and earthnut recall the unusual grow-ing habit; after fertilization, the flower stalks bend down so that their continuing growth pushes the ripening seedpods into the ground. The ripened pods then have to be harvested by digging them out of the soil.

The groundnut originated in Brazil, but it is now grown widely and in great quantities in many tropical countries. The amounts consumed as such are not considerable; they are eaten mostly as a snack, or in sweetmeats, or as peanut butter, made by crushing the nuts and adding salt and sometimes sugar. Nevertheless, in some tropical coun-tries, they are included in soups and in stews and so contribute signifi-cantly to protein intake. Mostly, groundnuts are processed for their oil, about 40% of their content. The oil is widely used for the manu-facture of margarine, and also in the home for cooking. Groundnut cake makes a good animal feed.

See also: Aflotoxins; Oils

Guar gum

Because it is not absorbed in the gut, guar gum has become more interesting with the increased interest in dietary fibre. It is produced from the seeds of a leguminous plant grown in the Indian sub-conti-nent, and also in the south-west of the USA. In small quantities, it has been used for a long time as a stabilizer.

Larger quantities of guar gum are sometimes used as a laxative. In these quantities, it has also been shown to act as an anorectic agent, and has been suggested as an aid to weight reduction.

See also: Fibre; Food additives; Obesity

Guava

Although consumed only in small amounts, mostly after canning, guava is noteworthy as a fruit with a high content of vitamin C. An average value is about 200mg/100g, which is three or four times as much as orange juice and matched or exceeded by very few fruits, notably the blackcurrant (200mg) and the West Indian cherry (850mg).

The guava tree, which grows to about 30 feet, is a native of the Caribbean but is now grown in many tropical countries. The fruit is the size of a small apple, bright yellow in colour with a soft juicy pulp containing many seeds.

H

Health foods

There are several sorts of the foods that some people consider health foods. They are claimed to be more wholesome than many of the conventional foods, in that they contain no harmful additives or contaminants; to have a higher nutritional value than the equivalent conventional foods, and to have positive and specific properties that increase the degree of health. Most if not all of these foods are referred to as 'natural foods'.

One category is foods grown without inorganic fertilizers (sometimes called chemical fertilizers) and without the use of herbicides or pesticides, then prepared without the addition of chemical preservatives. This category can be extended to include food from animals that have not been treated with hormones or antibiotics, and not confined indoors or in cages. Eggs from poultry reared in this way, or milk from cows similarly reared, are also sometimes considered to be health foods.

Another category of health foods includes those believed to carry some unique property that increases resistance to disease, or helps to cure common diseases, or simply improves health and so acts as a 'tonic'. Examples are yoghurt, royal jelly, the alga spirulina, and honey.

Finally, health food stores also supply a range of tablets, powders and solutions that contain extracts of herbs, or provide concentrated vitamins and mineral salts in a wide range of potencies.

The evidence that such foods are less harmful than conventional foods, or more beneficial, varies. Thus, no difference has been demonstrated in the nutritional value of crops grown with chemical fertilizers or organic fertilizers, that is, animal dung. Somewhat greater quantities of vitamin B_{12} are present in eggs from free-range hens than in those from battery hens. There are good regulations governing the use of pesticides, weed killers and preservatives, but hazards may exist if the regulations are not adhered to.

Apart from anecdotes that cannot be tested, there is no evidence that honey or any other of the special foods have properties not found in ordinary foods.

The advantages and disadvantages of vitamin supplements, protein supplements, preservatives and other additives are considered elsewhere.

See also: Cider vinegar; Honey; Tonic

Herbs and spices

The use of herbs and spices to impart flavour to foods is universal and has a long history. Spices consist of the whole or part of the seeds, bark, flowers or fruits of plants grown mostly in tropical countries; herbs are usually the leafy parts of plants grown in temperate climates. The flavour of these materials resides in the essential oils they contain.

Herbs were widely grown in British gardens in medieval times. They were used mostly as a means of imparting flavours to foods, but many were considered also to have important therapeutic properties for a variety of diseases; these were described in the various 'herbals' that have been written over several centuries. In addition, there has always been a high demand for spices in temperate climates, shown by the important and lucrative trade in spices brought to Europe from the countries of the east.

The direct nutritional value of herbs and spices is small, since they are used in such small quantities. Only one or two can contribute significant, but still small, amounts of nutrients: chillies are rich in ascorbic acid, and curry is rich in iron, but it is unlikely that they would contribute more than a milligram or two of these nutrients a day. Nevertheless, herbs and spices do have an indirect nutritional value. The starchy foods that constitute a large part of the diet of poor people tend to be low in flavour. Since such people do not have easy access to more expensive foods, such as meat or fish or eggs, that would increase the palatability of their diets, they add instead the available herbs and spices without which their diets would be exceedingly unattractive. It has been suggested, then, that the low total food intake of the poorest people would be even lower if they were not able to increase the palatability of their foods by the addition of herbs and spices to the bread or rice or maize that constitutes the major part of what they have to eat.

As well as imparting flavour to foods, spices and herbs have additional properties. One is that many of them have a preservative action, because they kill bacteria or at least prevent their growth. That is, they are bactericidal or bacteriostatic. Another property is that they may conceal the unpleasant taste of foods that have begun to deteriorate; this happens more readily in hot climates and may account for the more common use of spices with 'hotter' and stronger tastes in those areas.

These properties of spices, and particularly the property of adding palatability to otherwise insipid foods, have made spices highly sought after and occasionally very valuable. Pepper was used as currency in ancient Greece and Rome, and this continued for 1,500 years or more. During the middle ages, peppercorns were often literally worth their weight in gold. Although rent of a single peppercorn was indeed only nominal, rent was in fact often paid in peppercorns.

Some common herbs: balm, basil, borage, chives, fennel, garlic, horseradish, marjoram, parsley, rosemary, sage, thyme.

Some common spices: capsicum, chillies, cinnamon, cardamom, cloves, coriander, cumin, ginger, nutmeg, pepper, pimento, turmeric, vanilla.

See also: Appetite

Honey

Honey from wild bees has been known since prehistoric times, long before the introduction of bee-keeping, which probably began about 3000 BC. Honey was prized partly because of its high palatability, partly because of its rarity because the yields were so small, but chiefly because of its supposed contribution to health and well-being. It is praised not only in the Bible, but also in ancient Egyptian, Babylonian and other writings, and it was widely used in religious rites. It has always been endowed with unique properties: as an aphrodisiac, for the prolongation of youth, for the treatment of a variety of ills, and for the general restoration and maintenance of health. Even now, literature available in health food stores claims that it cures, or helps to cure, bronchitis, sore throat, anaemia, peptic ulcers and other digestive complaints, and kidney disease, as well as being a laxative and a diuretic.

Sadly, none of these qualities has been demonstrated in strictly controlled conditions, although there are still many people who firmly believe that they exist.

Bees make honey from the nectar of flowers, the chief constituent of which is sucrose; in addition, there are colours and flavours that vary according to the flowers from which bees have collected the nectar. In the production of the honey from nectar, much of the sucrose is converted to invert sugar. Apart from its water, honey is thus almost entirely a mixture of fructose and glucose, with a little unhydrolysed sucrose; less than 1% consists of mineral salts, protein, vitamins and other organic materials. The vitamin in the highest concentration is riboflavin, but even this is present in such a small quantity that one would need to eat 25kg of honey in order to provide the body with a day's requirement. Apart from these tiny amounts of salts, protein and vitamins, no other biologically active material has been found in honey.

See also: Health foods; Invert sugar; Sucrose

Hopkins, Frederick Gowland (1861–1947)

The contributions of Hopkins to biochemistry and to nutrition were many and far-reaching. Born in Eastbourne, on the south coast of England, he was fascinated with what could be seen through his father's microscope, and also took an interest in chemistry; otherwise, he was not at all outstanding in his school subjects.

After working briefly in an insurance office and with an analyst in the City of London, he took a degree in chemistry. Later, at the age of 33, he qualified in medicine. While still a student, he published a method for the assay of uric acid in urine. In 1898, at the age of 37, he went to Cambridge University as lecturer in chemical physiology.

Soon after he arrived in Cambridge, Hopkins isolated the amino-acid tryptophan from protein, and followed this by the demonstration that some of the amino-acids, including tryptophan, were dietary essentials. In 1906, in a very brief article, Hopkins mentioned his work that would lead to the discovery of vitamins. He showed that rats do not survive on a diet consisting of only protein, fat, carbohydrate and mineral salts, but do survive if small quantities of milk are added to the diet. The full paper describing this work was not published until 1912.

His other pioneer work in the biochemical field included the chemical changes occurring when muscles contract, and the mechanism by which the tissues carry out oxidation.

A new biochemical laboratory was built in Cambridge in 1924, with Hopkins as Professor of Biochemistry, which soon became probably the foremost in the world. Here he was surrounded by a group of scientists from many countries, of whom a large number became distinguished heads of departments of biochemistry around the world. All who worked with him were not only impressed by him, but came to love the small, modest and ever-helpful 'Hoppy'.

In 1929 he was awarded the Nobel Prize jointly with Eijkman, for their work leading to the discovery of the vitamins. He died in Cambridge in 1947.

See also: Eijkman; Vitamin history

Hormones

The co-ordination of the multifarious activities of the body is carried out by two systems of communication; they may be compared to communication between people by telephone and by radio. The first is the nervous system, through which messages are carried from one part of the body to another by conduction through nerves, just as telephonic messages are carried by conduction through wires. The body's second method of communication is by hormones, which are chemical substances put directly into the bloodstream by special organs. Although the 'messages' they carry now proceed to all parts of the body, they evoke a reaction only in those organs or tissues designed to receive them, just as radio messages are broadcast in all directions but are picked up only by apparatus tuned to do so.

Hormones are also called endocrines, or internal secretions. This refers to the fact that the organs or tissues that produce these secretions put them directly into the blood.

Most of the hormones are produced by special glands called the endocrine glands; some are produced by specialized cells distributed widely in an organ that has another quite different function.

The major endocrine glands are the thyroid, parathyroid, pituitary and adrenals. These endocrine glands may be contrasted with the exocrine glands, the secretions of which are passed along ducts to their destination. An example of an endocrine gland is the thyroid gland, which produces the hormone thyroxin. An example of an exocrine gland is a salivary gland which makes saliva and passes it along a salivary duct into the mouth.

There is one gland that has both endocrine and exocrine secretions. This is the pancreas, which has two quite different collections of cells.

Most of the cells produce pancreatic juice, which contains enzymes for digesting starch, protein and fat; this juice is delivered to the duodenum, the first part of the small intestine, through a duct that joins the bile duct as it enters the duodenum. In addition to these cells producing the digestive juice, there are clusters of quite different cells dotted throughout the pancreas. These islets of cells secrete a special hormone; it is easy to see how the hormone made by the islets derived its name, insulin.

In a sense, the testis and the ovary may also be considered as both exocrine and endocrine organs. On the one hand, they produce external secretions – containing the spermatozoa and the ova – that are delivered to their appropriate destinations by ducts; on the other hand, they produce the sex hormones, especially testosterone in the male and oestradiol and progesterone in the female.

See also: Adrenal glands; Insulin; Thyroid gland

Hydrolysis

The origin of the word indicates a loosening or separating by means of water. Many components of food and chemical compounds in the body are large molecules made up of smaller units linked together. When these are separated, the chemical action involved is a combination of the large molecule with molecules of water. An example is the hydrolysis that occurs when sucrose is digested. Chemically, this can be written most simply in this form

$$C_{12}H_{22}O_{11} + H_2O \longrightarrow C_6H_{12}O_6 + C_6H_{12}O_6$$
$$\text{sucrose} \quad \text{water} \quad \text{glucose} \quad \text{fructose}$$

In this instance, it might be added that although glucose and fructose have the same number of the same atoms, they are arranged differently in their molecules and so make up monosaccharides with different properties.

The digestion of much larger molecules than sucrose involves the use of large numbers of water molecules. This happens with hydrolysed protein, the result of a protein being broken down into its constituent amino-acids. A product commonly used in food manufacture is hydrolysed vegetable protein (HVP), which is put into various mixtures by manufacturers because it has a savoury taste somewhat like that of meat gravy.

See also: Amino-acids; Carbohydrates; Digestive juices; Invert sugar

Hyperplasia

An increase in the size of an organ because of an increase in the number of its cells. Examples of hyperplasia are the growth of the uterus and breasts during pregnancy. Apart from these examples, cell division is rare; if other healthy organs increase in size, it is usually because of an increase in size of each of the cells (hypertrophy).

Hypertrophy

The increase in size of an organ, such as a muscle because of exercise, is known as hypertrophy. It is caused by an enlargement of each of the cells of the organ, and not by an increase in the number of cells; the latter is called hyperplasia. The converse of hypertrophy is atrophy, in which an organ shrinks in size, often because of disease.

Hypoglycaemia

When the concentration of glucose in the blood falls considerably below its normal value of about 80mg/100ml, symptoms occur. The symptoms may also occur if the concentration of glucose falls extremely rapidly, even if it does not reach a particularly low value.

The people most likely to have an attack of hypoglycaemia are diabetics, who have injected their insulin, or taken their anti-diabetic drug by mouth, and have not followed it with their accustomed meal. It can also happen to some non-diabetic individuals who have taken some carbohydrate-rich food or drink, especially as sucrose or glucose; this can occur especially if the individual had previously not eaten for an unusually long time, or had been physically very active. Alcohol can also produce a reduction in blood glucose, enough to result sometimes in symptoms of hypoglycaemia.

The most likely time for hypoglycaemia to occur is about 2 hours after taking the appropriate food or drink. Immediately after ingestion, the glucose concentration of the blood normally rises, reaches a peak in about 45 minutes or an hour, and then returns to its previous level. There is, however, a tendency for it to fall to below this for a short time, before reverting to normal, and this excessive fall is most likely to occur if the original rise is rapid.

The symptoms of hypoglycaemia are a feeling of weakness, hunger, sweating, unsteadiness in walking and some mental confusion. People with such an attack have been known to have been accused of drunkenness. If the glucose concentration falls excessively, unconsciousness may occur and this is known as hypoglycaemic coma.

Some people believe erroneously that they suffer from hypoglycaemia; this is especially common in the US. However, unless this has been demonstrated by a glucose tolerance test, the diagnosis must be considered dubious. Symptoms of weakness and tiredness, even to the point of feeling quite exhausted, may be due to a variety of causes, both physical and psychological.

For someone who really does suffer from bouts of demonstrable hypoglycaemia, it may be necessary to make sure that it is not due to some rare condition, such as a tumour of the pancreas that produces an excessive amount of insulin. This would result in the gradual onset of hypoglycaemic attacks of increasing frequency in a previously normal person. For others, who develop hypoglycaemia occasionally in the circumstances described earlier, attacks are best prevented by avoiding foods or drinks containing mostly carbohydrate, especially if this is sugar. In particular, sugar-containing drinks or confectionery or alcohol on an empty stomach should be avoided. Meals should be taken at regular times, with no long intervals between them. A lump of sugar or a sugary drink taken during an attack will certainly relieve the symptoms very rapidly, but it may be laying the foundations for a further attack an hour or two later.

See also: Glucose; Glucose tolerance

I

Ice cream

Ice cream – presumably commercial ice cream – has been described as 'one of the triumphs of food technology'. It consists of a mixture of fat, the non-fat solids of milk, and sugar, together with emulsifiers, stabilizers, flavourings and colour; water amounts to about 60% of the weight of the finished product. Before it is frozen, the mixture is pasteurized and homogenized.

An additional and essential component of ice cream is air; ice cream has also been described as 'the only food product in which air is the principal ingredient'. The air in the ice cream makes up half or more of its volume; as a textbook for budding food scientists comments: 'As ice cream is sold by volume, this latter point is not unimportant!'

The air produces a fine foam, while the fat and the water combine as an oil-in-water emulsion. The emulsifiers and stabilizers, usually including gelatin, prevent the separation of the oil and the collapse of the tiny air bubbles constituting the foam. They also prevent the formation of large ice crystals, which would spoil the creamy smooth texture of the final product.

In the USA, the fat in a product sold as ice cream must consist of butter fat. In the UK, ice cream frequently contains vegetable fat, which may or may not be hydrogenated; only if the fat is butter fat may the product be called dairy ice cream.

See also: Emulsifiers and stabilizers

Infection

A disease caused by the invasion of the body by microbes, which remain there and multiply. The simple existence of microbes on the surface of the body, or in the alimentary canal, that do not enter into the body's tissues and so cause no ill effects, is not an infection.

Infestation

A disease caused by insects, ticks, mites or worms (helminths) that grow and multiply on the skin, in the intestine, or in the internal tissues of the body.

Inflammation

The reaction of the body to injury or irritation. It can therefore result from a kick on the shins, a burn from a hot iron, an infection, or from the constant rubbing of the big toe from wearing a pair of tight shoes. The inflammation of an organ is designated by the ending '-itis'; thus appendicitis, conjunctivitis, pancreatitis.

The four main characteristics were described nearly 2,000 years ago by the Roman medical writer, Celsus; they are redness, swelling, heat and pain – or, as every medical student is taught, *rubor, tumor, calor et dolor*. Inflammation serves the double purpose of protecting and healing, seen most clearly in a localized infection. The initial damage to the tissue releases a substance, probably histamine, that causes dilatation of the local small blood vessels. This accounts for the redness and heat. The dilatation of the capillaries allows a more rapid outflow of fluid into the tissues, and also a leaking of some of the plasma protein and some white blood cells, leucocytes, that normally cannot pass through the capillary walls. As a result, there is localized swelling. Because of this, pain arises, from pressure on the nerve endings and perhaps from irritation due to the release of irritant substances coming either from the materials causing the inflammation, or from the inflammation itself.

The white cells help in a protective role, acting as phagocytes, engulfing the offending micro-organisms or pieces of damaged tissue. If the damage or infection is slight, healing occurs quickly, first by the clotting of the released fluid, and later by the growth of new tissue. This at first is fibrous scar tissue, but if the damage is not extensive, the scar tissue will gradually be replaced by the normal tissue of the damaged part. Muscle and nerve cells, however, cannot be replaced, so that the fibrous tissue remains.

Healing may be prolonged if, for example, the infection persists, in which case pus may form. This consists of disintegrating tissue cells, perhaps with micro-organisms and exudate from the blood vessels. The pus may become surrounded by fibrous tissue, forming an abscess;

if this breaks through the skin or the mucous membrane of the stomach or intestine, an ulcer results.

These localized effects of inflammation may be accompanied by general effects. They include an increased body temperature and perhaps headache and vomiting; there is also an increase in the number of white cells circulating in the bloodstream (leucocytosis).

Inflammation may be acute or chronic. In acute inflammation, the onset occurs rapidly and progresses rapidly, and the increased number of white blood cells both locally and in the bloodstream consists mostly of granulocytes. Examples are appendicitis, pneumonia, and a boil on the neck. In chronic inflammation, the onset and progress are slower, the more numerous white cells are mostly lymphocytes, and the local centres of infection become more fibrous, the central tissue often dying and leaving cavities. Examples are leprosy and pulmonary tuberculosis.

See also: Lymphatic system

Inositol

Chemically an alcohol, inositol appears in the diet mostly as inositol hexaphosphate, otherwise known as phytic acid. Most bacteria and other micro-organisms cannot grow without inositol. Some animals need it too; for example, mice lose their fur if it is not included in their diet. It is not, however, required by human beings. Inositol is thus a vitamin for some species of living creatures, but not for man.

See also: Phytic acid; Vitamins

Insulin

In the body, the hormone insulin is produced by special groups of cells in the pancreas; these cells lie together in what are called the islets of Langerhans. It was the Latin for island, *insula*, which suggested insulin as the name for the hormone.

The actions of insulin are numerous, and affect profoundly the metabolism of the body's carbohydrates, fats and protein. Insulin is best known for its relationship with the disease diabetes, a disease that is now common and becoming commoner in affluent countries. It is caused either by the secretion of too little insulin from the pancreas, or by the resistance of the body's cells to the action of the hormone.

The most obvious action of insulin is in converting glucose from the blood into glycogen, which is then stored in the liver and the muscle cells. It also converts some of the glucose into fat for storage, and stimulates the synthesis of protein. In diabetes, glucose accumulates in the blood and some spills over into the urine.

Insulin is ineffective by mouth, since as a protein it is digested in the alimentary canal. It is therefore taken by diabetics by injection. If an excessive amount of insulin is injected, the effect is an excessive lowering of the glucose concentration in the blood; this is the condition known as hypoglycaemia.

Insulin is one of the smallest protein molecules known. Its composition has been determined, and it has been synthesized in the laboratory. This, however, has as yet no practical bearing on supplies of insulin, since only minute quantities have been made at vast expense and labour; insulin still has to be prepared from the pancreas of animals.

See also: Diabetes

Intelligence

There is no doubt that children who have been brought up in circumstances in which they have been inadequately fed suffer from diminished development, not only physically but also intellectually. However, before it can be concluded that this is due to their poor diet, it is necessary to examine whether some or all of their diminished intellectual capacity is due to the adverse factors that usually accompany poor feeding – factors such as lack of intellectual stimulus at home, inadequate or non-existent schooling, and frequent infection.

Careful recent work, mostly with rats in the laboratory, but also some work with young children, indicates that very early and continuing malnutrition may permanently retard intellectual development. However, it seems that a period of poor nutrition, for example because of illness, in a child who is usually well-fed will not affect its learning ability.

In the 1950s, it was suggested that the administration of the amino-acid glutamic acid to children in quite large quantities increased the intelligence by several points; this view was based on inadequately controlled trials, and has now been abandoned.

Intestinal bacteria

We are born with no micro-organisms of any sort in our alimentary canal, coming as we do from the germ-free environment of the uterus. Soon, however, micro-organisms take up their residence, entering the stomach and intestine with the food. At first there is a difference between breast-fed and bottle-fed infants; the former have a much higher proportion of lactobacilli and lactic acid streptococci, and the bottle-fed a more mixed range of bacteria.

Because of the huge numbers of bacteria that can be present, they are counted in powers of 10; 10^3 is $1,000$, and 10^6 is $1,000,000$. In the oesophagus the numbers are the same as in the food and saliva in the stomach the numbers are kept down by the acid to about $10^3 - 10^6$/gram of contents. The numbers grow from the point in the duodenum where the alkaline pancreatic juice and bile enter and neutralize the acid contents of the stomach. In the small intestine, there are about $10^5 - 10^8$ bacteria per gram, and this increases in the large intestine (colon) to $10^8 - 10^{11}$. In the faeces, 10% or 20% of the weight consists of bacteria; most of these are anaerobic and only $1-4\%$ are aerobic.

The vast numbers of bacteria in the colon actively affect the other materials in the gut. Firstly, they are mostly harmless bacteria and tend to keep down the number of pathogenic organisms entering the gut; without our resident population, we would be much more susceptible to intestinal infection than we are. Secondly, they synthesize vitamin K and perhaps also some of the B vitamins, making us less dependent on the amounts of these vitamins in the diet. If for any reason it is necessary to take anti-microbial drugs by mouth, these may reduce the amount of vitamins supplied by the bacteria and increase the amounts needed in the diet. Thirdly, the intestinal bacteria digest small quantities of some of the substances that constitute dietary fibre, and a part of these is then absorbed. Fourthly, the intestinal bacteria break down bile pigments and bile acids.

It is possible to change somewhat the relative proportions of the bacteria in the large intestine by, for example, including fairly large amounts of yoghurt in the diet. However, these changes are only temporary, and the bacteria revert to their original distribution when the intake of yoghurt ceases.

It is possible to breed and rear small animals in completely sterile conditions, so that they have no micro-organisms in the alimentary canal. The intestine of these so-called gnotobiotic animals has a very thin wall.

Commercial producers of pigs and poultry make use of the fact that the addition of small quantities of antibiotics to their feed accelerates their growth; there is so far no complete explanation of why this is so, although the intestinal bacteria are presumably involved.

See also: Aerobic/Anaerobic; Antibiotics; Yoghurt

Intravenous feeding

It is sometimes very difficult or even impossible for a patient to take food by mouth. The patient may be in a coma, or have a chronic fever, a chronic kidney disease, or extensive burns or other injury. Or there may be obstruction in the throat due to damage caused by the swallowing of a corrosive fluid, or due to cancer. In such circumstances, intravenous feeding may be carried out. This is also known as parenteral feeding, from the Greek words *para*, beyond or in addition to, and *enteron*, the intestine.

It is only since the middle 1960s that it has been possible to feed someone intravenously for any length of time. Before then, all that could be done was to supply water, salts and a limited amount of glucose for a short period. The difficulty arises from the fact that food when it is eaten is not the same as food when it has been digested, absorbed and modified, before it begins to circulate throughout the body. Digestion breaks down the larger molecules, so that it is not protein or starch or dextrin that is absorbed, but the small molecules of amino-acids or sugars. These products, as well as other small molecules already in the food, such as some sugars, salts and vitamins, are selectively absorbed into the blood vessels of the intestine. Not all substances are absorbed, and some are absorbed only to a limited extent.

The blood from the intestine, with its newly added materials, is carried to the liver; the liver then, as it were, decides which of the newly absorbed items are fit to go straight to the heart for distribution all over the body, and which need to be modified by the liver.

Thus, a nutrient solution that is to be put straight into a vein has to be more like the nutrient solution that gets into the blood from the intestine, and has then been passed as fit by the liver. Some of these requirements are readily recognized; some had to be discovered by experience. Here are some examples of both:

(1) The distilled water in which the solution is prepared very often causes a rise in temperature (pyrexia) in the patient; this is due to very small quantities of impurities (pyrogens) that still remain in the water. The preparation of pyrogen-free water needs special care.

(2) For an adequate source of energy, the most obvious source is glucose. However, a high concentration of glucose irritates the veins and may cause clotting (thrombophlebitis). On the other hand, if the solution is too dilute, it is difficult to get enough glucose into the patient without at the same time putting in too much water. Severely ill patients also often have impaired glucose tolerance. This may be overcome by adding fructose to the glucose solution, or a controlled amount of ethyl alcohol, or fat; all of these act as additional sources of energy.

(3) Fat presents a problem because it does not dissolve in the blood, and larger droplets could get lodged in a small blood vessel as an embolus and so impede the flow of blood. It is now possible, however, to obtain emulsions of soya bean oil or cotton seed oil with droplets not exceeding one micro-metre in diameter (one-thousandth of a millimetre).

(4) When intravenous feeding has to continue for more than a few days, the risk of producing thrombophlebitis can be reduced by using a large central vein rather than one of the superficial veins of the arm or leg.

(5) Protein requirements are met by a mixture of amino-acids. These are most conveniently prepared by the hydrolysis of a protein such as casein.

Because of all these advances, solutions for intravenous feeding are now readily available commercially.

Invertase

This enzyme is found in many plant tissues, as well as in intestinal juices of animals. An alternative name for invertase is saccharase or sucrase. It is sometimes convenient to make confections with sucrose, even if the final product needs to contain the less easily crystallizable invert sugar. To do this, invertase is mixed with the sucrose so as to produce the invert sugar after the manufacture is complete. Examples of confections made with invertase are some ice creams and sweets such as fruit pastilles, which need to have soft centres.

See also: Invert sugar

Invert sugar

Like all sugars, sucrose is optically active; it is dextro-rotatory, i.e. a solution of sucrose turns polarized light to the right. This is easy to measure, and the degree of 'turning' is used to measure the amount of sucrose in a solution. When it is hydrolysed by the enzyme invertase, or by acid, sucrose is split into the component monosaccharides, glucose (also known as dextrose) and fructose (also known as laevulose); as these alternative names show, glucose, like sucrose, is dextro-rotatory and fructose is 'left-turning' or laevo-rotatory. It so happens that the laevo-rotatory power of fructose is greater than the dextro-rotatory power of glucose, so that the mixture of equal amounts of the two sugars is laevo-rotatory.

The upshot is that the hydrolysis of 'right-turning' sucrose produces a mixture which is 'left-turning', so that the effect of the hydrolysis is to invert the direction of polarized light. This is why the product of hydrolysis of sucrose is called invert sugar.

Invert sugar is somewhat sweeter than the sucrose from which it is made. It does not crystallize as easily as sucrose does. Honey usually contains a high proportion of invert sugar, so invert sugar is used in making artificial honey.

See also: Honey; Invertase

Iodine

The adult body contains between 20mg and 50mg of iodine, and about 8mg of this is in the thyroid gland, which weighs only 25g or 30g. It is therefore much more concentrated in the gland than in the rest of the body. The iodine in the thyroid gland is almost entirely present as part of the two hormones, thyroxin and tri-iodothyroxine, which are especially concerned with the general metabolic activity of the body. Insufficient iodine in the diet causes simple goitre, and may cause cretinism and myxoedema.

The dietary requirements of iodine are not precisely known. The recommended intake is $150\mu g$ a day, that is, about one-seventh of a milligram. Most foods contain very little iodine; the main exceptions are sea fish and other seafoods. Freshwater fish contain only small quantities. In some countries iodized salt is available, to which iodide has been added to a level supplying about $100\mu g$ iodine in 5g.

IODINE IN SOME FOODS

μg per 100g

Apples	1.6	Halibut	52
Beef	2.8	Milk	3.5
Bread	5.8	Oysters	58
Cabbage	5.2	Pork	4.5
Cheese	5.1	Potatoes	4.5
Cod	146	Salmon	34
Eggs	9.3	Trout	3.1

See also: Thyroid gland

Iron

Iron forms part of a number of the substances, notably haemoglobin, that are concerned in transporting oxygen, or involved in the process of oxidation in all cells of the body. There is about 4g of iron in an adult body; about 2.5g in haemoglobin, 0.3g carrying out oxidation processes in the cells, and 1g as a store for emergency use in making iron-containing substances when required.

The red cells of the blood are continually breaking down and releasing their haemoglobin; the iron is removed from the haemoglobin molecule, and the rest of the molecule is converted into the pigments of the bile. The iron is retained in the form of ferritin, which acts as a store of iron for use when required. Consequently, the daily loss of iron in the normal adult man, almost entirely by excretion in the urine, is only one-tenth of 1mg, i.e. 100 micrograms. More is lost by women through menstruation and childbirth, and by any person young or old through acute or chronic haemorrhage.

Apart from severe blood loss, the total amount of iron that has to be replaced in the body, even for women during their reproductive life, is on average only 1 or 2mg a day. But although very few diets contain as little iron as this, anaemia due to iron deficiency is extremely common, especially in women, and especially in the poorer countries. The reason is that the absorption of iron from the diet is very poor.

One factor that affects absorption is the nature of the diet. In general, iron in vegetable foods or in eggs is not so readily absorbed as is the iron in meat. Vegetable foods contain phytates or are rich in phosphates, materials that form insoluble compounds with many iron compounds in the food. Meat, on the other hand, contains iron in a form that is absorbed without interference from other items in the diet.

The control of iron absorption is carried out by what is called the 'ferritin curtain'. When iron enters the cells of the intestinal lining (the mucosa), it can either proceed into the bloodstream, or be combined with a protein to produce ferritin. This remains in the mucosal cells; as these are constantly being shed, they carry the iron-containing ferritin into the intestine and so out of the body with the faeces.

An illustration of the effect of the nature of the diet on iron absorption is the common occurrence of severe anaemia among women workers in the UK in the latter part of the nineteenth century. The diet then had rather more iron, but it contained very little meat; most of the iron was present in the cereals and vegetables that constituted the major part of the diet.

The absorption of iron is also influenced by the body's need for it. With an intake of 10mg or so a day, a healthy adult man, or a woman past child-bearing age, is expected to absorb about 1mg, i.e. about 10%. When the need for iron is higher, as in growing children, in pregnancy or after haemorrhage, the body may absorb twice as much iron as usual, or more.

In spite of the limitations in the absorption of iron set by the body's needs, very large amounts in the diet can apparently increase the amounts absorbed. In South Africa, the use of iron vessels for cooking and home brewing of beer by many of the black population can result in a total daily intake of 100mg or more. Similar high consumption has been reported in chronic alcoholics in Boston in the US, and in cider drinkers in Normandy. As a result, iron is deposited in the liver as the compound haemosiderin. This may produce no ill effects; sometimes, however, it leads to cirrhosis of the liver.

IRON IN FOODS

Recommended daily intake (RDI) for moderately active man – 10mg

FOOD	PORTION	IRON, mg
Beef	100g	2
Liver	100g	8
Fish	100g	0.8
Egg	60g (1 egg)	1.2
Bread, wholemeal	30g	0.8
white fortified	30g	0.5
Cabbage	100g	0.4
Chocolate, plain	50g	1.2
Treacle, black	10g	0.9
Raisins	25g	0.5

The availability of the iron in different foods varies considerably, as explained in the text

See also: Absorption; Anaemia

J

Joule

The several forms of energy – electrical, chemical, physical work, heat and nuclear energy – have as their unit the joule. This is now used by scientists for the energy released by food in the body, rather than calorie, which is a unit only of heat.

The calorie and the joule are small units, so that it is customary in nutrition to use 1,000 calories (the kilocalorie, kcal) or 1,000 joules (the kilojoule, kJ). Quantities given in one of the units are readily convertible to quantities in the other if it is remembered that one calorie equals 4.18 joules.

James Prescott Joule was an English physicist who lived from 1818 to 1889, and who demonstrated the law of conservation of energy, that is, that energy may be converted from one form to another but does not disappear.

See also: Calorie; Energy

K

Ketosis

The complete oxidation of fat in the body results in the production of carbon dioxide and water. This process takes place in a series of steps; when it is not quite complete, some of the products of the partial oxidation accumulate. The two most common are acetoacetic acid and beta-hydroxybutyric acid. As these materials accumulate, there is also a production of acetone that comes from the breakdown of the acetoacetic acid; this and the acetone belong to a group of chemical substances known as ketone bodies.

Ketosis occurs in situations where most of the energy being produced by the body has to come from fat instead of mostly from carbohydrate. This happens in starvation, severe diabetes, or a diet very rich in fat. In starvation, the body uses up its relatively small store of carbohydrate within 2 or 3 days, and then has to use fat. In severe diabetes, the body is unable properly to metabolize carbohydrate. A diet very high in fat usually has little or no carbohydrate, and once again the result is ketosis.

A person with ketosis tends to have acetone in his breath, and this is readily recognized since it is the liquid constituent in most nail varnish, and is used itself for removing the varnish. Small children who have been sick for 2 or 3 days, and eaten very little, often develop ketosis.

It has been suggested that the development of ketosis is a measure of the efficacy of a weight-reducing diet. Manifest ketosis occurs in a diet that contains virtually no carbohydrate, and those who promote such a diet come to the quite absurd conclusion that it is dietary carbohydrate that produces body fat, whereas dietary fat is supposed to stimulate the metabolic removal of body fat.

The fact is that, in practice, a diet low in carbohydrate is inevitably a diet restricted in calories, and it is this, and not the ketosis, that leads to weight reduction in the obese.

A high degree of ketosis in a diabetic is an indication of the severity of the condition. This is partly because the acetoacetic and beta-hydroxybutyric acids are in themselves toxic, and partly because they induce severe acidosis. The effect may be to produce diabetic coma, and untreated this may be fatal.

It is unlikely that, in itself, mild ketosis is harmful; indeed, when it occurs in starvation, the ketone bodies serve as a source of energy for the brain after the carbohydrate stores have been exhausted.

See also: Acidosis; Brain; Diabetes; Famine; Fat; Obesity

Kidney

The kidney has several functions, including the conversion of vitamin D into its highly active form, the secretion of the hormone renin which prevents an excessive fall of blood pressure, and the production of the hormone erythropoietin, which stimulates the production of red blood cells. The most important function of the kidney, however, is in the control of the volume and composition of the blood. It does this by forming urine from the blood, which contains both the waste products formed in the body during metabolism, and any excess of the materials that have been absorbed from those taken above the body's needs. The waste products are mostly from the metabolism of protein, and include urea, uric acid, sulphates and acid (that is, hydrogen ions); the surplus consists mostly of water, sodium, potassium, chloride and acid or alkali.

Several different diseases may affect the kidneys. Many of them can be greatly helped by dietary measures. General impairment of kidney (renal) function can be mitigated by reducing the work they have to do, and this can be done especially by reducing the intake of salt and protein. If the capillaries in the kidney are damaged, protein may escape into the urine, and this may lead to a considerable loss of protein; in these circumstances, it will be necessary to increase rather than decrease the amount of protein in the diet.

The excretion of water and salt in renal failure is helped by the administration of diuretics; since they may also result in a loss of more potassium than is advisable, the diuretics are often taken together with a potassium salt. If diet and diuretics are not adequate, recourse must be had to dialysis by kidney machine.

See also: Dialysis; Lymphatic system; Sodium; Urine

L

Lactose intolerance

Ordinarily, lactose is digested in the small intestine by the enzyme lactase, and the glucose and galactose that result from this digestion are readily absorbed. If, however, there is an inadequate production of lactase, undigested lactose passes into the large intestine, where it is fermented by the bacteria with the production of lactic acid. This accumulation of lactic acid in the large intestine results in abdominal discomfort and diarrhoea when lactose is taken, the condition known as lactose intolerance.

Lactose intolerance occurs in malnourished babies or young children whose intestinal lining is not functioning well. It occurs too in older children and adults who are not Caucasian, that is to say, mostly in African, Asian or South American peoples.

The origin of racial lactose intolerance is not entirely clear. It may be a genetic difference. On the other hand, it may be that the custom of drinking milk, which is common among Caucasians, results in the continued production of lactase; many other races do not take much milk after infancy, so that the enzyme diminishes or disappears.

The intolerance can be tested by the administration of a solution of lactose, and then either noting whether symptoms appear, or whether the normal rise in blood glucose fails to occur. A more sensitive test than either of these is the appearance of an unusual amount of hydrogen in the breath; this comes from some of the fermentative activities of the intestinal bacteria on the unabsorbed sugar.

In practice, it is important to remember that intolerance demonstrated in these ways does not necessarily indicate that the individual cannot take milk at all. Most of those with intolerance revealed by the laboratory tests can take small quantities of milk with no untoward effect.

It is also necessary to realize that most sorts of cheese contain so little lactose that they do not produce symptoms of intolerance; the same is often true of yoghurt preparations in which much of the lactose has been converted to lactic acid.

See also: Allergy; Milk

Laetrile

This is sometimes called vitamin B_{17}; no doubt this strengthens its appeal to potential buyers, who have been persuaded that it is a cure for cancer. It is amygdalin, a chemical compound belonging to a group of substances that can release cyanide, and Laetrile can do so in the body. It is prepared from apricot stones, and has not been shown to have any effect in the body other than the possible toxic action from its cyanide. Its role as a cancer cure was invented in the USA, where for many years it was illegal to sell it. By pursuing court actions on the basis of freedom of choice, the manufacturers and distributors have now achieved the right to market Laetrile in several of the states.

See also: Cancer; Vitamins

Lathyrism

This is a condition caused by a toxin present in the pulse known as *Lathyrus sativus*.

It is common practice in many parts of North Africa and Asia to sow wheat together with *Lathyrus*. This ensures a good crop of wheat when there is adequate rainfall, since the wheat will then overgrow the pulse; on the other hand, a reasonable crop of *Lathyrus* will grow if the wheat fails because of a failure of the rains. Thus, it is in conditions of famine, where more than 50% of the diet is made up of *Lathyrus* and is continued for a long time, that the disease of lathyrism may result. This is an affection of the spinal cord, causing severe paralysis of the legs. The onset may be sudden and severe, with spasticity so that the knees are bent and the patient walks on tiptoe. Often the legs are crossed, resulting in 'scissors gait'. If the disease progresses, walking becomes impossible.

Lathyrism does not respond to any known treatment, and severe cases do not improve spontaneously. Mild cases may gradually improve, and some recover completely. The toxin in the *Lathyrus* seeds has been isolated and identified as beta-N-oxalylamino-l-alanine (BOAA). It is water-soluble and can be removed from the pulse when it is heated for an hour or so in water.

See also: Poisons in food

Lavoisier, Antoine Laurent (1743-94)

The founder of modern chemistry was born of a wealthy father in Paris, and studied science there. In 1766 he was awarded a gold medal from the Académie des Sciences, for his essay on the best way of lighting a town.

His chemical experiments led him to oppose the current phlogiston theory of Priestley (1733-1804), Black (1728-99), and others, and to announce that air consisted of two gases which he named oxygen and azote (later called nitrogen). Water, he maintained, consisted of a combination of oxygen and hydrogen. 'Fixed air' (carbon dioxide) was formed when carbon combined with oxygen, and the same fixed air was produced both during the respiration of a guinea pig and the burning of carbon in the air. With Laplace, he devised the ice calorimeter, into which he placed a guinea pig. This apparatus measured the amount of ice melted and thus the amount of heat produced, and this too was proportional to the amount of 'fixed air' produced by the animal.

Much of Lavoisier's scientific work was concerned with solving problems for the government. This included scientific improvement of agriculture, and devising a better system of taxation while he held the post of 'Fermier Général' of taxes from 1768.

During the Revolution, his liberal ideas as well as some of his scientific statements displeased Marat and others. He was arrested, sentenced to death and guillotined in 1794. His friends remarked, 'It took only a few seconds to cut off his head; a hundred years will not suffice to produce one like it.' The official view, it is said, was 'La république n'a pas besoin de savants' (The Republic does not need scholars).

See also: Energy

Lawes, John Bennet (1814-1900)

Lawes was born in Rothamsted, in England, to a wealthy family of landowners. At home, he carried out experiments on the chemistry of drugs, but also studied chemistry at University College, London, where he met Joseph Gilbert. At the age of 21 he inherited the family estate, and extended his experiments on plants. He began to experiment with what came to be known as chemical fertilizers. By 1843, Lawes had discovered and patented the manufacture of fertilizers by the treatment

TRAITE
ÉLÉMENTAIRE
DE CHIMIE,
PRÉSENTÉ DANS UN ORDRE NOUVEAU
ET D'APRÈS LES DÉCOUVERTES MODERNES;

Avec Figures :

Par M. LAVOISIER , de l'Académie des Sciences, de la Société Royale de Médecine, des Sociétés d'Agriculture de Paris & d'Orleans, de la Société Royale de Londres , de l'Institut de Bologne , de la Société Helvétique de Basle , de celles de Philadelphie, Harlem, Manchester, Padoue , &c.

TOME PREMIER.

A PARIS,

Chez CUCHET, Libraire , rue & hôtel Serpente.

M. DCC. LXXXIX.

Sous le Privilège de l'Académie des Sciences &. de la Société Royale de Médecine.

of bone ash and various phosphate minerals with sulphuric acid, and set up a factory for producing them.

With the profits of the factory, he instituted at Rothamsted the first agricultural research institute in the world. He persuaded Gilbert to join him, and thus began a partnership that lasted for more than half a century.

Their work with plants was mostly concerned with the effects of different sorts of fertilizer, including animal manure, on different crops. Their work with animals was concerned with the effects of different feed composition on the growth of animals and the composition of their carcases. They demonstrated that nitrogenous materials, mostly protein, were not necessary for work, in direct contradiction to the opinion of Liebig. They also showed that carcase fat could be produced not only from the fat in the diet of the animals, but also and chiefly from the carbohydrate.

A few years before he died, Lawes set up a trust fund to secure the survival of the Rothamsted Experimental Station.

See also: Gilbert; Liebig

Lecithin

Lecithin is important in the body as a group of substances that help to emulsify fats, and thus aid in their transport from one part of the body to another. Like fats, the various lecithins have a general structure based on glycerol; however, instead of having all the three relevant positions in the glycerol molecule occupied by fatty acids, it has two positions so occupied and the third occupied by phosphate to which choline is attached. It thus belongs to a group of compounds known as phospholipids. Lecithin also exists in some foods, especially egg yolk. This is why egg yolks are used when making emulsions of oil and vinegar in the production of mayonnaise and similar foods.

Although lecithin performs an essential role in regard to fat transportation in the body, it is not essential in the diet because it is readily manufactured by the body.

See also: Absorption of fat; Choline; Emulsifiers and stabilizers

Die Grundsätze

der

Agricultur-Chemie

mit Rücksicht

auf die in England angestellten Untersuchungen.

Von

Justus von Liebig.

Braunschweig,

Druck und Verlag von Friedrich Vieweg und Sohn.

1855.

Liebig, Justus von (1803–73)

One of the most prolific chemists of the nineteenth century, Liebig was born in Darmstadt, Germany. He was appointed Professor of Chemistry at Giessen University (now the Justus von Liebig University) when he was 21. There he set up a students' laboratory, the first in Europe, in a disused military barracks. He was a pioneer in agricultural chemistry, demonstrating that the mineral salts found in the soil were essential to plant growth, that the growing crops depleted the soil of these essential materials, and that the fertility of the soil could be restored if the salts were restored either by natural decay or by the addition of the mineral salts.

Liebig's work on animal and human nutrition led him to differentiate the components of foodstuffs into 'plastic nutrients', which contain nitrogen, and 'foods for respiration', which were derived from carbohydrates and fats. In opposition to the French school, he suggested that the fats in the body could be derived from dietary components other than fat, and that they contributed to the maintenance of animal heat. He drew up tables of the nutritive values of food based on their nitrogen content. Liebig accepted the view of Lavoisier that respiration involved the oxidation of substances in the body, and was responsible for the heat and carbon dioxide produced by the body. Much of Liebig's writing was based on theory rather than experiment, but he exerted considerable influence on the development of food chemistry and body metabolism. He died in Munich in 1873.

See also: Energy; Meat extracts

Lind, James (1716–94)

James Lind was born in Edinburgh. He entered the Royal Navy as surgeon's mate in 1739; by 1743 he had been promoted to the rank of surgeon to HMS *Salisbury*. He developed a wide concern for the hygiene of sailors, and insisted on proper provision for clothing, bathing, good ventilation and adequate supplies of pure water.

Lind is remembered especially for having shown that scurvy can be cured and prevented by the administration of orange juice or lemon juice. This he did in what was in effect the first controlled clinical trial ever carried out, and described in his *Treatise of the Scurvy*, first published in Edinburgh in 1753. While HMS *Salisbury* was cruising in

A

TREATISE

OF THE

SCURVY.

IN THREE PARTS.

CONTAINING

An inquiry into the Nature, Causes, and Cure, of that Disease.

Together with

A Critical and Chronological View of what has been published on the subject.

By *JAMES LIND*, M. D.

Fellow of the Royal College of Physicians in *Edinburgh*.

EDINBURGH:

Printed by SANDS, MURRAY, and COCHRAN.
For A. MILLAR, in the Strand, *London*.
MDCCLIII.

the English Channel, there was – as so frequently happened – an outbreak of scurvy on board. In May 1747, Lind took 12 sailors who had developed scurvy, and divided them into 6 pairs. Each day, a pair received either a quart of cider, or drops of sulphuric acid, or vinegar, or sea water, or two oranges and a lemon, or a mixture of garlic, mustard seed and other ingredients commonly used as medicine at the time. He described the result thus: 'The consequence was, that the most sudden and visible good effects were perceived from the use of the oranges and lemons; one of those who had taken them being at the end of six days fit for duty . . . the other was the best recovered of any in his condition.'

The treatise was also remarkable both for Lind's superb and very critical review of the many authors who had written on the subject earlier, and for his most clear and detailed clinical description of the disease.

In spite of his outstanding work, it took the Admiralty 42 years to introduce the daily ration of 'lime' juice (probably in fact lemon juice), thus abolishing scurvy from the Royal Navy. The issue of lime juice continued until well into the present century, and was responsible for the American use of the word 'Limey' to describe not only the members of the Royal Navy but British citizens in general.

In 1748 Lind left the Royal Navy and returned to Edinburgh, where he went into medical practice. In 1758 he was appointed physician in charge at the new Hasler Naval Hospital in Portsmouth. He retired to Edinburgh in 1783 and died there in 1794.

See also: Citrus fruits; Scurvy; Vitamin C

Linoleic acid

This is one of the essential fatty acids (EFA). It is readily converted into arachidonic acid, the EFA that the body uses. It occurs in both animal and plant foods, and especially in some vegetable oils such as the oils from maize, cottonseed, soya bean and sunflower seed; coconut oil contains very little. It contains 18 carbon atoms, and its two double bonds qualify it as being a polyunsaturated acid.

See also: Arachidonic acid; Essential; Fatty acids; Oils

Lipoprotein

Much of the fat (triglyceride) in the bloodstream is carried in an emulsified form as tiny droplets of lipoprotein. These are compounds made up of triglycerides, cholesterol, phospholipids (mainly lecithin) and protein. They are for convenience put into four classes, which are separated by their density. Thus, if the blood plasma is spun in a high-speed centrifuge, the lipoproteins will separate from the watery part of the plasma, and the droplets with the lowest density will be at the top of the fatty layer while those with the highest density will be at the bottom of this layer.

The very lightest section are called the chylomicrons, and these are the droplets of fat that enter the bloodstream during absorption from the intestine. They are made up mostly of triglycerides with very little of the other constituents. The next group are the very low density lipoproteins (VLDL); they consist of about 50% triglyceride, with about 20% cholesterol. The low density lipoproteins (LDL) are made up of only 10% triglycerides, but are rich in cholesterol. Finally, the high density lipoproteins (HDL) contain 50% of protein, very little triglyceride and about 20% each of cholesterol and phospholipid.

For the last 30 years or more it has been known that people who have an increased risk of developing coronary disease tend to have an increase in the concentration of cholesterol and triglyceride in their blood. More recent work has shown that this susceptibility to coronary disease is better indicated when there is a low amount of cholesterol bound to HDL and by a high concentration of total cholesterol.

See also: Absorption of fat; Coronary heart disease

Liver as food

There was a time when liver was widely recommended as a highly nutritious food, and many people – especially children – ate it or were compelled to eat it because it was supposed to be 'good for you'. Pork and beef livers especially have a strong taste and are somewhat tough; calves' liver is more popular and some adults find it quite attractive. Nevertheless, liver is now not consumed by many people, at least not as a separate dish.

Partly this is because, like other offal, much of the liver of cattle and pigs is used for petfood. Partly, liver finds its way as one of the components of a number of composite manufactured foods.

Liver from poultry is consumed separately only in small quantities, as a delicacy. Pâté de foie gras, made from the fatty liver of force-fed geese, is very much a dish for gourmets and is very expensive.

Liver is especially rich in iron, in vitamins A and D, and in several of the B vitamins. It was this last quality that was responsible for the considerable part played by liver in the discovery, separation and identification of these vitamins, and particularly the role of vitamin B_{12} in the cure of pernicious anaemia.

Compared with ordinary meat, which is muscle, liver contains a high proportion of cells; the nuclei they contain give rise to purines in the body, so that liver is one of the foods that gouty people are advised not to eat.

See also: Anaemia; Minot; Vitamin B_{12}; Vitamin history

Liver function

The liver is an intensely active organ and an important organ for storage. Its activities include the manufacture of bile, the detoxification of some of the harmful materials that appear in the body, and the metabolism of fat, carbohydrate and protein. It stores iron and copper and the fat-soluble vitamins. Whether its high concentration of some of the B vitamins can be considered storage, or whether they are needed for the considerable metabolic activity of the liver, is not known.

Detoxification is usually carried out by chemically converting a harmful material into a harmless one. For example, the first product of the metabolism of amino-acids that are not required for protein synthesis is ammonia, which would be dangerous if it were allowed to accumulate. The liver converts the ammonia to urea, which is relatively harmless and is rapidly excreted by the kidney before it can reach any dangerous quantity. The liver is also capable of detoxifying small amounts of other substances which may be present in the food, or enter the body unintentionally.

See also: Bernard; Bile

Locust bean

Known also as carob or St John's Bread, the locust bean grows mostly in Mediterranean regions. It belongs to the Leguminosae, like the pulses. The bean is up to 8 inches long, about 1 inch wide and not more than $\frac{1}{2}$ inch thick. It is dark brown or black in colour, and has a hardish, sweet pulp in which the seeds are embedded. It is harvested mostly for animal feed, although it is said to have been the food on which St John the Baptist fed in the wilderness. Carob gum is also extracted from it and added to foods and cosmetics as a thickener and emulsifier, or made into size for textiles.

The carob seed was the original standard carat for weighing diamonds; the standard is now fixed more precisely at 205mg.

Longevity

There are two ways in which people think of longevity. One is in terms of the maximum lifespan of individuals, demonstrated by our interest in people who reach the age of 90 or even 100. The other way is to consider the expectation of life; how long on average can a newborn baby be expected to live, or a man or woman of 50 or some other specific age?

As to long life, it has often been claimed that there is a spectacularly high number of centenarians in some parts of the world, including Georgia in the USSR, the Andes in Ecuador, and in the Hunza province of Pakistan. Interestingly enough, these are mostly fairly inaccessible places where there are no reliable records of dates of birth, or where close local inquiry fails to discover the claimed number of old people. Discussions with centenarians themselves will always elicit some comment upon the role of diet in determining their longevity; these anecdotes, however, tend to identify quite opposing dietary regimes.

Perhaps the best-known food recommended for a long and healthy life is fermented milk, such as yoghurt, especially if made with *Lactobacillus bulgaricus*. This notion was promoted particularly by Metchnikoff (1845–1916), a Russian working in the Pasteur Institute in Paris, who later was awarded the Nobel Prize in Medicine for his other bacteriological research. There is, however, no justification for the claim that yoghurt prolongs life.

The average expectation at birth is clearly much influenced by the numbers dying in infancy or early childhood. The fall in the death rate at these early ages is the chief cause of increasing the average expectation at birth of US males from about 50 years at the beginning of the century to about 70 years now. On the other hand, there is little change in the expectation of life from middle age onwards; in 1900, men aged 50 had a life expectancy of about 21 years, and now this has risen by only 5 years or so. When one looks at still higher ages, there is no evidence that there has been any increase in the maximum age people can attain.

These examples illustrate the effects of increasing affluence on longevity; what is difficult to do, if not impossible, is to isolate the separate changes that accompany increasing affluence in a way that makes it possible to quantify the extent to which each contributes to increasing longevity. As populations become less poor, there is less hunger and malnutrition, better housing, improved working conditions, improved sanitation and increased medical services. Such changes, which have occurred as it were spontaneously in the past, are now deliberately combined in attempts to raise the living standards in poor countries; programmes to improve nutrition are always accompanied by measures to improve hygiene, eliminate infection and infestation, and institute sewage disposal.

However, it does not follow that affluence results in improvement in nutritional status. Much has been said recently about the possibly harmful effects of some of the characteristics of the diets in affluent countries. These include excessive intakes of energy, fat, sugar and salt, and the presence of additives and contaminants. If one or more of these factors is responsible for significant increase in diseases such as some sorts of cancer or coronary heart disease, a potential improvement in life expectancy at middle age is being thwarted by a deterioration of life expectancy through nutritional error.

It is to answer some of these uncertainties about the role of nutrition in life expectancy that experiments with animals have been carried out. The best known of these were with rats, studied during the 1930s and 1940s, in which the effect of severe restriction of total food intake was investigated. The results purport to show that there is a considerable increase in survival time, in one study from some 650 days to about 950 days. Apart from the obvious impossibility of persuading people to accept such dietary restriction, or imposing it in a civilized society, there are serious flaws in the design of these experiments. For example, no account was taken of the reproductive capacity of the rats, of the numbers that die at or around birth, or during the many months before the animals are counted as being in the experiment.

The conclusion is that we are still not certain what sort of diet will ensure maximal life expectancy, nor do we know whether this diet will also ensure maximal growth and maximal vigour. Common sense perhaps suggests that there should be a way of eating that ensures both good health and long life; there is, however, no general agreement about what this way is, but again common sense suggests the approach described in the entry 'Dietary instinct'.

See also: Old age; Yoghurt

Lusk, Graham (1866–1932)

The son of a distinguished obstetrician, Graham Lusk was born in Bridgport, Connecticut. When it was realized that the boy had impaired hearing, the father decided that he should be trained as a physiological chemist rather than as a clinician. Graham first studied in the United States, and then went to work with Voit in Germany.

He returned to America in 1891, and held posts in Yale and Bellevue Medical Schools. In 1909, he was appointed to the Chair of Physiology at Cornell University Medical College, from which he retired only a few weeks before his death in July 1932.

His first research work was on the disturbances in carbohydrate metabolism in dogs made diabetic with the chemical phloridzin. In 1906 he published his book *The Science of Nutrition*. In Cornell, it became possible for him to enlarge his research programme, and in particular to continue the work on energy metabolism he had begun with Voit. A respiration calorimeter was constructed, in which with du Bois and other colleagues he could study the energy metabolism of children and dogs. He worked especially on specific dynamic action, measuring the effect of the ingestion of amino-acids, carbohydrates and other food components on the metabolic rate. The subsequent series of publications on clinical calorimetry are now recognized as being the solid foundation for studies on energy metabolism, and included the confirmation by D. du Bois and E. P. du Bois of the work of Rubner on the relation of the basal metabolic rate to the surface area.

See also: Carbohydrates; Diabetes; du Bois; Energy; Rubner

Lymphatic system

Although we always speak of the blood transporting food, oxygen and other materials to the cells in different parts of the body, and of the blood removing waste products and carbon dioxide from the cells, this is an incomplete picture. The blood does not itself get to each cell. What happens is that the blood passes along the arteries from the heart into smaller and smaller arteries, then into still smaller vessels called arterioles and finally into tiny vessels, the capillaries, which have exceedingly thin walls through which a filtered part of the blood passes. The capillary walls act as a semi-permeable membrane, allowing only the smaller molecules to pass through. This 'filtered' blood, called tissue fluid, consists of water in which there are salts, vitamins, hormones, oxygen and other reasonably small molecules, but none of the red blood cells or the blood platelets, and almost none of the proteins which are mostly quite large molecules. It does contain a few of the white cells, which as it were squeeze their way through the pores in the walls of the capillaries. As this tissue fluid washes past the cells, they take what materials they need from it, and pass into it materials they do not need.

The question that then arises is what now happens to the tissue fluid? Clearly, it cannot just go on flowing out of the blood circulation, but has to get back somehow. This it does in two ways. Some of it simply enters other capillaries, so that in effect it is flowing out of some of the capillaries, washes around tissue cells, and then enters other capillaries. But not all of the tissue fluid does this. Some of it enters a different system of vessels, called the lymph vessels. Unlike the blood system, this does not constitute a circulatory system. The lymph vessels begin as narrow, blind tubes, which join into larger and larger tubes, and end in two fairly large vessels that open into two of the main veins in the body, the subclavian veins at either side of the neck. Thus, the fluid that has left the capillaries as tissue fluid gets back into the circulatory blood system either directly by entering other capillaries, or by being picked up by the lymphatic system and getting into the blood system through the lymphatic vessels.

Like veins, the lymphatic vessels have valves at intervals; the lymph in them, like the blood in the veins, passes along the vessels by intermittent pressure of the muscles lying near them. Because of the valves, the fluid is pushed in one direction, but cannot be pushed in the other.

At intervals in the lymphatic system there are the lymph glands or lymph nodes, in which there is, as it were, a maze of lymph vessels. These act as a filter, especially for infecting organisms. The nodes lie in groups, especially in the axillae, in the groin, around the neck, at the elbow, and in the abdomen. When infected, the glands become inflamed and may be swollen and painful.

In the digestive system, the lymph vessels are especially concerned with the absorption and transport of the fat.

See also: Absorption of fat

M

Macrobiotics

In the early 1900s, George Ohsawa, a Californian Japanese whose original name was Sakurazawa Nyoiti, suggested that the Zen Buddhist philosophy should be applied to the determination of what constitutes the most healthy diet. He accordingly selected the appropriate foods on the principle of yin-yang; yin was exemplified by acidity, potassium, sugar and fruits, and yang by alkalinity, sodium, salt and cereals. He considered the ratio of 5 : 1 of yin to yang to be the perfect balance, and this balance is found in the perfect food, brown rice.

Brown rice was the final level in the 7 levels of diet in the macrobiotic regime. Five of the 7 diets are vegetarian, as shown in the Table. Mostly, the diets to be consumed are those on levels 1–6; level 7 is to be followed for 10 days at a time, and in periods of illness. A person who is following a mixed Western diet is expected gradually to give up meat according to what are called levels − 3 to − 1, before beginning on level 1 of the macrobiotic regime.

DIETARY REGIMEN FOR LEVELS OF MACROBIOTIC DIET
On all levels, fluids are to be taken sparingly

LEVEL	CEREAL	VEGETABLE	SOUP	ANIMAL	FRUIT	DESSERT
7	100%	—	—	—	—	—
6	90%	10%	—	—	—	—
5	80%	20%	—	—	—	—
4	70%	20%	10%	—	—	—
3	60%	30%	10%	—	—	—
2	50%	30%	10%	10%	—	—
1	40%	30%	10%	20%	—	—

The macrobiotic diet has been adopted by many young people in Western countries, especially in the United States; it has led to several instances of malnutrition, and a few deaths. Its claim to be based on Zen Buddhism is challenged by adherents of that school.

See also: Health foods

Magnesium

Most of the 25g of magnesium in the adult body is present in the skeleton. There is, however, some magnesium in the cells of all the tissues. It is, after potassium, the most concentrated cation (that is, positively charged ion) within the cells. It is an essential part of many of the body's enzyme systems.

Because it is part of the chlorophyll system of green leaves involved in photosynthesis, it is found in almost all foods as it moves through the food chain. The typical Western diet provides 200–400mg of magnesium a day; about two-thirds of this comes from vegetables and cereals. The Americans put the daily allowance at 350mg for an adult; the UK gives no figures for magnesium.

Dietary deficiency in man is never seen. Conditioned deficiency of magnesium occurs, however, as it does of potassium, in persons with chronic diarrhoea, or in whom there has been excision of part of the small intestine. It may also occur in chronic alcoholism, because of excessive excretion of magnesium in the urine. The effects of deficiency are depression, muscular weakness, vertigo and convulsions.

Deficiency of magnesium may occur in lambs and in cattle, where it gives rise to 'grass tetany'. It has been suggested that this hypo-magnesaemia might be caused by a high intake of phytate in young pasture, which would reduce the absorption of the magnesium in the diet.

Maize

Unlike the other cereals, the wild grass from which maize is derived now seems to be extinct. It is called Indian corn because it was origi-nally cultivated in central America; in the United States it is known simply as corn. It is mostly golden in colour, but it can also be almost white, or red or blue or brown. It still plays a large part in the diets of central and south America and in parts of Africa; it is only recently that it has become less important in the US and in southern and eastern Europe. It was at one time a common enough food in eastern Europe to be given the name Turkey wheat.

Very large quantities are grown in the United States in what is known as the 'corn belt', stretching through Ohio, Illinois, Indiana, Missouri, Kansas, Iowa and Nebraska; the corn is mostly used for animal feed. Some, however, is used for the manufacture of glucose and corn starch, or fermented for the production of alcohol. The small quantities still consumed in the US are chiefly in the form of cornflakes as a breakfast cereal, or as a sort of porridge known as grits or hominy grits.

Maize grows and matures quickly and can give a high yield. When it constitutes a large proportion of the human diet, its use is associated with the development of pellagra. This disease does not, however, occur in countries such as Mexico, where the tortillas are made from maize mixed with lime water; this increases the availability of nicotinic acid, deficiency of which produces pellagra. Modern advances in plant breeding have resulted in the production of varieties with a higher content of protein and more sugar, with lower starch. These hybrid varieties are being introduced in an increasing proportion in those countries where maize is a staple food.

See also: Casal; Cereals; Goldberger; Nicotinic acid; Pellagra

Malic acid

One of the acids found in fruits, especially apples, but also tomatoes and plums, is known as malic acid because *malum* is the Latin word for apple. In its pure form, it is sometimes added by food manufacturers, together with other acids, to soft drinks, confectionery and ice cream to increase their fruity taste.

See also: Apples

Malthus, Thomas Robert (1766–1834)

Born in Guildford, Surrey, young Robert Malthus was educated mostly privately by his father before he entered Jesus College, Cambridge, where he was elected Fellow of the College in 1793. Malthus was impressed by William Godwin's (1756–1836) publication of *Political Justice* (1793) and *Enquirer* (1797). Godwin looked forward to a millennium of quality and prosperity; Malthus, however, disagreed strongly with Godwin's conclusions. In 1798, in reply to Godwin, Malthus published anonymously his famous book, *An Essay on the Principle of Population as it affects the future Improvement of Society.* In this, he puts forward the thesis that unchecked population grows geometrically (i.e. 1, 2, 4, 8, 16, 32 . . .), whereas means of subsistence, especially food supplies, grow arithmetically (i.e. 1, 2, 3, 4, 5, 6 . . .).

This was not consistent with the optimistic conclusions of Godwin; the natural checks to population growth were war, disease and famine. The only other check would be sexual abstinence, which Malthus considered impractical. He wrote: '. . . the great obstacle in the way to any extraordinary improvement in society, is of a nature that we can never hope to overcome. The perpetual tendency in the race of man to increase beyond the means of subsistence, is one of the general laws of animated nature, which we can have no reason to expect will change.'

The vigorous discussion that followed the publication of *An Essay on the Principle of Population* made Malthus realize that he needed to set out his views much more carefully; he travelled extensively, with friends, through Europe, getting information for a second edition; this he published in 1803.

Malthus died in 1834, and was buried in Bath.

See also: Population

Manganese

Manganese is one of the essential mineral elements. Deficiency has not been described in human beings, but does occur in poultry; it has also been produced experimentally in rats. The effects are diminished growth, interference with reproduction, anaemia, and changes in the nervous system and bones. The average Western diet contains about 5mg a day; it is found mostly in cereals and vegetables, and tea is a particularly rich source.

See also: Mineral elements

Margarine

Margarine was introduced in 1869 by the French chemist, Mège-Mouries (1817–80), who took out a patent on a product made from beef fat, milk and cow udder. As the demand for this alternative to butter increased, other sources of fat were sought. This was supplied at the beginning of the twentieth century by the invention in Holland of the process of hydrogenation of vegetable oils. These were much more plentiful and thus cheaper than meat fat; hydrogenation made the liquid oils harder, so that they more resembled the animal fats they were intended to replace.

The process of hardening is performed by passing hydrogen, in the presence of nickel as a catalyst, through the oil which contains poly-unsaturated fats. The effect is to increase the amount of hydrogen in the molecules of fat, making them more saturated. The oils used today include those from the cotton seed, maize (corn oil), soya, sunflower, coconut, groundnut and whale; the proportion of these that is used is determined chiefly by their current price to the manufacturer, as well as by the sort of final product desired. Colouring matter, emulsifying agent, salt and perhaps antioxidants are added during manufacture, and some brands contain up to 10% of butter. Legally, in the UK margarine must contain added vitamins A and D, and it must not have more than 16% water, which is about the same proportion as in butter.

Some soft margarines, but not all, contain a higher proportion of their original polyunsaturated fatty acids, and so are useful as part of a diet designed to reduce the concentration of cholesterol in the blood. Many people, however, mistakenly believe that all margarines, and certainly all soft margarines, will do this. The process of hydrogenation also changes the chemical structure of some of the fatty acids in the oils, so that they are converted into what is called the 'trans' form from their normal 'cis' form. There is a continuing discussion by nutritionists whether this transformation affects the way they act in the body, and particularly whether they are harmful.

Margarine in the United States is usually called oleo-margarine. For many years, chiefly through the influence of the dairy industry, it was illegal in some states to colour the product, so that its white colour made it less appealing to the consumer as an alternative to butter. Some manufacturers attempted to overcome this disadvantage, at least partially, by selling the margarine together with a small amount of separately packed colouring material. This legislation was abolished in 1950.

COMPARISON OF MARGARINE AND BUTTER

Quantities in 100g

	MARGARINE	BUTTER
Fat	81g	82g
Water	up to 16g	15.4g
Energy, kcal	730	740
Vitamin A (retinol equivalent)	900μg	750μg
Vitamin D	8μg	0.8μg

See also: **Butter; Coronary heart disease; Fatty acids; Oils**

Meals

The habit of eating meals at particular times is very much a practice that has arisen with the advent of civilization. So long as man was a hunter and food gatherer, he mostly ate when he found his food. If there was more than he and his family needed, he was able to some extent to put food aside for later, but before the advent of controllable fire, the food was not easily preserved and so deteriorated.

The question that is now much discussed is the extent to which it is necessary to have meals regularly and at pre-set times. The general answer is that there appear to be no ill effects when people eat at the times they themselves prefer. It is, however, also worthwhile to consider particular aspects of food frequency. One question commonly raised is whether it is necessary to have breakfast, by which is usually meant something more than a slice of toast and a cup of coffee or the equivalent. A series of experiments carried out in the United States in the 1940s is often quoted as demonstrating a distinct deterioration in performance by midday in children and workers who were not given breakfast. There are, however, flaws in those experiments, and other research workers have not been able to substantiate their results.

Another question is how many meals one should take a day, and how much should be taken at each meal. Of the very large number of possibilities, one definite result has emerged from research studies. This relates to the consumption of the same daily amount of food taken either in 1 or 2 large meals, or in 4 or 5 smaller meals. The former procedure results in a slight gain in weight and a small increase in the blood concentration of triglyceride. These results have been shown in experiments both with human subjects and with laboratory rats.

It is often believed, especially by parents, that a hot meal is necessarily more nutritious than a cold meal is. In particular, it is supposed that a hot cereal for breakfast is the best way for a child to start a cold day, or a hot soup in the evening to nourish or warm him. The temperature of a meal, however, contributes virtually nothing to its nutritional value; the additional energy would be unlikely to amount to more than 10 kcal or so. It is easy to construct a nutritionally poor hot meal consisting of clear soup, spaghetti bolognese, sponge pudding and a cola drink; it would be equally easy to construct an excellent cold meal consisting of a sandwich with beef, a salad of tomato and coleslaw, fresh fruit and a glass of milk.

Meat

The word 'meat' is used mostly to denote the edible muscle of animals, particularly of mammals and birds; it can also include the heart, liver and some other viscera. Historically, and in poetical writing, the word is extended to mean food in general, as in the expression 'One man's meat is another man's poison', or as in Shakespeare's 'Upon what meat doth this our Caesar feed/That he is grown so great?' The word 'bread' is similarly used both in the particular and in the general meaning.

There are many species of animals that provide flesh for human consumption. Excluding fish, the commonest in Western countries are sheep, cattle, pigs and chickens; however, dozens of other animals are used in different parts of the world and at different times. They include camels, horses, donkeys, goats and buffaloes, geese, ducks, turkeys and guineafowl, as well as monkeys, hedgehogs and dogs. Nor is man confined to eating the muscle and some of the viscera of mammals and birds; in several parts of the world snails and insects are consumed, both as regular food and as a delicacy.

It seems that man and his immediate ancestors have been meat eaters for 5 million years or more. As a result, they had a considerable advantage over those cousins that remained largely vegetarian, in that meat provided a much more concentrated source of energy and nutrients than did shoots, leaves and fruits. They were therefore able to spend less time searching for food, with more time to develop the skills and crafts that determined their unique transition to makers and users of tools.

Meat is a desirable item of diet for most people. However, it is in most circumstances a more expensive or rarer commodity than are plant foods, so that its consumption is greater in wealthier populations; the average in the UK is now about 130lb a year, and in the US about 200lb a year. The average consumption is much lower in the poorer countries, but here too most of those who can afford to buy it, do so. There seems to be an inherent demand for meat that is usually limited by the ability to pay for it. This view is supported by the number of people whose culture or religion requires them to be vegetarians, but who begin to eat meat if they become sufficiently affluent. There is also the fact that vegetarian foods are often made to look and taste like meat-containing foods, and are often given names normally used for such foods: for example, nut cutlet or vegetable hamburger.

The common demand for meat has often been taken to demonstrate a physiological demand for an increased intake of protein. What in fact it demonstrates is nothing more than that most people like to eat meat when it is available.

The attractiveness of meat lies mostly in its texture and taste. Older animals yield less tender meat because of the increase in connective tissue. Tenderness also depends on the presence of some fat, especially between the muscle fibres. The 'conditioning' of meat increases its tenderness; this is achieved by keeping it for some days during which enzyme action produces some digestion of the meat and thus some degree of softening. This is particularly true for very lean meat, such as game, which has less fat than does meat from farm animals.

The energy supplied by meat depends largely on its fat content, so that 100g may supply as little as 100 kcal or as much as 400 kcal.

Whereas the amount of protein is always around 20g per 100g, the amount of fat can vary between 3g and 40g.

The protein in meat has a high biological value. In addition, meat is a good source of iron and zinc, but it contains little calcium, as has been discovered many times in zoos, where carnivorous animals such as lions have developed rickets when fed meat without the bones they would have chewed in their native environment. Most of the B vitamins are present in flesh, but very little of the fat-soluble vitamins.

Apart from the flesh, many of the viscera are used as human food. Liver and kidneys are excellent sources of vitamins A and D, as well as of the B vitamins and a little vitamin C and protein. All offal, including liver and kidneys, contains a great number of cells and hence of nucleic acid. This gives rise to uric acid during metabolism, so that offal is often restricted in patients with gout.

Cooking makes meat fibres contract and expel some of their fluid contents; the weight of a piece of beef, for example, can be reduced by about 20% when it is cooked. The fluid constitutes the gravy and contains the 'extractives', consisting of salts, especially of potassium and phosphate, amino-acids, creatine and the water-soluble vitamins. Concentrates of this gravy are used for making meat extracts, such as Oxo and Bovril, although the process results in the destruction of much of the thiamin. Various other substances are added to some of the proprietary preparations of meat extracts, and salt is added as a preservative. It used to be thought that such extracts, particularly the first well-known one, Liebig's extract, were highly nourishing, but in fact they add little to the nutritive value of an ordinary diet in the quantities in which they are consumed.

Because most people find the taste of meat highly desirable, and because it is usually relatively expensive, there are very many made-up foods in which meat is 'stretched' by the addition of other components. Sausages, meat pies, haggis, stews and bolognese sauce are a few of the large number of such dishes. Other methods of satisfying the demand are the use of otherwise unattractive parts of the animal in preparations such as corned beef, and the addition of textured vegetable proteins to meat products. The former practice was well described by Upton Sinclair in his novel *The Jungle*.

See also: Appetite; Neolithic revolution; Vegetarianism

Meat extracts

In the manufacture of corned beef, minced meat is extracted with boiling water, and is then separated and concentrated. In its contact with the meat, the water dissolves much of the soluble constituents of the meat, which consist of nitrogen-containing substances such as creatine, urea, peptides, amino-acids and purines, the water-soluble vitamins and potassium and phosphate salts. These are also the sorts of components that gravy contains when meat is cooked in the home; one of them is likely to be glutamate, which as MSG is used a great deal to enhance flavours.

When commercial meat extracts are made, a high concentration of salt (sodium chloride) is added in order to preserve them.

Meat extracts are either used to add flavour to cooked foods, or made up as a drink. Although very tasty, the amounts used are small, so that their contribution of nutrients, chiefly some of the B vitamins, is also small. The extracts, however, are powerful stimulants of salivary and gastric secretions, and are sometimes given in order to stimulate the appetite of convalescents.

The method of producing the extracts was developed by Justus von Liebig, the famous German chemist. 'Liebig's Meat Extract' was then produced commercially, followed by a number of other brands, including Oxo and Bovril.

See also: Liebig

Medium chain triglycerides (MCT)

The common triglycerides contain chiefly fatty acids with 16 or 18 carbon atoms. The short chain fatty acids (butyric and caproic), with 4 and 6 carbon atoms, occur less commonly in ordinary foods, as do the medium chain triglycerides (MCT) such as caprylic and capric acids, with 8 and 10 carbon atoms. One of the few rich sources of MCT is coconut oil, from which preparations are made for medical purposes. MCT are used in the treatment of jaundice and other affections in which the common dietary fats are not well absorbed. This is because MCT are soluble in water and thus do not require the presence of the bile salts for their absorption, as do the triglycerides that contain the long chain acids.

See also: Bile; Fatty acids

Megavitamin therapy

Since normal bodily functions require the correct balance of essential substances such as vitamins, it has been suggested that an imbalance can be an important cause of a diminished lifespan and a number of diseases such as the common cold, cancer, schizophrenia and heart disease. From this it is claimed that a very large intake of ascorbic acid, or some other vitamin, or a combination of vitamins, will restore the balance and so will be important in prolonging the lifespan, in preventing several diseases, and in curing these diseases if they have occurred. This concept was largely the brainchild of the distinguished American scientist, Dr Linus Pauling, who was awarded the Nobel Prize for his research in chemistry. Pauling introduced the term 'orthomolecular medicine' to describe the megavitamin theory based on this supposed restoration of the body's chemical balance.

The quantities of the vitamins recommended are extremely high: for example, Dr Pauling suggests that the proper requirement of vitamin C to induce perfect health is 3g a day or more, which is at least 100 times the intake of 30mg recommended by the authorities in the UK.

Although some medical practitioners have used this therapy, especially in the US, the few properly conducted tests that have been carried out have failed to demonstrate any convincing benefits other than those attributable to a placebo effect. For example, children with Down's Syndrome have not shown the improvement for which claims have been made. Moreover, large doses of even the water-soluble vitamins, those of the B group and vitamin C, may not be without danger. For example, megavitamin doses of vitamin B_6, recommended for premenstrual tension or for fluid retention, have produced disturbances of movement and sensation.

See also: Vitamins

Mellanby, Edward (1884–1955)

Edward Mellanby was one of the most important contributors to our early knowledge of the vitamins. After graduating in physiology at Cambridge, his first appointment was with F. G. Hopkins, whose work in nutrition influenced what became Mellanby's main area of research.

He went on to qualify in medicine, and then became lecturer and later Professor of Physiology at King's College for Women, London University. This became Queen Elizabeth College, and Mellanby's research there on vitamin D initiated an interest in nutrition that culminated in the establishment of the renowned Department of Nutrition at that college.

Mellanby next became Professor of Pharmacology at Sheffield University, and later secretary of the Medical Research Council.

His most important work was the induction of rickets in puppies on a diet deficient in 'fat-soluble A', and its cure with cod liver oil. He also showed that cereals, especially before milling, have a rachitogenic (rickets-producing) effect, due to what Mellanby called a toxamine; this was later shown to be phytate. He maintained that the effect was due to a deficiency of vitamin A, and that there was no separate vitamin D. He was also convinced that vitamin A deficiency was involved in the causation of several diseases, including respiratory infections, toxaemia of pregnancy and some neurological conditions such as sub-acute degeneration of the cord. These views, many of which were later proved wrong, do not undermine the value of his pioneer experimental work.

In 1946 Mellanby drew attention to the toxic effects of flour that had been treated with agene. As a result, this treatment to accelerate ageing of flour was prohibited.

See also: Ageing; Hopkins; Phytic acid; Vitamin D

Metabolism

The total of all the chemical reactions that are going on in the body is known as metabolism. The term may also be used in a more restricted way, for example to refer to the metabolism of fat.

Since all the metabolic reactions of the body end up by releasing energy, the total is sometimes referred to as energy metabolism. In the end, they involve the oxidation of food components, and produce heat. Because of this, the energy metabolism of the body may be assessed by measuring either the amount of heat the body is producing, or the amount of oxygen it is using.

See also: Basal metabolism

Microbes

Living organisms that cannot be seen by the naked eye, sometimes called micro-organisms or germs, are often colloquially called microbes. Only a few of the very many sorts of microbes cause human disease, that is, are pathogenic to human beings. Among the vast majority of microbes that do not cause human disease, some have commercial uses in the manufacture of foods such as beer and cheese, or in the manufacture of leather, and some cause disease in animals but not in man. The various groups of pathogenic microbes are proto-zoa (causing, for example, malaria), fungi (e.g. athlete's foot), bacteria (e.g. tuberculosis, diphtheria) and viruses (e.g. measles). New groups of microbes have also been identified during the past few years; an example is mycoplasma, one species of which causes atypical pneu-monia in human beings.

Milk

People have for long consumed the mammary secretion of a variety of animals. These are almost invariably domesticated vegetarian animals, and include the cow, buffalo, camel, goat, reindeer and sheep, and occasionally the mare and the ass. By far the greatest proportion of milk comes from the cow, although in India and eastwards to the Philippines, as well as in parts of Africa, milk comes mostly from the buffalo. Different species produce milk with quite different amounts of the major components – carbohydrate, protein and fat (see Table). The high proportion of fat in reindeer milk is exceeded by that in whale milk, which reaches 35%.

Cows' milk is widely consumed in its liquid form; however, much is distributed in dried form, especially as aid to developing coun-tries.

The carbohydrate in milk is entirely lactose, which for some people limits its consumption because of lactose intolerance. The protein is a mixture of casein, amounting to about three-quarters of the total; the rest is mostly lactalbumin.

The fat in cows' milk contains more of the short chain fatty acids than does that of human milk, and less of the polyunsaturated acids, notably linoleic acid. It has a wide range of vitamins; it has little vitamin C but a high content of riboflavin. The vitamin C slowly diminishes with time, but the riboflavin is sensitive only to daylight, especially strong sunlight. Milk in colourless bottles exposed to sunlight can lose 50% of its riboflavin within a few hours.

The major mineral element in milk is calcium. A pint of milk, about 600ml, contains some 700mg. It has also reasonable amounts of other mineral elements except iron. An infant, especially one born prematurely, is likely to become anaemic if fed beyond the age of 4–5 months largely on milk with no added source of iron.

In relation to the calories it supplies, milk has a wider range of essential nutrients, in more worthwhile amounts, than most other foods. However, it is not only human beings who find milk an excellent source of nutrients; many micro-organisms can flourish in milk. Since some of these may be pathogenic, it is necessary to take precautions to ensure that milk is safe for human consumption. The commonest contaminant used to be the bacteria of bovine tuberculosis sometimes present in the milk of cows with this disease. Another disease of cows that could contaminate milk was brucellosis, the organism of which produces undulant fever. Many people, especially children, used to develop tuberculosis, especially of the bones, and this often resulted in long periods of hospital treatment and considerable deformity. Other diseases too could be carried by milk infected by organisms transmitted from, for example, people who were handling the milk.

Milk is now one of the safest foods, because almost all milk sold in developed countries has been heat treated. The only exceptions in the UK are small quantities available from supervised farms, which are allowed to sell their milk only directly to individual customers and not to dealers for resale.

The commonest form of heat treatment is pasteurization, in which the milk is heated to well below boiling point for a short time. This kills pathogenic organisms, but other bacteria, including some lactobacilli, will survive. Cooled, pasteurized milk will therefore keep fresh for a few days, but not indefinitely. However, a very short treatment at a temperature higher than that used for pasteurization gives UHT milk (ultra-heat treatment), which, in sealed containers, will keep for several months even without refrigeration. Pasteurized milk has a detectable flavour, and UHT a somewhat more marked flavour. Sterilization produces quite a distinct flavour; the milk is heated for a significantly longer time than for the processes of either pasteurization or ultra-heat treatment, but, unlike these processes, there are no prescribed processes or times for sterilization.

The average consumption of milk in the UK is about 4–5 (2¼–3 litres) pints a week.

Milk is an emulsion, that is, the fat is dispersed in tiny droplets as globules. It is this that gives milk its white colour. The fat droplets tend to rise to the surface, but they do not coalesce. As a result, after a time, the upper part of the milk is visibly separated from the rest by what is sometimes called the cream line. This separation can be prevented by the process of homogenization. It consists of forcing the milk through a very small orifice, which breaks up the larger fat globules into smaller ones. As a result, the size of the globules, which in fresh milk ranges from $1–18\mu$m (1μm = one thousandth of a millimetre) is now much more uniform, between $1–2\mu$m. This makes homogenized milk look whiter and taste creamier than it does before processing.

Skimmed milk still contains almost all of the protein, lactose, mineral elements and water-soluble vitamins that were present in the milk. Because it is a by-product in the manufacture of butter, and because it is readily dried, it is available in large quantities at quite low prices. For this reason and especially because it is a highly nutritious food, dried skimmed milk forms a large and important part of the food aid sent to developing countries.

Milk may be dried by evaporation of the water, by allowing it to drip on to heated rollers, or by the more expensive method of spraying it into a chamber into which heated air is passed. Roller-dried milk does not reconstitute as well as the more expensive spray-dried milk, and some of the protein may be damaged by the heat.

COMPOSITION OF SOME MILKS

Amounts in 100ml

	PROTEIN g	FAT g	CARBOHYDRATE g	ENERGY kcal
Cow	3.5	3.5	5.0	65
Buffalo	4.3	7.5	4.5	105
Camel	3.7	4.2	4.0	70
Ewe	6.5	7.0	5.0	110
Goat	3.7	5.0	4.5	75
Mare	1.3	1.2	5.5	30
Reindeer	10.5	22.5	2.5	250
Human	1.1	6.2	7.5	70

Evaporated milk is reduced by heat until it reaches about half its original volume. Condensed milk is concentrated somewhat more, to about one-third of its volume, and has had sugar added to it.

See also: Lactose intolerance; Pasteurization

Millet

There are several species of this rapidly growing cereal, which can be harvested within 10 or 11 weeks of sowing. It is grown especially in India, in parts of Africa, and in the Altiplano plateau of the northern Andes in South America. In spite of its rapid growth, it is not as attractive in taste as rice or wheat. Since it has no gluten, it cannot be made into bread, but is used either as a gruel or is made into flour and cooked as flat cakes rather like tortillas or chapatis. For these reasons, it is being replaced in many places by other cereals. Nevertheless, it constitutes a major item of food in many parts of the world.

Sorghum vulgare is grown especially in India, in some areas of which it is known as juar; in South Africa, it is often known as kaffir corn, and in West Africa as guinea corn. Among other species are *Chenopodium* in South America and *Panicum* in China, Japan and parts of Arabia and Africa. The species known as teff is found exclusively in Ethiopia. Millet in North America is grown for animal feed and not as a food for human consumption.

See also: Cereals

Mineral elements

Some of the essential nutrients – the proteins and the various vitamins – are organic molecules of varying complexity and configuration; all of these are made up of atoms of carbon, hydrogen and oxygen, and some include nitrogen and occasionally phosphorus and sulphur. The mineral elements, on the other hand, can be present in the diet in all sorts of compounds, but most commonly they appear as simple salts.

About 25 mineral elements are present in the body, in very different quantities. However, the fact that an element is present does not necessarily imply that it has some special function to perform and that it therefore needs to be supplied in the diet. A few appear to be present fortuitously, simply because they are picked up from the soil by plants and so appear in the food chain; they are then not essential nutrients.

The Table gives a list of the elements found in the body, and whether they are known to be essential nutrients, that is, whether the body needs to receive supplies of the element in the diet.

Deficiency of some of the elements is seen in farm animals or occasionally in intensively reared poultry. These deficiencies occur far more readily than does deficiency in human beings; this is either because the feed prepared for the animals has not been designed to include all the nutrients required, or because the soil and thus the pasture is naturally deficient, or because livestock is fed for many years on the same pasture, so that it becomes depleted of one or more of the required mineral elements. Examples that have occurred include phosphorus deficiency in cattle, copper deficiency in sheep, and manganese deficiency in poultry.

If an element is part of a tissue or a compound that is itself essential, then it is clearly needed in the diet, at least during the process of growth. It will also be needed by adults if there is a constant loss from the body in the urine or through the skin. This is true, for example, of sodium, calcium and iron. Some elements, however, are not known to be a constituent of any essential bodily component, but are nevertheless known to be essential in the diet because deleterious effects result from a diet lacking them. If an element is required in very small amounts, and if it is likely to be present in most foods usually eaten by human beings, its essential nature can be demonstrated only in animals in laboratory conditions.

In some instances, it has been necessary to use the most sensitive new methods of analysis, the construction of specially purified foods and special containers, the elaborate filtration of the air, and the siting of the laboratory as far as possible from industrial areas, before it is possible to demonstrate that animals do not thrive on diets free from a particular element. An example of such an element is nickel. Because of the difficulty of carrying out the necessary experiments, and because of the continuing improvements in techniques, it may be that elements now considered not to be essential will have to be reclassified.

The amount of an element that is needed is determined by studying the effect of varying the amounts of it in the diet. In animals, these diets are fed for a long period, and the growth and health of the animals are assessed as well as the state of the organs after death; the requirement is the amount in the diet that just prevents observable ill-effects. In human subjects, such experiments cannot be continued for long periods lest they result in permanent harm. For this reason, balance experiments are performed, in which different amounts of the elements are given for only a few days at a time; the requirement is taken as the minimal amount that prevents net loss to the body.

The amounts of the different elements required by the body vary considerably. Those required in quite small amounts are referred to as the trace elements, but the cut-off point is not universally agreed. Many experts include zinc among the trace elements, but not iron, although the body requires about the same amounts of each in the diet – some 10–15mg a day.

As with all the other soluble constituents of the body, the amounts of the mineral elements carried by the blood tend to be kept fairly constant. There are two main ways by which this is effected. One is by variation in the amount excreted in the urine; this is what happens to sodium, potassium and phosphorus. These elements, especially sodium, are usually absorbed from the diet in amounts greater than those required, so that excretion of the excess enables the body to regulate the concentration in the blood. The second way in which a constant concentration is achieved is by regulating the amount absorbed from the gut; the unabsorbed excess is then simply excreted in the faeces. An example is iron.

Both of these methods work well when intake is within limits, which differ for different elements; beyond these limits, the adequacy of the regulatory mechanism fails. When sodium intake falls, urinary excretion falls, but when intake is very low, some excretion still occurs and the body loses sodium. When iron intake rises, faecal excretion rises, but when intake becomes very high, some increased absorption does occur and the body accumulates iron.

It has been suggested that deficiencies of zinc and some other mineral elements can be detected by measuring the amounts in the hair. It is, however, doubtful whether this is at present a practical and reliable procedure. Firstly, the quantities of the minerals in the hair are extremely small, so that both the hair sample and the materials and apparatus used for the assay require a degree of preparation beyond the capacity of any but the most sophisticated laboratory. Secondly, there is as yet not enough information about the quantities that can be considered normal and those that can be considered indicative of deficiency.

MINERAL ELEMENTS IN BODY

CERTAINLY ESSENTIAL			
Calcium	Ca	Nickel	Ni
Cobalt	Co	Phosphorus	P
Copper	Cu	Potassium	K
Fluorine	F	Selenium	Se
Iodine	I	Silicon	Si
Iron	Fe	Sodium	Na
Magnesium	Mg	Vanadium	V
Manganese	Mn	Zinc	Zn
Molybdenum	Mo		

POSSIBLY ESSENTIAL		NOT ESSENTIAL	
Arsenic	As	Aluminium	Al
Chromium	Cr	Boron	B
Tin	Sn	Cadmium	Cd
		Lead	Pb
		Lithium	Li
		Mercury	Hg
		Strontium	Sr

The Table gives the chemical symbol for each element.

Some of the elements may have to be transferred to a different column from the one indicated, as research reveals more information.

See also: Dietary requirements; Nutrient balance tests

Mineral oils

Mineral oils are derived from the crude oil found in the earth and consist mostly of mixtures of hydrocarbons, which contain only hydrogen and carbon in their molecules. The crude oil is separated in refineries into a large number of products; these range from gases and highly volatile petroleum, through diesel and lubricating oils, to solid materials such as paraffin wax.

The best known example of a mineral oil that may enter the diet is liquid paraffin. Taken regularly and in large amounts as a laxative, it can lead to deficiency of the fat-soluble vitamins, because it dissolves these from the food during its passage through the gut, and carries them out of the body. The use of mineral oils in food is strictly limited, because there is evidence that tiny droplets of oil may be absorbed and deposited in the liver. It is also possible that small amounts of the impurities the oils contain may be carcinogenic, so that those few that are permitted have to be of the highest purity.

Wax is allowed on Gouda and Edam cheeses; some mineral oil is sometimes used on the skin of citrus fruit. It is permitted on some dried fruits in order to keep them moist.

Mineral waters

Water that comes from natural springs has long been thought to have special properties in maintaining or restoring health. Whatever their origin, such waters contain only very small quantities of mineral salts. They may also be carbonated, that is, contain carbon dioxide gas; occasionally, the waters as they arise from the springs have had carbon dioxide added to them before the water is bottled. The salts are mostly the chloride, carbonate, bicarbonate and sulphate of sodium, calcium and magnesium; occasionally, iron salts are also present, and rarely hydrogen sulphide with its characteristic unpleasant odour.

There is, however, a considerable variation in the amounts of these and other dissolved solids. Some have as much as 3.5g/litre, and some less than 0.1g; the higher quantities are more likely to affect the taste.

It is commonly supposed that, as well as containing salts and other constituents to promote health, mineral waters are less likely to cause illness because they are free from bacteria. They certainly are most unlikely to contain pathogenic organisms, but that is also true of tap water in any advanced country, and indeed in public water supplies in most countries. As for non-pathogenic organisms, there are just as many in still mineral waters as in tap water; carbonated waters do contain fewer of these harmless bacteria, presumably because some sorts of bacteria are less likely to survive in the presence of carbon dioxide.

There has been a rapid increase in the consumption of mineral waters in the 1980s. There are several possible reasons for this: people

DIRECTIONS

FOR

IMPREGNATING WATER

WITH

FIXED AIR;

In order to communicate to it the peculiar Spirit
and Virtues of

Pyrmont Water,

And other Mineral Waters of a similar
Nature.

By JOSEPH PRIESTLEY, LL.D. F.R.S.

LONDON:

Printed for J. Johnson, No. 72, in St. Paul's
Church-Yard. 1772.

[Price One Shilling.]

may dislike tap water in which chlorine can be tasted, they may believe that it contains lead, they may not wish to drink water to which fluoride has been added, or they may find repugnant the knowledge that much tap water has been recycled several times through human and animal bodies.

In the early part of this century, some waters were claimed to have radioactive properties. In Iran, this is no longer listed on the bottle, but as recently as the 1970s it was possible to be served mineral water in a bottle that had not been replaced and still had the claim for radioactivity printed on it.

One of the lesser-known publications of Joseph Priestley (1733–1804), the discoverer of oxygen, is a short book published in 1772 in which he demonstrates how to make carbonated water by the production of carbon dioxide from chalk to which sulphuric acid has been added, and then passing the gas into ordinary tap water. He did this because of claims that the natural carbonated mineral water from the German spa town of Pyrmont was a cure for scurvy, on the theory that the curative action of vegetables and fruits was that they fermented in the body and produced carbon dioxide. Priestley's objective was to persuade the British Navy to use this as an alternative to supplying fresh fruits and vegetables to their personnel.

See also: Scurvy

Minot, George Richard (1885–1950)

The term pernicious anaemia now seems melodramatic because its treatment has become simple and effective during the last 50 years or so, and especially during the last 30 years. This transformation of a disease that was almost invariably fatal is due to the work of several people, including Minot.

Minot was born in Brookline, near Boston, Massachusetts, in 1885. He graduated in medicine and worked mostly in the Harvard Medical School as Professor of Medicine. He was also director of the medical research laboratories in Harvard and held consultancies in several other hospitals.

His research interests had always been on the problems of blood diseases. The work of Whipple (1878–1976) on the usefulness of some dietary constituents, especially liver, in the treatment of the anaemias led Minot to try liver on his private patients with pernicious anaemia. The encouraging results led him, with Murphy (b. 1892), to continue research with patients in the Peter Bent Brigham Hospital in Boston. The effects of half a pound of liver a day were so striking that they were able to convince the medical profession in a way that the work of Whipple had not been able to do.

It was not until 1948 that vitamin B_{12} was isolated and shown to be the principle that prevented or cured pernicious anaemia. Nevertheless, by that time the disease had long ceased to be the virtual death sentence it was before the work of Whipple, Minot and Murphy, who in 1934 shared the Nobel Prize for Medicine.

Minot died in his birthplace in 1950.

See also: Anaemia; Liver as food; Vitamin B_{12}

Molasses

The extraction of sugar from the sugar cane involves a series of processes that begin with the crushing of the cane to obtain the juice, adding small amounts of water to the crushed cane to extract more sugar, removing some of the impurities by the addition of lime, and then boiling the solution so as to concentrate it. The sugar now begins to crystallize, and the mass is centrifuged so as to separate the crystals from the thick sugar solution. This is now further concentrated and again centrifuged, and the process then repeated once more. By now it is reckoned that it is not worth attempting to evaporate the solution yet again to get another batch of crystals, and in any case crystallization is now difficult to achieve. All of the sugar solutions produced in this way are known as molasses.

The molasses from consecutive boilings are increasingly brown in colour, and contain less cane sugar (sucrose) and more other sugars and other components. Sometimes, the lighter products are known as syrups and the darker products as treacle or black treacle; the American name for the latter is blackstrap molasses. Golden syrup is a brand name made from an undisclosed process, and the product is described on the container simply as 'Partially inverted refiners syrup'.

With the decreasing amount of sugar in the darker molasses, there is an increase in the amount of mineral elements. Nevertheless, the quantity of, for example, calcium and iron is very small. The same is true for other nutrients, such as some of the more stable B vitamins.

It is believed by many people that its content of nutrients makes blackstrap molasses a worthwhile source of mineral elements and perhaps of other nutrients. However, a significant amount of nutrients would be obtained only if a large amount of sugar and consequently of calories was taken at the same time. To get the daily needs of iron, one would have to eat about 4oz (more than 100g) of blackstrap molasses, and this would provide more than 70g sugar and about 280 kcal; there would also be a gram or so of protein and small traces of some of the B vitamins. The same number of calories from wholemeal bread would come with about half as much iron, but it would also have about 12g of protein and quite appreciable quantities of several B vitamins.

So far, we have been concerned with the molasses from the sugar cane. Molasses from the sugar beet is not used for human consumption because it is extremely bitter. Most of it goes into animal feed and a small proportion of it is used for the fermentative production of citric acid and other materials.

See also: Quantities; Sucrose

N

Neolithic revolution

Man is the only animal that deliberately produces most of his food from the soil by tilling, sowing and reaping, and from domesticated animals. The discovery of food production by agriculture is known as the neolithic revolution. It seems to have taken place independently but not simultaneously in several parts of the world; the exact dates are not known, but excavations of some of the sites date them at about 8000 BC. The ape-like creature that adopted the erect posture and then made and used tools emerged over one million years ago. The neolithic revolution of about 10,000 years ago began a period of man as a food producer that has lasted less than 1% of the time since he emerged as what can reasonably be called 'man'.

Among the earliest crops to be sown were probably accidentally discovered hybrids of the wild grasses that, by later selection, became the cereals, including the barley and the wheat used for early bread-making. At other times, and in other sites, plants with storage roots and tubers became the first cultivated foods.

The earliest animals to be domesticated seem to have been dogs, for protection and for hunting; horses, sheep, goats, pigs and cattle were also domesticated and were used both as draught animals and for food. In some areas, chicken, geese and other birds were additional sources of food.

This food production resulted in a revolution in man's social and cultural development. Instead of a nomadic existence because of having to move on when food sources diminished, people were tied to the land that produced their food. If they lived in a fertile area and if the climate was favourable, they created permanent settlements. The production of food usually yielded more, and more reliable, supplies than did hunting and gathering, while the less mobile existence allowed for storage from season to season. There were thus periods of relative leisure while the crops were growing, or between harvest and sowing, during which there was time for painting, story-telling, and other social and cultural activities. The conditions were also favourable for a rapid increase in population. The neolithic revolution, in more senses than one, sowed the seeds that resulted in the changes we know as civilization. A straight line can be drawn from the people who first deliberately cultivated the soil, to Michelangelo, Newton, Picasso, penicillin and the nuclear missile.

In general nutritional terms, it seems that the neolithic revolution led to a decreased intake of protein, especially animal protein, a decreased intake of fat, and a considerable increase in the proportion of carbohydrate, especially starch and dietary fibre.

See also: Cereals; Omnivorous

Neoplasia

The growth of an organ, or on to an organ, is known as a tumour (a swelling). If the growth consists of normal cells, it is a benign tumour. If, however, it consists of abnormal cells, it is a malignant tumour, or neoplasm, or cancer. The characteristic of a cancer, apart from its abnormal cells, is that it tends to grow into the adjoining normal tissues, that is, to invade them, and to disperse some of its cells through a vein or a lymph vessel so that they act as seeds and set up secondary growths or metastases in other parts of the body.

See also: Cancer

Nicotinic acid (Niacin in US)

This vitamin occurs usually in the form of the amide, nicotinamide (niacinamide in US). Unlike most of the other vitamins, as a chemical substance it has been known for more than 100 years, although its role as a vitamin was recognized only in 1937. One reason for the delay is that it was not until 1928 that pellagra was finally accepted as being caused chiefly because of a vitamin deficiency; further delay occurred because no animal could be made to develop a disease that was recognizably the same as human pellagra. However, some nutritionally defective diets did produce a condition in dogs called 'black tongue', which resembled some aspects of pellagra. This condition was found to be cured by nicotinic acid extracted from liver, and soon after this nicotinic acid was found to be effective in the treatment of human pellagra. Nicotinic acid was thus identified as what had previously been known as the P-P (pellagra-preventing) factor.

Like most of the other members of the B group of vitamins, nicotinic acid, or more properly its derivative nicotinamide, plays a vital part in the metabolic reactions of the body; in particular, it is concerned with the processes of oxidation.

The vitamin can be produced in the body from the amino-acid tryptophan, which is a constituent of most proteins. However, this conversion is not very efficient, so that it requires about 60mg tryptophan to produce 1mg nicotinic acid. To take account of this, the amount of nicotinic acid in a food is given as 'nicotinic acid equivalent', in which allowance is made for the quantity of tryptophan. The contribution of tryptophan is sometimes considerable: 100ml of milk contains about 0.08mg of nicotinic acid, but the tryptophan in the milk proteins contributes 10 times this amount, so that the 'nicotinic acid equivalent' of 100ml of milk is about 0.9mg.

In the opposite direction, the nicotinic acid in some foods, notably cereals, is chemically combined in a compound called niacytin, and this makes it largely unavailable to the body. The vitamin is released when cereals are treated with alkali, as when lime is added to maize in the making of tortillas.

Since the body can readily convert the acid into the amide, it usually does not matter which is used for the treatment of deficiency. This is not true, however, when large doses are taken, because the acid, but not the amide, causes flushing due to dilatation of the blood vessels of

---

NICOTINIC ACID IN FOODS

Recommended daily intake (RDI) for moderately active man – 18 mg nicotinic acid equivalents (NAE)

FOOD	PORTION	NICOTINIC ACID EQUIVALENT, mg
Beef	100g	4
Fish	100g	3
Liver	100g	10
Bread, wholemeal	30g	1.8
Bread, white fortified	30g	1.0
Yeast, dried brewers'	5g	2
Yeast extract	5g	2
Coffee, instant	5g	1.5

The availability of the nicotinic acid in different foods varies considerably, as explained in the text

---

the skin. Other blood vessels are also dilated, so that nicotinic acid in these doses has been used in the treatment of the atherosclerotic disease of the leg arteries, peripheral vascular disease. Some doctors have also given large doses of the acid for reducing high concentrations of blood lipids.

Cooking does not have much direct effect on the vitamin, except that, being water-soluble, some of it can be lost by extraction in the cooking water if this is plentiful and is not used, for example, in soup or gravy.

See also: Amino-acids; Casal; Goldberger; Maize; Pellagra

Nitrates/Nitrites

The addition of potassium nitrate (saltpetre) or sodium nitrate (Chile saltpetre) as a means of preserving foods, especially meat, has a very long history. This process of curing is used in the production of ham, bacon, pickled tongue, corned beef and some sausages.

During the process, the nitrate is reduced to nitrite; for this reason, some manufacturers add nitrite, or a mixture of nitrite and nitrate, directly to foods. Nitrites prevent the growth of many micro-organisms; the most important of these, because the most dangerous, are the bacteria that cause botulism. In addition, the nitrates and nitrites introduce new flavours, partly directly and partly because of the chemical changes they induce in the meat. They also combine with the meat haemoglobin, which tends to go brown in stale meat; the new compound has the more attractive bright red colour.

Other compounds, called nitrosamines, are formed by the combination of the nitrate with substances present in the food known as amines. Experiments have shown that animals can develop cancer when fed nitrosamines in quantities vastly greater than those present in cured meats. Although the amounts that may be added are controlled by legislation, there seems at present no intention of banning the use of nitrates and nitrites.

Babies are especially sensitive to nitrate, which in some areas can be found in tap water in amounts that may cause concern. There is always some nitrate in tap water, but it can be significantly increased by the general use of chemical fertilizers in the field that may drain into the water supply; these contain nitrogen in the form of nitrates, and ammonium salts which can form nitrates. Because babies have little acid in their stomachs, a higher proportion of nitrate is converted into nitrite, and this can react with the baby's haemoglobin so that it is no longer able to carry out its function in transporting oxygen. Special water is available in areas where the local tap water is known to have an abnormally high content of nitrate; in addition, most manufacturers of baby food do not add nitrate or nitrite to their products.

See also: Cancer; Food additives

Novel protein foods

In the world as a whole, the commonest deficiency of a particular nutrient has long been held to be a deficiency of protein (which, for some unknown reason, was called protein malnutrition rather than protein deficiency). Thus, since the 1940s, a major concern of many nutritionists and governments, and of some commercial organizations, has been the search for an inexpensive source of protein that could be used as a food, or as a food additive, in those countries of the Third World where conditions such as kwashiorkor commonly occurred.

Because of this view, a joint committee of FAO and WHO was set up, called the Protein Advisory Group, or PAG. At the same time, three or four very large commercial organizations and many academic departments began to explore the possibility of mass production of high-protein foods. Those that have been, or are, under investigation include the harvesting of plankton, the extraction of protein from green leaves, or the cultivation of micro-organisms. The micro-organisms investigated are algae, bacteria, fungi and yeast, grown on inexpensive substrates such as molasses, crude oil, or methyl alcohol produced from natural gas.

These well-meaning plans soon began to run into several problems not appreciated at the outset. One was that the cost of the projects was much greater than had been forecast; partly this was due to the need for extensive tests to ensure that the proposed new food was not harmful when part of a continuing diet. Another problem was the insufficient appreciation that the new food must be accepted into the habitual diet, and not simply accepted when offered once or twice. It had been widely believed that people whose diet was short of protein would accept a rich protein source into their diet because of some sort of nutritional instinct. In spite of well-known examples to the contrary, such as the fact that people who developed beri-beri did not give up polishing their rice, it was believed that the abolition of protein deficiency required only that protein-rich food be made available at low cost. The fact is that people may try a new food once or twice, but will not eat it habitually if it does not appeal to their taste or fit into their pattern of eating. This is true however high its nutrient content; the nutritional value of a food that is not eaten is precisely zero.

It was also not recognized originally that the problem was not really a deficiency of protein in the diet; it was much more a deficiency of energy, that is, of food in general. When energy intake is inadequate, more than the usual amount of dietary protein is used by the body as a source of energy rather than to supply the amino-acids necessary for rebuilding tissue protein. Thus, protein deficiency and energy deficiency are closely linked. It follows too that in these circumstances an increase in dietary energy, even without an increase in dietary protein, can often make good a deficiency of protein and not only a deficiency of energy.

These considerations have resulted in a decreased emphasis on producing foods especially rich in protein, and an increased emphasis on producing palatable foods that, like all foods, should have a reasonable nutrient density. Again, the recognition of the link between the requirements for energy and for protein led to the abandonment of the term protein malnutrition, and the introduction of the term protein-calorie malnutrition (PCM), and more recently protein-energy malnutrition (PEM).

See also: Algae; Appetite; Dietary instinct; Population; Protein-energy malnutrition; Unconventional foods

Nucleoproteins and nucleic acids

All living cells, except mature human red blood cells, have nuclei which contain nucleoproteins, consisting of nucleic acids bound to different proteins. The nucleic acids are of two main types. Ribonucleic acids (RNA) occur mostly outside the nucleus of the cell, and are concerned chiefly with controlling the manufacture of the body's proteins, including its enzymes. Deoxyribonucleic acids (DNA) occur inside the cell nucleus, and are concerned in the hereditary character of the individual, and in transmitting these characters to its offspring.

The body has no difficulty in producing the DNA and RNA it requires, so that it is not necessary that they be present in the diet. On the other hand, they do occur in foods that are very cellular, such as fish roe, kidneys, liver and brain. Because DNA and RNA contain purines in their molecules, they give rise to uric acid in the body; this is why the cellular foods are often restricted in patients with gout.

See also: Gout; Phosphorus

Nutrient balance tests

One of the ways in which one can determine whether a diet is providing an adequate quantity of a particular nutrient is to measure the balance of intake and output of the nutrient.

Consider a nutrient such as calcium, one of the essential mineral elements. So long as a person is having enough, or more than enough, to meet his physiological needs, the amount taken in the food will be equal to the amount excreted – in the faeces, urine and sweat. There will, that is, be a balance between calcium intake and calcium excretion: between calcium gain and calcium loss. The only exceptions to this will be a rapidly growing child, or a pregnant woman, or a person whose body is repairing a sizeable wound. In these instances, some calcium will be retained in the body, so that excretion will be less than intake, a condition that is known technically as a positive calcium balance. On the other hand, if an adult's intake of calcium is less than its excretion, he will be in negative calcium balance, indicating a diet that is inadequate in calcium.

The same situation applies to the other essential mineral elements, and to water. It also applies to protein, for although the protein not used by the body is itself not excreted, the nitrogen it contains is excreted. Moreover, by far the largest proportion of the nitrogen intake is that found in protein, and so constitutes by far the largest proportion of the nitrogen excretion. Thus, the measurement of nitrogen intake and excretion is a measure of nitrogen balance, so that it can be used to identify an adequacy or deficiency of protein in the diet.

One of the uses then of the balance method is to discover whether the diet being consumed provides enough of the nutrient under investigation. It can also be used as a method of assessing the requirements of the body for this nutrient. A person is given a diet complete in all the nutrients except the one being investigated. It will be found that the amount of the nutrient excreted exceeds the amount in the diet. This amount is then increased, and again the amount excreted is measured after sufficient time for the body to adjust. The procedure is repeated until a level of intake is reached that is the minimal amount that produces a balance. This intake then is the minimal requirement of the nutrient. Alternatively, one can begin with a diet containing more of the nutrient than is required, and reduce this at intervals until intake falls below excretion.

It is not possible to use this method directly for the vitamins, since any amount that exceeds requirements tends, at least in part, to be metabolized, and the metabolic products excreted are either difficult to identify, or do not accurately reflect the quantities of unused vitamin. On the other hand, there is a method that depends on measuring urinary output of the vitamin, or of its major metabolic product, which can still give a reasonable indication as to the adequacy of the current dietary intake. The method is based on the idea that, if the habitual intake of a vitamin exceeds the body's requirements, the tissues contain as much of the vitamin as they need, i.e. they are saturated. If then a large amount of the vitamin is taken, some of it (or some of its metabolic product) will spill over into the urine. On the other hand, if the habitual intake has been below requirement, all or most of a large dose will be absorbed by the 'unsaturated' tissues, and retained in the body, so that there is little if any left to be excreted in the urine. By this means, it has for example been found that a healthy adult is saturated with vitamin C when the average daily intake is something like 50–60mg a day.

See also: Dietary requirements

Nutrient density

When food is available that people can afford, they will eat enough to meet their energy ('calorie') requirements – and perhaps even more; the only important exceptions are illnesses, including anorexia nervosa, and the unavailability of foods that are appetizing. Since, however, the body requires a diet that supplies adequate nutrients as well as adequate energy, people need to choose the right sorts of foods as well as the right quantities. In simple terms, this may be stated as choosing foods that bring with them a reasonable supply of nutrients in relation to their calories. Thus, if a particular food is eaten in an amount that supplies 20% of the body's energy needs, it would be a 'good' food in respect of, say, protein if it supplied at least 20% of the body's protein needs.

This assessment of the nutrient quality of a food is referred to as its nutrient density. It is calculated, as we have seen, by finding whether the proportion of the body's needs for energy carries with it the same proportion of its needs for a particular nutrient, or series of nutrients. In mathematical terms, the nutrient density is the content of the nutrient in 100g of food expressed as a proportion of the RDI (Recommended Daily Intake) of that nutrient, divided by the energy content in 100g, expressed as a proportion of the RDI of energy

$$\frac{\text{Nutrient in 100g}}{\text{RDI of nutrient}} \div \frac{\text{Energy in 100g}}{\text{RDI of energy}}$$

If the figure obtained for nutrient density is greater than 1, then in respect of that nutrient the food has a high nutrient density.

Values of nutrient density do not help in assessing the value of a total diet, which is best done by calculating the total amounts of energy and of the nutrients consumed in, say, a typical week, and comparing these totals with the RDI values. Nutrient densities are however of use for comparing the comparative nutritional values of items used as alternatives within a diet: a slice of bread or a piece of cake; 100g meat or 100g baked beans; a boiled egg or 25g Cheddar cheese.

Nutrients

The items in food that are not used for producing energy ('calories'), or not only for that purpose, are the nutrients. Specifically, they are the vitamins, linoleic acid, mineral elements and protein – or more correctly, the amino-acids. In describing the nutritional value of a food, it is therefore necessary to describe its content both of energy and of nutrients.

Nutrition

The field of nutrition can be defined briefly as the study of the relationship between people and their food. It asks, and attempts to answer, questions relating to food production and processing, factors that determine food choice and ways in which this may be changed, the nutrient value of foods, the effects of excess or inadequacy of food or of particular nutrients, and the role of diet in causing or preventing or curing disease. It thus requires a knowledge of some aspects of physiology, biochemistry, clinical medicine, psychology, sociology and epidemiology.

Nutrition education

Nutrition is taught at several different levels.

(1) *Nutrition education of the public:* It is now evident that people do not necessarily choose a correct diet, even if the appropriate foods are available and people can afford to buy them. Dietary instinct alone, that is, does not ensure the correct dietary choice. The improvement in such diets requires a change in behaviour, and this is the objective of programmes of nutrition education. Although nutrition education is part of health education, it presents difficulties that do not exist, for example, in the attempts to stop people smoking or to undergo immunization against some specific infectious disease.

It is often imagined that nutrition education, like other aspects of health education, consists simply in instructing people about nutritional needs, the nutritional values of foods, and the ways these should be chosen so as to provide a nutritious diet. But the imparting of knowledge does not guarantee the appropriate change in behaviour. Only a few of the many programmes of nutrition education of the public have been evaluated, even fewer evaluated in terms of changed dietary behaviour rather than in terms of acquisition of knowledge, and almost none has in fact been found to have succeeded in changing dietary behaviour. Most people in Western countries know that eating sticky confectionery and sugar promotes dental decay, or that eating excessive amounts of food leads to overweight, but the high prevalence of tooth decay and obesity indicates that knowing is not necessarily doing.

One major problem is that there are several sources of nutritional information, and they are often inconsistent and even contradictory. Talks on the radio or television, or articles in newspapers or magazines, tend to be the most reliable in content, but are not always so. Information from food manufacturers is usually factually correct, but sometimes misleading. It is indeed arguable whether good feeding practice is best encouraged by the current emphasis on describing nutrients, their actions, the effects of deficiency, and the nutrient content of common foods; the chief dietary fault, especially in Western countries, is the over-consumption of nutritionally undesirable foods. It is the reduced consumption of these undesirable foods rather than the increased consumption of desirable foods that can be expected to restore the primary role of food instinct in determining choice.

(2) *Nutrition education for health workers*: Nurses, doctors and other workers have to give nutritional advice as part of their professional activities. It is widely believed by the public that these trained people are the ones who are best qualified in nutrition and especially able to give practical advice on how to maintain health and how to accelerate healing of disease by nutritional means. Unfortunately, medical and para-medical students are rarely taught much about nutrition, and what they are taught tends to have little bearing on what practical advice they should give.

(3) *Dietitians and nutritionists*: The training of those who intend to be professional dietitians or nutritionists is now carried out in a few universities and colleges in the UK. The first courses in Europe for dietitians began in London University in 1931, in what later became Queen Elizabeth College; the first course in Europe leading to a degree in nutrition was begun in the same college in 1953. Several other European countries now have schools of nutrition, and in America there are many universities that have courses for both dietitians and nutritionists.

See also: Appetite; Dietary instinct; Dietitian; Nutritionist

Nutritionist

A nutritionist is someone who is knowledgeable in the science of nutrition and applies this knowledge to promoting health, advising on diets for particular individuals or groups, conducting dietary and nutritional surveys, and carrying out research into aspects of diet.

See also: Dietitian

Nuts

From a nutritional point of view, it is reasonable to consider several sorts of nuts together, since they have a similar nutrient content; chestnuts and coconuts are considered elsewhere. One ounce (about 25g) of shelled almonds, Brazil nuts, cashew nuts and walnuts provides about 140 kcal, 4g of protein, 13g of fat, 2g of carbohydrate and 2g of fibre. The protein, like that of cereals, is low in lysine. There is also about 1mg of iron, 0.3mg of thiamin, and 0.2mg of nicotinic acid; other vitamins and important mineral elements are present in only small quantities, and there is no vitamin B_{12} or C.

These nuts are often considered, for example by vegetarians, as a rich source of protein because they contain about 15% of protein. However, they also contain about 50–60% fat, so that the nutrient density in terms of energy is lower than all but the fattest cuts of meat. Thus, 100 kcal from nuts comes with perhaps 3g of protein, whereas 100 kcal from an average slice of beef comes with 8–10g of protein. Again, it is not difficult to eat a couple of small boiled eggs, providing about 15g of protein and 300 kcal; it would, however, be difficult to eat 100g of almonds and Brazil nuts, also providing about 15g of protein, but with some 550 or 600 kcal.

Botanically, groundnuts are not nuts.

See also: Groundnuts; Quantities

O

Oats

Oats, a cereal that grows well in a temperate climate, contain little gluten, and so are not suitable for making bread. Milling removes the husk, but usually leaves the germ. Oatmeal has about 12% of protein and about 8.5% of fat, both higher than in other cereals. The high fat content is responsible for the relative ease with which oatmeal becomes rancid. Rolled oats are more convenient than oatmeal for making porridge. They are produced by crushing the grain between heated rollers so that it is partially cooked, and the enzymes that accelerate rancidity are destroyed. Uncooked oats, mixed with sugar, nuts and dried fruit, make the Swiss breakfast food muesli, which is taken with hot or cold milk.

Johnson's *Dictionary of the English Language*, published in 1755, has the famous definition of oats: 'A grain, which in England is generally given to horses, but in Scotland supports the people.'

Oats now play a smaller part in the diet of Scotland, but are still made into oatcakes and sometimes mixed and cooked with water and milk and possibly a little whisky.

Roasted oats have been used in France, it is said, as a substitute for vanilla.

See also: Cereals

Obesity

Obesity is the condition in which an individual accumulates an excessive amount of body fat. The body of an average adult man contains about 12% of fat, and that of an average adult woman about 25%. It would usually be assumed that a person is obese if there were more than 20% of fat present in a man or 30% in a woman. On the other hand, for most people, the existence or otherwise of obesity can be determined fairly readily by looking at oneself, without clothes, in a full-length mirror.

Commonly, the assessment of whether an individual is obese or not is by determining body weight. The Table gives the latest UK figures for the 'normal' weights of men and women of different heights. It must be remembered, however, that a greater weight than average may be the result of well-developed muscles, as in athletes, rather than an excess of body fat.

Fat accumulates in the body when more food is consumed than is used. It is usual to refer to both the amount consumed and the amount used in terms of their energy, expressed in lay language as calories, or in professional language as joules.

In simple terms, then, it can be said that fat accumulates when caloric input exceeds caloric output. This is usually interpreted as saying that people will become overweight, and perhaps obese, if caloric intake exceeds caloric need; that is, if they eat more than they require.

If this were true, a person whose weight remains constant over long periods, with an average intake of say 2,500 kcal a day, would have had unconsciously to control his food intake within a very narrow range, since a surplus of intake over needs by only 1%, that is 25 kcal a day, would result in an accumulation of 2lb of fat in a year, or 20lb in 10 years. A constant weight would then require a most sensitive mechanism to regulate precisely the amount of food eaten to the number of calories expended.

This seems highly unlikely. It is much more likely that there is at least some degree of adaptation in the number of calories the body can lose so as to match the number of calories consumed. Thus, the body would not simply be matching caloric input to caloric output, but also modifying caloric output to help match caloric input. Such a mechanism, in which both sides of the equation can be altered, would bring caloric balance into line with other balance mechanisms, such as the control of the body's temperature or of the body's fluid content. The degree to which this adaptation occurs is probably not very great, and is certainly not easy to measure; no doubt it also varies from person to person. The adaptation to an intake somewhat greater than requirements is one aspect of thermogenesis.

Obesity then will arise when more food is consumed, in terms of calories, than the calories the body expends. The total amount of calories produced is the sum of those produced by basal metabolism, by physical activity, and by thermogenesis.

All this may be summarized by saying that a calorie intake above requirements is a necessary but not sufficient condition for the production of obesity.

Having said that obesity arises when caloric intake exceeds caloric expenditure rather than caloric requirement, it is still necessary to ask what is the reason for this eating to excess. In some people there may be some physiological disturbance, possibly hormonal, that results in an uncontrollable disturbance of eating behaviour. For the majority of people, however, it seems to derive from a greater than normal desire to achieve the pleasure of eating. Here it is useful to distinguish between hunger and appetite. Inquiry among overweight people usually reveals that it is only particular foods that are taken to excess and that are found to be especially tempting. Mostly, they are manufactured foods or drinks, often items that are sweet or contain alcohol. The reason for consuming them is not to satisfy hunger through their caloric content, but to derive pleasure irrespective of their caloric content.

It is still not certain what role heredity plays in producing obesity. The difficulty is that the fat child of fat parents may result simply because of the undesirable eating habits adopted by the child. However, studies with identical twins brought up separately suggest that a small part of the tendency towards obesity is genetic.

Few comprehensive studies have been made of the prevalence of obesity. If it is defined as a body weight of more than 20% above the standard weight for height, then obesity affects about one-third of the adults in many Western countries. There is general agreement that it has increased in these countries during the last 50 years or so, and also that it is now more common in infants and young children than it used to be.

In Western countries, it is commoner in the lower economic classes than in the higher classes, and also commoner in women than in men. In the higher classes, it is the men who tend to put on excessive weight, and their wives who keep to the current fashion of being slim. Thus, one factor that determines the presence or absence of obesity is the expectation of other people in the class to which one belongs.

Disadvantages of obesity: Obesity in Western countries, especially among upper-class women, is considered undesirable chiefly for aesthetic reasons. Among men, the concern about being fat is less common than in women, and usually induced by considerations of health; the simplest statistic is that a middle-aged man who is 10kg (25lb or so) overweight can expect to die four years earlier than one of normal weight.

Specifically, there are several diseases associated with overweight. Excessive weight may produce varicose veins and osteoarthritis of the knees, hips and spine. Accidents are more common in obese individuals, as are gall-bladder disease, high blood pressure, angina pectoris and heart failure. Perhaps the most common complication is diabetes, which in turn may lead to kidney failure and blindness. In overweight women, infertility is more common; if they do become pregnant, they are more likely to have toxaemia, and more difficulty during childbirth. Children suffer from not being able so easily to join in games and from being teased by their peers.

Prevention: The prevention of obesity should ideally begin in infancy, so that a child is brought up without becoming accustomed to sweet foods and drinks. This incidentally serves another equally important objective, in that most of these foods are poor in nutrients as well as rich in calories. A conscientious mother will not only avoid feeding her child with inappropriate foods, but will see that they are not normally found on the table, or better still in the house.

Cure: The suggested cures for obesity exist in great numbers and in great variety, as is evident from the large number of books and articles about the subject. This is another way of saying that they are mostly ineffective as a long-term cure, although they may satisfy those who wish to lose weight for a special occasion. Permanent weight reduction can be achieved only by permanently reducing food intake, or by permanently increasing caloric output through increasing physical activity, or by both. In practice, it seems even more difficult to persuade overweight people to increase activity than to reduce food intake.

The multiplicity of diets recommended for weight reduction occurs because of the multiplicity of foods and drinks that contribute to caloric intake. If the diet is designed for permanent weight reduction, that is, as a permanent new pattern of eating, it needs to be nutritious as well as reduced in calories. It needs also to consist of foods that are readily available, and preferably of foods enjoyed by the whole family. Nevertheless, in so far as the diet that has caused the obesity was one freely chosen by the individual to suit his preferences, any diet designed for weight reduction is bound to be less attractive either in quality or quantity. It is therefore important that the individual accept this from the outset, rather than resist any change because it involves some degree of hardship. It is in the hope of being able to lose weight while continuing to eat as before that the obese so persistently demand some anorectic agent or other aid to slimming that eliminates the necessity of changing the diet. It is possible that some harmless stimulant to thermogenesis may one day be discovered that will help to reduce overweight without the need to limit caloric intake more than a little, if at all.

Many doctors believe that it is important to change the way over-

GUIDE LINES FOR BODY WEIGHT, IN POUNDS
(Royal College of Physicians, 1983)

MEN

HEIGHT (ft ins)	ACCEPTABLE AVERAGE	ACCEPTABLE RANGE
5 2	123	112–141
5 3	127	115–144
5 4	130	118–148
5 5	133	121–152
5 6	136	124–156
5 7	140	128–161
5 8	145	132–166
5 9	149	136–170
5 10	153	140–174
5 11	158	144–179
6 0	162	148–184
6 1	166	152–189
6 2	171	156–194
6 3	176	160–199
6 4	181	164–204

WOMEN

HEIGHT (ft ins)	ACCEPTABLE AVERAGE	ACCEPTABLE RANGE
4 10	102	92–119
4 11	104	94–122
5 0	107	96–125
5 1	110	99–128
5 2	113	102–131
5 3	116	105–134
5 4	120	108–138
5 5	123	111–142
5 6	128	114–146
5 7	132	118–150
5 8	136	122–154
5 9	140	126–158
5 10	144	130–163
5 11	148	134–168
6 0	152	138–173

weight people eat as well as what they eat. This has resulted in an increased emphasis on behaviour modification.

See also: Anorectic agents; Appetite; Behaviour therapy; Body fat; Thermogenesis; Thyroid gland

Oedema

The water in the body normally makes up about 60% of its volume, that is, about 40 litres. Of this, some 3 litres are in the blood, 12 litres in the tissues between the cells, and 25 litres in the cells themselves. The 12 litres of tissue fluid are filtered out of the narrow, thin-walled capillaries, leaving the protein in the blood; it then flows around the cells and returns to the blood through other capillaries and through lymph vessels. The outflow is largely caused by the pressure of the blood in the capillaries, and the inflow partly because of their low blood pressure but chiefly because of the osmotic pressure in the capillaries, due mostly to the protein they contain.

Ordinarily, the amount of tissue fluid is fairly constant. If, however, the pressure in the capillaries is too high, or the osmotic pressure of the blood too low, there will be an excessive amount of tissue fluid formed. This may show itself as a swelling of the limb or other part of the body, or the accumulation of fluid in the abdomen or other body cavity; this is known as oedema. Severe oedema is called dropsy, although this is now rather an old-fashioned term.

Here are some examples of oedema. When you stand for a long time, or sit still, for example in an aeroplane, your feet are likely to swell. This is because the blood flow back to the leg veins from the heart is lessened, because of the cessation of the 'massaging' action of the contracting muscles that normally help to keep the blood moving. If the muscles are not contracting and the blood not being properly removed from the veins, the result is an increase in pressure in the capillaries and so an increase in tissue fluid. Similarly, varicose veins can lead to oedema in the legs, again because the veins are not very effectively doing their job in helping the return journey of the blood from the legs.

In heart failure, the heart is working with less than its usual efficiency in getting the blood circulating, so that again it tends to back up in the veins. The resulting accumulation of tissue fluid takes place in all the tissues of the body; however, because of gravity, the resulting oedema will tend to accumulate in the legs again, but if the person is lying down, there may be some swelling in the back. In addition, fluid may accumulate in the abdominal cavity; this is known as ascites.

To the nutritionist, two of the causes of dropsy are of special interest. One is the oedema of starvation or in kwashiorkor; this is caused chiefly by the lack of dietary protein, which results in a fall in the protein content of the blood and hence its osmotic pressure. The second cause that specially interests the nutritionist is the accumulation of salt in the blood. This happens particularly in kidney disease, but also to some extent in heart failure. The result is an excessive amount of salt in the tissue fluid and therefore an increase in the water that goes with it. For these reasons, restriction of salt is a common feature of the treatment of these two conditions.

See also: Famine; Kidney; Protein-energy malnutrition; Sodium

Offal

The word was originally off-fall. In meat, it referred to the entrails or intestines, but it now includes everything removed when dressing the carcase, leaving only the muscle and bone. It therefore now refers to the tail, heart, liver, spleen, pancreas, thymus, tripe, kidneys, brain and tongue. Many of these items are richly cellular and are therefore often restricted in the diet of patients with gout.

In the milling of flour, offal is the bran and germ, that fraction of the wheat berry that is removed before white flour is made.

See also: Liver as food

Oils

The best description of 'oils' is the dictionary definition: they are liquids that have a smooth and soft feel, and are not soluble in water. Some oils are known as essential oils; these are volatile, and have a smell and flavour that enable them to be used as flavouring agents and in perfumes.

Edible oils are triglycerides that unlike those in butter or lard are liquid at ordinary temperatures, above, say, 10°C (50°F). Most of these oils are produced from plants; the best-known are from cotton seeds, corn (maize), coconuts, groundnuts (peanuts), olives, palm nuts, rape seeds, safflower seeds, sesame seeds, soya beans and sunflower seeds. The largest production is of soya bean oil, but there has recently been a great increase in the production of rape seed oil. Unlike most of the other sources of edible oils that grow in tropical or sub-tropical or Mediterranean climates, rape is easy to grow in temperate climates such as those of Canada and Northern Europe. Rape seed oil contains erucic acid, a fatty acid with 22 carbon atoms that, in large quantities, damages the heart muscle in animals; new varieties of rape have, however, been developed, with seeds containing only 2% of erucic acid compared with 40% in the older varieties.

The oils are produced by crushing or pressing the nut or seed, and sometimes additional oil is extracted by alcohol. The oil is then refined by neutralizing the free fatty acids they contain, and washing with water. Most oils tend to have a high proportion of polyunsaturated fat, compared with the low proportions present in solid fats from land animals. On the other hand, there is also a high proportion of poly-unsaturated fats in marine animals, that is, in fish and whales. Because of the high content of these acids, most edible oils readily become rancid, chiefly through oxidation to aldehydes and ketones, and hy-drolysis to fatty acids; this is more likely to happen if the oils have not been adequately refined. Rancidity is accelerated by the presence of metallic ions, and is inhibited by vitamin E and by some additives such as butylated hydroxyanisol (BHA) or butylated hydroxytoluene (BHT). In some highly unsaturated oils such as linseed oil, the effect of oxygen on thin layers of the oil results in 'hardening', which is a combination of oxidation and polymerization.

The oils are also partly decomposed by heating. Repeated mild heating reduces the amount of vitamin E and of the polyunsaturated fatty acids, and increases the content of oxidized products. It has often been suggested that the accumulation of such products, for example in oil used for repeated frying, can be harmful to health, but this has never been demonstrated. Strong heating of oils produces an acrid product with the appropriate name of acrolein.

Not all edible oils, however, are rich in polyunsaturated fats. Olive oil has a high proportion of oleic acid, which has one double bond; this is thus mono-unsaturated, but not polyunsaturated. Cocoa butter, palm kernel oil and coconut oil have a relatively low proportion of polyunsaturated fats and a relatively high proportion of saturated fats.

The residue remaining when the oil has been removed from the seeds contains protein, often in substantial proportions; this oil cake or seed cake forms an important feeding stuff for farm animals.

The edible oils contain vitamin E, but, with one exception, no other vitamin. The exception is red palm oil, which is a rich source of carotene. The palm seed (nut) is the source of two different oils; the fleshy outer part contains the red palm oil, and the hard inner part contains the colourless palm kernel oil.

See also: Antioxidants; Cooking fats; Fatty acids; Food preservation; Vitamin E

Old age

The increase in the expectation of life in affluent countries is not so much that there has been an extension of the natural lifespan, but that many more babies, children and young people now survive into adulthood compared with the numbers surviving in earlier times; it was the numerous deaths at an early age that reduced average longevity.

In the UK, the proportion of people over the age of 65 has more than doubled during the last century, and – unless there is some catastrophe – is likely to reach 14% or 15% of the total population by the year 2000. Surveys in Britain have indicated that just over 3% of people of this age have definite clinical signs of malnutrition; more than 10% have low concentrations of haemoglobin and other components of the blood, which also suggests dietary inadequacy. If one accepts a figure of only 3%, there would be at least 200,000 malnourished elderly people in Britain at the present time.

The uncertainties of determining nutritional requirements are greater for the elderly because of the greater difficulties of measuring dietary intakes and especially of the paucity of information on nutrient requirements from experiments with elderly volunteers, from blood analysis and from physical examinations. Nevertheless, the conventional view is that the undoubted lower energy requirement of the elderly compared with the middle-aged does not extend to a lower requirement of nutrients. This is to be interpreted as accepting that the elderly require less total food but containing a higher proportion of nutrients, that is, their food should be of a higher nutrient density than that recommended for the middle-aged. This could be achieved by reducing the intake of foods of low nutrient density, such as confectionery, soft drinks, cakes and biscuits, and increasing the proportion of such foods as milk, eggs, meat and fish, fruit and vegetables. Those dietary surveys that have been done with the elderly find that they do eat less than younger people, but they eat the same foods in roughly the same proportion.

See also: Longevity

Olive oil

Olive trees grow mostly in the Mediterranean region, and have been cultivated since biblical times. The trees are small, grow slowly and can live for hundreds of years still bearing fruit. Whereas the olives for pickling and eating may be harvested either unripe or ripe, only the purplish ripe fruit is used for the manufacture of olive oil. It has a characteristic taste and is preferred by many people for cooking and use in salads, although it is relatively expensive. It is also used in small amounts for making high-class soap; it used to be used in canning fish, but the less expensive oils are now used. Olive oil contains a high proportion of the fatty acid, oleic acid, which has one double bond. It is thus a 'mono-unsaturated acid', and neither increases nor decreases the concentration of cholesterol in the blood.

See also: Fatty acids; Oils

Omnivorous

There are a very few species of animals that can eat almost any plant or any animal. These omnivorous (all-devouring) species include the rat and the pig, as well as man. Being omnivorous has one great biological advantage, in that these animals are not restricted by their diet as to where they can live. Other animals can live only in areas where their more limited diet is available; for example, the koala eats the leaves from only a few of the many varieties of eucalyptus trees, and has never made its home other than in the Antipodes. Pigs, rats and man, on the other hand, can be found in virtually every country in the world.

As well as having this advantage, however, an omnivorous animal presents a unique problem. Animals that are not omnivorous rarely suffer from nutritional deficiency provoked by the wrong choice of foods; if their usual foods are not available, they may go hungry, or even starve, but they will not eat other foods that may or may not provide all the essential nutrients. On the other hand, omnivorous animals may readily be tempted to eat such foods; man in particular is able to make foods that may be eaten whether or not they are wholesome or nutritionally adequate, and irrespective of the availability of more appropriate foods.

See also: Appetite; Dietary instinct; Neolithic revolution

Organic

In chemistry, the term originated as a description of a general characteristic of chemical substances found only in living organisms. It transpired that most of these contained carbon atoms in their structure, and organic chemicals now refers to all those containing carbon, except cyanides and carbonates.

In relation to foods, organic describes those grown without the use of chemical fertilizers or pesticides; only fertilizers derived from animals or plants are permitted. The term is sometimes extended to include animals reared without antibiotics or hormones, or foods prepared without the addition of synthetic colours, flavours or preservatives, and having undergone only minimal refining.

Osmotic pressure

If a salt solution is put into a pig's bladder, and this is then suspended in water, some of the water will enter the bladder, but the salt will not pass out of the bladder into the surrounding water. The bladder is semi-permeable, allowing water but not salt to pass through; it is as if the salt pulls water into the bladder in order to dilute the solution, and so reduce the difference in the salt concentration inside and outside the bladder. This 'pull' of the salt solution is the osmotic pressure. It can be arranged that a tube is fixed to the bladder in such a way that the solution rises in it as water enters. Thus, like a barometer, the height to which the solution rises will be a measure of pressure; when it stops rising, the pressure of the column in the tube pushing downwards has become equal to the osmotic pressure pulling water inwards.

The blood capillaries are permeable not only to water but also to salt, glucose, urea, and other small molecules; they are, however, not permeable to the proteins of the blood, which are appreciably larger molecules. It is these proteins then that determine the osmotic pressure of the blood. They are responsible for holding water in the blood vessels. If the amount of albumin and other proteins in the blood falls, there will be an excessive 'leaking' of water, salt and other dissolved materials into the tissues, and the result will be dropsy or oedema. Famine oedema occurs because the lack of food causes a fall in the concentration of blood albumin.

See also: Oedema

Osteomalacia

A deficiency of vitamin D combined with a deficiency of calcium produces in adults a disease called osteomalacia. It used to be common in the Far East, but is less common now. Especially prone to the disease were women whose bones were depleted of calcium by repeated pregnancy. Characteristics of the disease are pain, which may be very considerable, and extreme distortion of the bones. This is especially true of the backbone, the ribs and the legs, and the woman may end by being stunted and so crippled as to be unable to walk.

A different disease met with in adults, especially among the elderly, is osteoporosis, which is also caused by a demineralization of the bones, but in a somewhat different way that can be differentiated from the bones of osteomalacia by X-ray. Instead of a general diminished density which produces less of a shadow on the X-ray, the bones in osteoporosis have a somewhat moth-eaten appearance. The chief result is that the bones are exceptionally brittle and liable to be fractured with less than normal trauma. Particularly common is fracture of the thigh bone (femur) in the narrow neck that is attached to the pelvis.

There is no generally recognized cure for the condition. Various treatments have been tried, including the administration of the male sex hormone or of calcium salts. However, since people with osteoporosis may also be suffering from some degree of osteomalacia, treatment with vitamin D as well as calcium is often recommended, and some degree of improvement may be achieved.

See also: Bone; Calcium; Vitamin D

Oxalic acid

Most foods have less than 10mg oxalic acid or oxalate in 100g; a few, notably unripe tomatoes and some varieties of strawberries, may have between 10mg and 20mg. However, beetroot has about 100mg in 100g, parsley about 150mg, and rhubarb and spinach between 300mg and 600mg. Quite large quantities are present in the leaves of rhubarb, and these may be enough to cause poisoning by damaging the lining of the mouth and stomach, and interfering with the action of the nerves and muscles.

In the small amounts normally present in foods, the only importance of oxalic acid is that it combines with calcium in the diet and so reduces the amount of this mineral element that can be absorbed.

As well as deriving oxalate from the diet, the body can synthesize it from citric acid. Some urinary stones contain calcium oxalate, as well as other calcium salts, but it is not known to what extent this is derived from dietary oxalic acid or from excessive synthesis. Nevertheless, if a person is known to excrete an excessive amount of oxalate in the urine, or to have had kidney stones containing oxalate, it is reasonable to restrict the consumption of spinach and rhubarb, as well as chocolate and cocoa.

See also: Calcium; Poisons in food

Oxidation

When a candle burns, or when the cut surface of an apple or a potato darkens, chemical reactions are taking place in which components of the candle, or of the apple or potato, undergo a change by combining with the oxygen in the air. These components are undergoing oxidation. None of the reactions will take place in a vacuum, or if the oxygen in the air has been used up, or prevented from reaching the cut surface.

The burning of the candle clearly produces energy in the form of heat and light. Less obviously, the darkening of the apple or potato also produces energy, but at a much slower rate. The fact that, without air, animal life is not possible, demonstrates that the oxygen in air is needed also to provide animals with the energy for their essential living processes. This was neatly demonstrated by John Mayow (1643–79), who showed that both a burning candle and a living mouse use up the same component of air, after which the air supported neither the burning of the candle nor the life of the mouse. These experiments, however, were virtually forgotten for 100 years, until the work of Priestley and Lavoisier.

Within the body, the production of energy is carried out chiefly by the oxidation of glucose, fat and amino-acids, derived from food. These oxidations occur at a controlled rate, determined ultimately by the energy needs of the body. In some instances, the energy is released in stages, and the early stages may take place anaerobically, that is, by chemical changes not requiring oxygen. Thus, muscular movement first involves the conversion of glucose into lactic acid, a reaction that is anaerobic. Later, the lactic acid is oxidized with the release of more energy.

Usually, anaerobic reactions release much less energy than do aerobic reactions; for this reason, when glucose is converted into lactic acid, much more glucose is used in producing a given amount of energy than would be used if the glucose were oxidized. This apparent wastage, however, is so to speak corrected in the next stage, when a small amount of the lactic acid is oxidized and releases enough energy to convert the rest of the lactic acid back into glucose. As a result, only about one-fifth of the glucose that has taken part in these reactions is, in the end, oxidized.

All this adds up to the fact that oxidation is the essential activity that keeps the cells and the tissues alive, and ultimately the body itself. This is why we breathe, and why we die if we cannot breathe, or if the blood ceases to bring oxygen to the eseential organs like the brain.

See also: Aerobic/Anaerobic; Energy

P

Palm oil

The importance of the oil palm, which is a major source of edible oils, derives from the fact that its yield per acre is greater than that of any other source of animal or vegetable fat. It originated in West Africa, but is now cultivated in several tropical countries where there is heavy rainfall; it does not require a particularly good soil. Major production is now in Malaysia and Indonesia, as well as in central and western Africa. Fruit-bearing begins when the palm is 5 years old, and the maximum yield continues from about 10 years until the tree is 50 years old.

The fruit consists of a skin surrounding a fibrous pulp, within which is the seed or kernel. Both the pulp and the kernel contain oil. The oil from the pulp is orange-coloured, because of its high content of carotene. Most of this oil is consumed locally in stews and other dishes; the rest is exported and some is added to margarine for its colour. The palm kernel oil is pale yellow, and almost all is exported to be used in making margarine and soap.

See also: Carotene; Margarine; Oils

Pangamic acid

This is sometimes known as vitamin B_{15}. Like Laetrile, sometimes known as vitamin B_{17}, pangamic acid is not in fact a vitamin. That is, it does not have the characteristic feature of a vitamin as a dietary substance that is essential for the preservation of complete health. It has been suggested that it is of value in the treatment of some cardiovascular and rheumatic diseases, but this has not been demonstrated. The substance itself occurs in many foods containing several of the B vitamins – liver, yeast, and many seeds.

Its chemical name is N-di-isopropyl-glucuronate.

See also: Vitamins

Pantothenic acid

As the name implies, this vitamin is found almost universally in foods; the exceptions are the processed foods such as sugar, fats and oils. Like many of the other members of the B group of vitamins, it is a co-enzyme involved in several metabolic processes in the body. Deficiency in rats results in failure to grow, and greying of the hair. Deficiency does not ordinarily occur in human beings; it has, however, been produced in volunteers given a specially constructed diet. People with grey hair have taken pantothenic acid by mouth, or applied it directly to their hair; their optimism has not, however, been rewarded.

Papaya

The fruit of the tropical papaya or paw-paw tree usually resembles a rather small elongated melon. Its most interesting feature is that it contains the enzyme papain, a protein-digesting enzyme which is sometimes used to tenderize meat. The leaves of the tree also contain some of this enzyme, and are occasionally wrapped around meat and left for some time to make it tender. The enzyme is unusually resistant to heat; most enzymes are destroyed when heated to 45°C or 50°C, but papain works best at a temperature of 80° or so. Because of this, it continues to tenderize meat as its temperature is raised in the early stages of cooking, but it too is destroyed above 80°.

Papain is sometimes included in pharmaceutical preparations designed for the treatment of indigestion, but it is doubtful whether it has any beneficial action.

The papaya fruit itself gained a great deal of publicity in the early 1980s, when it appeared, together with pineapple, as an important ingredient in the popular and incredible Beverly Hills Diet for Weight Reduction. The reason was the absurd notion that foods that are not digested are converted into body fat, so that the inclusion of papaya and pineapple helps to digest foods and thus prevent this undesirable but quite fictitious process.

See also: Digestibility; Enzymes; Obesity

Para-amino-benzoic acid

Known also by the much simpler acronym PABA, this is one of the substances that is a vitamin for some organisms but not for man. The fur of rats becomes grey when PABA is absent from their diet, and many sorts of bacteria cannot grow without it. The sulpha drugs have a chemical structure similar to that of PABA, and they act by blocking the access of PABA to the bacteria, so that they die. PABA is part of the more complex molecule folic acid, which is a vitamin for man.

See also: Vitamins

Pasteurization

As its name implies, pasteurization is a process derived from the discovery of the French chemist, Pasteur (1822–95), that foods such as milk deteriorate much more slowly if they have been heated. The process is now carried out for the dual purpose of destroying pathogenic (i.e. disease-producing) organisms in a food, and for increasing its keeping quality. It happens that most pathogenic organisms are more readily destroyed than are non-pathogenic ones, which is why pasteurized milk is safe to drink but will still go sour after a time. The effect of pasteurization of milk on health is best seen in the dramatic fall in bovine tuberculosis, which affects especially bone, in the UK and USA since the 1930s. There has been a similar fall in the less common disease of brucellosis.

The process is now used for foods such as milk, beer and fruit juices. The standard for milk is a temperature of 63–66°C for 30 minutes, or 72°C for 15 seconds; the apparatus is designed so that both heating and subsequent cooling are extremely rapid.

Ultra heat treated (UHT) milk is first homogenized and then heated to at least 132°C for one second. It is usually packed in cartons and will keep for several months, even without refrigeration, if the carton is kept sealed. Sterilized milk is homogenized and put into bottles before being heated to 104–113°C for 15–40 minutes. Provided the bottle is not opened, the milk will keep for many months.

See also: Milk; Food preservation

Pears

Like apples, pears are fruits that are technically known as pomes, the fleshy part developing from the coat of the ovary. Cultivated pears are derived from the wild pear, *Pyrus communis*, which grows in many European countries, especially in the south. They are also found in America and in China. It is more difficult to produce new varieties of cultivated pears than of cultivated apples, and so fewer varieties are seen.

The flesh of the pear is characterized by its content of small, slightly gritty particles. These are made up of cells having thick, hard walls, the so-called stone cells. The wood of the pear tree, especially of the wild pear, is hard and has a beautiful grain, so that it is much in demand by furniture makers.

Pellagra

Now far less common that it was as recently as the 1930s and 1940s, pellagra is a disease that was endemic in many countries in which there was severe poverty combined with a diet consisting largely of maize. The features of the disease are dermatitis, diarrhoea and dementia, so that it was called the disease of the three 'Ds'. It was described first in the middle of the eighteenth century by Casal, who drew attention to its occurrence in northern Spain. It occurred too in southern France, Italy and the Balkans; later, it spread to Egypt and southern Africa. In the southern United States, it appeared after the Civil War and spread rapidly among the blacks and poor whites; even as late as 1940, there were still some 4,000 deaths due to the disease. Since that time, the disease has virtually disappeared in the United States, where improved living standards have reduced the dependence on maize as an important part of the diet; it is, however, still seen in southern Africa and parts of Asia.

The symptoms of pellagra begin with weakness, loss of weight, depression and irritability, and a characteristic redness of the skin of the face, neck and other exposed parts of the body. It was this latter symptom that led to the Spanish name, quoted by Casal, 'mal de la rosa'. The tongue is red and swollen, and diarrhoea is often present although constipation may be present instead. The mental signs are usually severe depression rather than the dementia included as one of the three Ds. The mental disturbances are often severe enough for the patient to be taken to a mental hospital. The redness of the skin may give way to cracking and exudation, or more slowly to the production of thickened, darkened skin that resembles chronic exposure to sunlight. It is from this that the modern name of the disease derives, *pelle agra* being Italian for rough skin. The appearance of the skin around the neck is known as 'Casal's collar'. Signs of other nutritional deficiencies, especially of riboflavin, are often found to accompany those of classical pellagra. Untreated, the weakness and mental deterioration progress, and death may ensue.

The cause of pellagra has produced much discussion and not a little confusion. Casal himself thought that a poor diet was largely responsible, but this was disputed by many of his successors. It was, for example, suggested that the victims had inherited a poor constitution that made them especially susceptible to the disease. When it was accepted that the diet played an important role in causing the disease, and that the main constituent responsible was maize, some held that it was because the maize was contaminated with mould, or alternatively that the whole diet was deficient in protein.

The work of Goldberger in the 1920s and 1930s led to nicotinic acid being identified as the major 'pellagra-preventing' factor (P-P factor), but there are in fact three features of maize that determine its central role in producing pellagra. Firstly, it does not contain much nicotinic acid, although white bread, oats and rye contain less. Secondly, the vitamin in maize is present in a bound form as niacytin, from which the nicotinic acid is not released in the alimentary canal. It is, however, released when maize is treated with an alkali; this explains why pellagra has always been rare in Mexico, where the maize is mixed with lime before being made into tortillas. The third reason for the association of pellagra with maize-eating is that the body can make nicotinic acid from the amino-acid tryptophan, but this is lacking in the protein of maize, zein. In the usual Western diet, about half of the nicotinic acid in the diet comes from tryptophan, mostly from the proteins of meat, milk and eggs.

Treatment of pellagra with nicotinic acid (or nicotinamide) produces relief of the gastro-intestinal features within days or a week or two; the mental features recede more slowly, if at all. Unless the general diet is improved as well, treatment with the pure vitamin alone may leave a residue of pathological changes due to other deficiencies, for example, the cheilosis and the ocular and perigenital features of riboflavin deficiency.

See also: Antivitamins; Casal; Goldberger; Maize; Nicotinic acid; Vitamin history

Pemmican

For expeditions, or for iron rations in the services, pemmican is often carried as a concentrated food. It is made from a mixture of dried meat and fat. It keeps well because it contains only 3–4% water, and it may be flavoured with herbs and spices to make it more attractive. If it contains, as it often does, about equal quantities of protein and fat, 100g of pemmican will provide between 500–600 kcal.

Peptic ulcers

Gastric ulcers and duodenal ulcers are known as peptic ulcers. They are of special interest to the nutritionist both because of the suggestion that diet plays a part in causing them, and because of the considerable effort that has gone into devising special diets for treating them.

Like ulcers of any other part of the body, ulcers in the stomach or duodenum begin with an inflammation of its surface (mucous membrane or mucosa). This gradually breaks down until there is an open sore. Occasionally, it extends more and more deeply into the wall of the organ, until it opens one or more blood vessels, or it extends right through the wall and perforates it. In the former instance it leads to bleeding, which may be very slight and cause nothing but gradual anaemia, but may be extensive and cause death unless surgical intervention can stop the bleeding. In the second instance, it almost certainly produces peritonitis, which is inflammation of the suspending membrane of the abdominal viscera. This may or may not be curable, but immediate surgery is certainly necessary to stop the further entry of gastric or duodenal contents into the abdominal cavity.

The cause of the ulcers is uncertain, although it is perhaps surprising that the mucosa is ordinarily able to resist the combined action of the quite strong hydrochloric acid and pepsin being secreted by the stomach. It is rare for ulcers to be found in the lower part of the duodenum, below the point of entry of the common bile duct conveying the alkaline bile and pancreatic juice, which neutralizes the acid gastric juice.

Gastric ulcers are uncommon in the poorer countries of the world; they have also become less common in Western countries since the end of the Second World War. Duodenal ulcers are, however, as common in some poor countries as they are in Western countries; moreover, in the West, their prevalence seems to have increased recently. While the exact cause of duodenal ulcers is unknown, some associated factors have been identified. There is, for example, an hereditary factor, as shown by its being more common among relatives of those known to have the disease; it is also more common in those belonging to blood group O. Of the environmental factors, smoking increases the risk of developing duodenal ulcers.

As to diet, it is said that irregular and hasty meals predispose to peptic ulcers. Caffeine, alcohol and spicy foods are known to irritate the gastric mucosa, and increase the secretion of gastric juice; they are therefore assumed to increase the chances of developing an ulcer.

Most discussion still revolves around dietary treatment. Until recently, there were several special diets recommended, each with the name of the doctor who had first developed it, with smaller or greater variations upon the same principles. These principles were a regime beginning with little other than milk and eggs, leading to a gradual increase in size and complexity, but continuing with small and frequent meals, and the avoidance of spicy and fried foods. The result could have been called 'white menus', in which typical meals were something like steamed fish with mashed potatoes, followed by a milk pudding. However, it was found that patients who were allowed a much more liberal diet did just as well, so long as they trained themselves to recognize and avoid particular foods that produced symptoms, and continued to avoid spicy foods and to restrict their intake of alcohol, especially on an empty stomach. According to one carefully controlled investigation, however, a high proportion of patients reported a reduction of symptoms with a diet in which only carbohydrate-rich foods were restricted, and this diet was shown to reduce the secretion of both acid and pepsin in the gastric juice. This recalls the fact that, in the early years of this century, 'carbohydrate dyspepsia' was a commonly diagnosed condition.

See also: Digestive juices; Dyspepsia; Inflammation

Peptones

When proteins are being digested, the long chains of amino-acids of which they are composed are broken down into smaller and smaller chains until the amino-acid units are released. There is thus a progression from protein through peptones to polypeptides and finally amino-acids. There is no clear demarcation between peptones and polypeptides, and indeed there is a tendency to use the term polypeptide to indicate all the compounds that contain several amino-acids, but a smaller number than in the original undigested protein.

See also: Amino-acids

pH

pH is a way of expressing how acid or how alkaline a solution is. It derives from the fact that the degree of acidity, or alkalinity, depends on the number of hydrogen ions present in the solution.

We can understand the situation best if we begin by considering pure water, which is neutral, that is, neither acid nor alkaline. In these circumstances, while most of the water is present as molecules of H_2O, a very small part is split into ions – hydrogen ions with a positive electrical charge, and the same number of hydroxyl ions with an equal negative charge. These ions are represented by the notation H^+ and OH^-.

The amount of hydrogen ions in a litre of water is one ten-millionth of a gram. This can be written as $\frac{1}{10,000,000}$g, or, more simply, $\frac{1}{10^7}$g, or even more simply, 10^{-7}g. An acid solution has more hydrogen ions than pure water has; for example, it may have 10 times as many, or 1 in 1,000,000, or 10^{-6}g in a litre. But even writing 10^{-6} for the amount of hydrogen ions is rather clumsy; if someone were to tell you that the acidity of vinegar is 10^{-3}, or the acidity of gastric juice at a particular time is 10^{-1}, or the acidity of a cola drink is 10^{-5},

EXAMPLES OF pH VALUES

	pH
Lemon juice	2.4
Vinegar	2.9
Cider (dry)	3.3
Tomato juice	4.2
Milk (fresh, pasteurized)	7.0
Bicarbonate of soda (1g in 100ml water)	8.1
Washing soda (1g in 100ml water)	10.0

you would soon find yourself thinking only of the small number after the minus sign in 10^-.

If that number is more than 7, the solution is alkaline. Thus, an alkaline solution would have an amount of hydrogen ions considerably less than one ten-millionth of a gram in a litre; for example, it might have one hundred-millionth of a gram, or 10^{-8}, so that the pH is 8.

This is what pH is – it is, so to speak, that small number that comes after 10^-. In mathematical terms it is the negative logarithm (to the base 10) of the hydrogen ion concentration in gram ions per litre.

See also: Acidosis; Buffer

Phenylketonuria (PKU)

The essential amino-acid, phenylalanine, is needed for building up body protein and for making the hormones adrenaline and thyroxine. In producing these substances, some intermediate substances are formed called phenylketones. Occasionally, babies are born with a genetic defect in which there is none of the enzyme necessary for the complete metabolism of phenylalanine. The result is that the phenylalanine that is contained in most food proteins accumulates, together with the phenylketone intermediates; these can then be detected in the blood and in the urine. They are, however, harmful when they exceed very tiny amounts, and they can produce damage to the brain so that mental deficiency ensues.

The condition must be detected and treated soon after birth in order to prevent brain damage, and many countries routinely test all week-old babies for the presence of the phenylketones in the urine or excess of phenylalanine in the blood. The treatment is to restrict the intake of protein, so that it provides just enough phenylalanine to allow for proper growth but not enough to produce brain damage. As the child grows older, he is able to take special foods free from phenylalanine. It is necessary to check the blood from time to time; tolerance to phenylalanine in the blood usually increases so that it may be possible gradually to revert to an ordinary diet by the time the child is 8 or 10.

The routine testing of newborn babies suggests that about 1 in 8,000 have the condition.

See also: Amino-acids

pH of blood

The pH of blood is about 7.4, and it varies very little. It rarely becomes more alkaline than pH 7.6, or more acid than 7.1.

The constancy of the pH of the blood, and hence of the fluids that bathe the body's cells, is achieved by a combination of mechanisms. The first is rapid but limited; the second is slower but unlimited. The rapid method is achieved by the presence in the blood of buffers; substances like phosphates, bicarbonates and blood proteins can as it were mop up acids and alkalis, thus allowing only a very small change in pH. If there were no other method, the buffers might eventually be used up, but this does not happen because of the second, slower and unlimited mechanism. This involves two processes. One is carried out by varying the amount of carbon dioxide, which is acid, in the air expelled from the lungs. The second is by varying the amount of acid or alkali excreted in the urine.

See also: Buffer; Kidney; pH; Urine

Phosphorus

The body of the average adult man contains about 700g of phosphorus. As with calcium, a great part of this is in the skeleton, where it is present mostly in the form of apatite, a phosphate of calcium. However, while only 10g or less of calcium are in the other tissues of the body, more than 100g of phosphorus are found outside the skeleton. The reason for this is that phosphorus plays an essential part in many more bodily functions than does calcium. As phosphate, it is concerned with the absorption of glucose in the gut, and with the metabolism of glucose, fat and protein by the cells of all the tissues. Lecithin, and other compounds of phosphorus with fatty acids, are involved in the integrity and properties of the membranes of all the cells, with the covering sheath – the myelin – of the nerve fibres, and in the transport of fat. The nuclei of all the cells of the body contain nucleic acids, which are compounds of phosphorus, and which are part of the DNA that carries the genetic properties of the cells.

The concentration of phosphorus in the plasma tends to remain constant; the normal amount is between 3 and 5mg/100ml blood. Because of the wide range of living activities in which phosphorus is engaged, it is present, chiefly as phosphate, in all animal and vegetable organs and so in almost all foods. The average intake is about 1,500mg a day, and dietary deficiency of phosphate in human beings never occurs. On the other hand, cattle may develop deficiency because of a shortage of phosphate in the soil. That plants needs phosphate is well recognized, since it is a constituent of many fertilizers.

Probably because of its occurrence in brain and nerve tissue, it has for long been a popular belief that taking more phosphorus in such preparations as bone-ash or glycerophosphates improves one's health, acting as 'tonics'. One manifestation of this is the notion that 'fish is good for the brain', because fish as well as the brain have a rather high concentration of phosphorus compounds. In P. G. Wodehouse's stories, when Jeeves had an especially good idea for getting his master Bertie Wooster out of one of his scrapes, Bertie would say with admiration, 'I see that you've been at the sardines again, Jeeves.' Unfortunately, there is no evidence that the consumption of phosphate, in fish or in any other food, has any effect at all, beneficial or detrimental, on any organ of the body.

See also: Bone; Lecithin; Nucleoproteins and nucleic acids; Phytic acid; Polyphosphates

Phytic acid

Phytic acid is a compound of inositol and phosphoric acid. It occurs partly as the acid and partly as salts such as calcium phytate in plant foods, especially in the bran of cereals, and in pulses and nuts. It readily combines with metal elements including calcium, iron and zinc, and if these are present in only marginally adequate amounts in the diet, phytic acid may reduce their availability sufficiently to cause deficiency. There are, however, three ways in which this hazard is in practice reduced. In the UK, flour for bread-making, except, illogically, wholemeal flour which contains the highest amount of phytic acid, has to have calcium carbonate added to it in amounts more than enough for all the phytic acid present to be converted to the insoluble calcium phytate. Secondly, the yeast used for proving dough contains an enzyme, phytase, that breaks down much of the phytic acid. Thirdly, the body gradually adapts to a high amount of phytic acid in the diet, perhaps by an increase in the amount of phytase in the intestine, so that after a time its effect in reducing the availability of calcium and other elements diminishes.

See also: Absorption; Antivitamins; Baking; Calcium; Mellanby; Yeast

Pica

The eating of items that are not food is found in many parts of the world. Eating earth (geophagia) is, or was, common in some communities, including the southern United States, the Caribbean and parts of Austria. Other non-foods sometimes eaten include coal, paper, vaseline and toothpaste.

Pica occurs frequently among children, who may chew paint from their cots or cosmetics from their parents' bedroom; clearly this may be hazardous. It is also found among pregnant women, who may have an uncontrollable urge to eat or chew some non-food such as wood or vanishing cream, although they are more likely to crave some unusual, expensive food.

It has often been suggested that pica is an unconscious expression of attempts to correct a nutritional deficiency. A pregnant woman demanding peaches when they are not in season is, it is suggested, indicating that she lacks vitamin C; it is not clear, however, why she does not then demand an orange, which is much more readily and far more cheaply available. Again, the fact that many of those who eat earth are anaemic is taken to indicate an instinctive desire to increase their supplies of iron. It is, however, more likely that the geophagia is a cause of the anaemia rather than the result, and occurs because of the reduction of the availability of dietary iron which becomes bound to some of the substances in the earth.

The word *pica* is Latin for magpie, the bird that picks up and eats, or tries to eat, a wide range of items, not all of which are properly food.

See also: Pregnancy

Pineapple

From the point of view of its nutrients, there is nothing special about the pineapple to distinguish it from most other fruits; in particular, its consumption is so small that its contribution to the body's average nutrient supply is almost negligible. It does, however, have one interesting property that it shares with papaya but with very few other fruits. The pineapple contains an enzyme that digests protein, called bromelin, the action of which resembles that of the enzyme papain from papaya. This is the reason why it was included as an important item in the nonsensical Beverly Hills diet, published in 1981.

See also: Papaya; Obesity

Pitta

As a typical bread, pitta is eaten chiefly in Greece, Turkey, Iran and the Arab countries. It is traditionally made with wholemeal or high extraction wheat flour, but white flour is sometimes used. It is allowed to ferment somewhat, so that when it is baked as flat cakes it tends to rise slightly, leaving a cavity in the middle. Often, the pitta is opened down one side and stuffed with various foods, especially vegetables and pickles. This is known as falafel.

Placebo

The word *placebo* is Latin for 'I shall please'. A surprisingly large number of people report an improvement in their symptoms when they have taken what they believe is an effective medicine, even though it is something as simple as coloured water or a pill consisting of nothing but a little flavoured sugar. Sometimes the subjective relief of discomfort or pain is accompanied by objective improvement, such as restoration of the ability to walk in a paralysed individual.

It is also possible to elicit what might be called a negative placebo effect. When a new drug is being tested for its efficacy, care is taken to record any possible adverse effect. Quite frequently people given a perfectly innocuous substance complain that this has been responsible for giving them a headache or making them vomit or keeping them awake.

The importance of these psychological effects is the need to be aware of them when testing a new drug, or when assessing the claimed benefits or harmfulness of some new diet or dietary supplement. In the history of medicine, there are countless examples of what we now know are quite useless drugs or other treatments that were believed to be effective largely on the basis of enthusiastic endorsement by people claiming relief from their ailments, if not indeed complete cures. For this reason, modern testing of a new treatment involves the careful selection of a control group of patients, who are matched with those to be treated. The matching of the control subjects involves choosing individuals of the same age, sex, class and other characteristics that might possibly influence their response. The tested patients will receive the drug or other treatment; the control patients will receive a placebo that is not in appearance or taste very different from this. For ethical reasons, patients will be told in advance the way the test is planned, and that they will be placed at random into one or other of the groups; it will depend entirely on chance whether they receive the new treatment or the ineffective placebo, but they will not be told which. They are promised that, in due course, they will be told what the test revealed about the efficacy of the drug, so that their doctors will be able to prescribe it if it turns out that the drug can usefully contribute to their treatment.

Since the investigators themselves, however careful and scientific, can unconsciously be affected in assessing how good the treatment is, it is usual for the distribution of the patients into the treatment group or placebo group to be done without the knowledge of those who will assess the result of the treatment. Thus, neither the patient nor the assessor knows whether or not the patient is getting the treatment. Such an arrangement is what is known as the double blind test or trial.

Plankton

In the upper layers of bodies of fresh and sea water are numerous tiny living organisms. Some are plants (phytoplankton) which are mostly diatoms and other algae; some are animals (zooplankton), often protozoa and tiny shrimps. They form the beginning of a food chain; a simple example is seen at the Poles, where the phytoplankton are eaten by the zooplankton, mostly the small shrimp known as krill, and this in turn is the main source of food for the whale.

It has for long been suggested that the mixed plankton could be harvested and used directly as human food. The Japanese have been active in research in this field; however, it is still quite expensive to harvest and prepare it in any quantity, and it is not known how well it will be accepted.

See also: Novel protein foods; Unconventional foods

Poisons in food

The consumption of particular foods may produce ill effects in a variety of ways. Some foods are in themselves harmful; in addition, foods that are innocuous can become contaminated so that they carry with them the potential of causing harm.

Among the foods that are inherently harmful are those that affect a minority of people who are especially sensitive. Sometimes this is a true food allergy, sometimes it is a reaction by people who have a biochemical abnormality, as in coeliac disease, favism, or lactose intolerance.

It has been pointed out that some of the foods to which people are most commonly allergic, or hypersensitive in other ways, are those that have become available since the introduction of agriculture, that is, have relatively recently been added to man's diet. The suggestion is that the human family has not had enough time to adapt, through selection, to these foods, notably cereals and milk.

There are, however, some foods with constituents that are universally harmful. This may occur when unusually large amounts of a food are eaten, while smaller amounts are harmless. Examples are nutmeg (which contains myristicin), bitter almonds (cyanide), sprouting potatoes (solanine), and rhubarb, especially the leaves (oxalic acid). Other foods may contain enough of a toxic substance to produce ill effects, even when they are eaten in amounts that would not be considered excessively large. In Western countries, one thinks especially of some sorts of mushrooms and toadstools; in other countries there are the vetch lathyrus, polar bear liver because of its high content of vitamin A, and cassava that has not been well cooked. Some people might consider whole grain foods as being in a sense toxic, because the phytic acid they contain may induce deficiency of zinc and other elements.

Foods may be contaminated with chemical substances, either accidentally or intentionally. In many countries, pesticides or insecticides on fruit or seeds, or hormones in meat, are used in ways laid down by regulations designed to prevent poisoning. Accidental intake of pesticides, sometimes fatal, has occurred most often during manufacture or in careless use by workers on the farm. Occasionally, death has occurred through the consumption of seeds of grain treated with fungicide, but which have been used as food either by accident or in times of severe food shortage or bought from a dishonest source.

Foods may cause harm through being contaminated with living organisms. Beef or pork may be infested with tapeworm, and pork with the worm that causes trichinosis, but the compulsory inspection of meat in abattoirs has virtually eliminated this and other infestations in Western countries. Proper cooking of meat is an additional safeguard.

More commonly, food is infected with micro-organisms. This usually occurs with meat or meat products, but egg and milk dishes may also be contaminated; the microbes are most commonly introduced by the people who handle the food. The commonest organisms are bacteria of the Salmonella group. The most dangerous members of this group are typhoid and paratyphoid, which are also fortunately the least common, especially in temperate countries. Other types of Salmonella are responsible for most of the outbreaks of food poisoning occurring in these countries, varying in severity from a short-lived bout of mild diarrhoea and vomiting, to a more prolonged and more severe attack that may be fatal.

Food poisoning may be caused by the toxins produced by bacteria. The toxin from staphylococci can be produced in food in sufficient amounts to cause vomiting and diarrhoea, sometimes severe enough to cause symptoms within a few hours of consumption of the food. Food is most easily infected with staphylococci through being handled by persons who have skin infections, such as boils, caused by this organism. The most serious disease produced by toxins in the food, now fortunately rare, is botulism. The organism involved produces spores resistant to ordinary cooking, and these can then grow in anaerobic conditions, such as in tinned meat that has been inadequately processed.

Unpasteurized milk may carry infectious organisms, derived either from the cow or from people who handle the milk. Bovine tuberculosis is now rare, not only because of pasteurization but also because vigorous steps to control and in some countries to eliminate the disease from cattle have been very effective. In the UK, similar measures have been taken to eliminate brucellosis, which gives rise to undulant fever. In the days when milk was dispensed from open vessels, almost any sort of pathogenic organism affecting those who handled the milk could be passed on to the consumers.

Thus, eating and drinking can be hazardous. The hazards are reduced by the actions both of the authorities and of the consumer. Legislation controls the kinds of materials that may be used in food production, including additives, and also ensures the inspection of food and its preparation for sale. The consumer is responsible for the hygiene in the home, which ensures that the risk of infection is minimized by proper handling, storing and cooking of food.

See also: **Bacteria**

Polyphosphates

Added mostly to meat, to poultry and to meat products such as sausages and ham, polyphosphates are chemical substances that tend to preserve the colour and reduce spoilage. They also make the product more tender by increasing the amount of water it can hold. Since water adds to the weight of the product, manufacturers are tempted to use polyphosphates for this purpose; putting water into meats, like putting air into ice-cream, costs the manufacturer very little.

See also: **Food additives**

Population

For at least a minimal existence, people need clothing and shelter, but above all they need food. This is why nutritionists have to concern themselves about the current rapid growth of the world's population in relation to the current and future supplies of food.

The population of most species tends to remain constant when considered over a long time, but fluctuates very much in between. The number of births is always high enough to produce a considerable increase in population, were it not for the fact that the number of deaths too tends to be high. The fluctuations in numbers occur mostly because of changes in the number of deaths because of lack or plenty of food, or occurrence of or freedom from natural disasters.

The human population probably did not change much before the neolithic revolution, when agriculture was introduced. It is likely that there was then a slow increase, but this has since accelerated considerably, as the Table shows. The cause was a reduction in the death rate; in the prosperous countries it has fallen from 33–40 per 1,000 population to around 10–12 per 1,000. The causes of this fall are not entirely clear; they include better food supplies and distribution, but particularly improved hygiene, and thus a considerable decrease in infectious disease. New medical treatments such as antibiotics have had a relatively small effect on death rates.

The fall in death rates in the wealthier countries was followed by a considerable fall in birth rates, but this lagged behind; it took 200–250 years before the birth rates approached the low death rates. At present, then, there is only a slow growth in population in the affluent countries, with birth rates only a little above the death rates of 12 or less per 1,000. In the poorer countries, however, there has been a more recent and much more rapid fall in death rates, and only the beginning of a fall in birth rates, so that population growth has been very rapid and continues to be greater than it is in the prosperous countries. In the world as a whole, the present annual rate of population growth is 1.7%, with an increase of more than 70 million people each year.

Several of the poorer countries are making efforts to reduce their birth rates in order to reduce the pressures on food and other resources. This is done largely by making arrangements for the ready availability of physical or oral contraceptives, or by encouraging vasectomy. The Chinese encourage parents to have only one child by a variety of financial incentives and by the creation of a climate of social disapproval. Such policies are often not very successful. This is because people do not find it easy to relate the very personal decision to have sexual intercourse and to interfere with its normal biological consequence of pregnancy, with what must be considered an impersonal nationally planned population policy.

Meanwhile, efforts are being made to increase the supply of food and to improve its distribution. Supplies of conventional foods such as cereals are being increased by the development of higher-yielding strains, irrigation or drainage of land, application of fertilizers, and the use of mechanical equipment. In some areas, the effects have been dramatic enough to have earned the name 'The Green Revolution'. However, the total effect has been disappointing, in that the measures require a high capital investment, and the benefits have mostly been in increasing the wealth of the small already affluent section of the population in the developing countries.

As well as increasing the supplies of conventional foods, much has been done in the search for unconventional foods such as novel proteins. This too has run into unexpected difficulties, largely because of insufficient attention having been paid to the acceptability of the new foods.

Finally, there has been little progress in ensuring the distribution of food according to needs. It is still true that food production is deliberately curtailed in some countries, while food availability is woefully inadequate in others. It is even true that food production within some countries would be more than enough for its own poorly fed portion of the population, but it does not reach all of them. The problem of adequate purchasing power, both for whole countries and for sections of the population of one country, still escapes solution, though it has been on the agenda of the United Nations and its specialized organizations for several decades.

HOW POPULATIONS GROW

BIRTH RATE PER 1,000	DEATH RATE PER 1,000	ANNUAL GROWTH OF POPULATION %	NUMBER OF YEARS FOR POPULATIONS TO DOUBLE
35	34	0.1	700
40	34	0.6	115
40	30	1.0	70
35	15	2.0	35
30	10	2.0	35
20	10	1.0	70
15	10	0.5	140
10	9	0.1	700

These figures have been chosen to demonstrate the way population growth has occurred in the industrialized countries, and is occurring in developing countries, as extreme poverty gives way slowly to affluence. At first, there is a similar high rate of both births and death, so that the population remains more or less constant. The first sign of decreasing poverty is a small rise in birth rate, which remains at this higher level while the death rate begins to fall, so that there is a slight increase in population. The death rate falls further and now the birth rate begins slowly to fall; meanwhile, there is an even more rapid growth in population. Finally, the continued fall in birth rate begins to slow population growth; in due course, death rate and birth rate are only slightly different, or indeed are the same. Now the population grows only very slowly, if at all.

CHANGES IN WORLD POPULATION

YEAR AD	WORLD POPULATION MILLIONS	YEARS FOR POPULATION TO DOUBLE
0	200	
		1,500
1500	375	
		300
1800	750	
		100
1900	1,500	
		60
1960	3,000	
		35
1995 (projected)	6,000	

Figures for current world population cannot be precisely determined; earlier figures are even less accurate, and those before about 1500 AD are only very approximate.

POPULATION IN DIFFERENT AREAS OF THE WORLD 1978

	POPULATION MILLIONS	BIRTH RATE PER 1,000	DEATH RATE PER 1,000	RATE OF INCREASE %	YEARS TO DOUBLE
WORLD	4,219	29	12	1.7	41
Africa	436	46	19	2.7	26
Asia	2,433	30	12	1.9	36
North America	242	15	9	0.6	116
Latin America	343	36	9	2.7	26
Europe	480	15	10	0.4	173
USSR	261	18	9	0.9	77
Oceania	22	21	9	1.2	58

See also: Fertility; Malthus; Neolithic revolution; Novel protein foods; Unconventional foods

Potassium

There is about 140g of potassium in the body, most of it inside the cells. With roughly an equivalent amount of sodium outside the cells in the inter-cellular tissues and blood plasma, these two elements are responsible for maintaining the proper distribution of fluid within the body.

Dietary deficiency of potassium virtually never occurs, since it is present in almost every food, especially those of vegetable origin. Excess in the body occurs only if excretion is impaired, for example by kidney failure. Deficiency occurs only with such conditions as chronic diarrhoea, or occasionally when people take very low-calorie formula diets over long periods. Deficiency may also be produced by the prolonged use of particular kinds of diuretics; many of these are now prescribed together with potassium salts.

Curiously, either deficiency or excess of potassium may cause muscular weakness and abnormalities of the heart.

Because the body's potassium is slightly radio-active it is possible to assess the lean mass, that is, the weight of the body's cells, by the use of a whole body counter.

See also: Basal metabolism; Sodium

Potatoes

With its considerable and secure place in the diets of most developed countries, it is difficult to appreciate that it is only about 200 years since the potato (*Solanum tuberosum*) became a common food beyond its original home in the Andes, from Colombia, through Ecuador, Peru and Bolivia, to the Patagonian end of Chile. It was brought first to North America and soon to Spain during the sixteenth century; it then spread northwards, and became especially popular in Ireland. It was an excellent alternative to cereals, because it produces more food in terms of energy than they do. This made it a particularly valuable crop during the recurrent famines, which in England continued at least until 1800. In Scotland its use was opposed by ministers of the Presbyterian church up to the end of the seventeenth century, on the ground that it was not mentioned in the Bible. In Ireland its popularity became so great that it was a major staple food; thus, when the potato crops failed because of blight in 1845, 1846 and 1847, nearly one million people died and many emigrated, especially to the United States.

In some European countries there was more resistance to this unaccustomed food from the New World. The French chemist, Antoine Parmentier (1737–1813), who later carried out a great deal of re-

TRA·ITÉ

SUR

LA CULTURE ET LES USAGES

DES POMMES DE TERRE,

DE LA PATATE,

ET DU TOPINAMBOUR.

PAR M. PARMENTIER.

Publié & imprimé par ordre du Roi.

Villemin

A PARIS

Chez BARROIS, l'aîné, Libraire, Quai des
Augustins, N°. 19.

M. DCC. LXXXIX.

Avec approbation de la Société Royale d'Agriculture,

search on food, became very impressed by the potato, which was his main item of diet during five years of captivity by the Prussians, beginning in 1748. Later he persuaded Louis XV to try this new food, especially as an alternative to cereals when the crops were scarce. It is said that he overcame the reluctance of the people to accept this new food by asking the king to provide a military guard around the field where he grew his royal crop, so impressing the people with its great value and therefore its desirability. Thereafter, the popularity of the potato in France was assured. The association of Parmentier with the potato is still maintained by the use of his name on menus as a description of a soup that contains potato. Through his promotion of the potato during the 1770 famine, Parmentier was awarded the Besançon prize.

The major constituent of the potato is water, which makes up some 75% of its weight. Most of the solid matter is starch, but there is also about 2% of a high quality protein, and some of the B vitamins. There is also a reasonable amount of vitamin C, which is especially high in new potatoes. In the UK, about one-third of the average intake of vitamin C comes from potatoes, and it is said that, if this food were not consumed, there would be a high prevalence of scurvy among the British population.

Because of the high water content, the energy value is low, so that one would have to eat a lot of potatoes in order to contribute significantly to energy needs. This would result, however, in a significant intake of protein and other nutrients. Thus, 1kg of boiled potatoes could readily be consumed in a day, providing about 800 kcal. This amount of energy would be accompanied by 16g of protein, 3mg of iron, nearly 1mg of thiamin and 8mg of nicotinic acid; the vitamin C content would be some 40mg if they were old potatoes, and as much as 150mg if they were new potatoes.

There are two special features of the potato that contribute to its popularity; these are that it can, with care, be stored for several months, and that it can be cooked in very many different ways.

The green part of the potato plant contains solanine, which is toxic. Solanine also appears when old potatoes begin to sprout. The effects are to produce nausea and vomiting, and abdominal pain.

Not everyone has held the potato in high esteem. Brillat-Savarin (1755–1826), the famous gastronome, wrote: 'I appreciate the potato only as a protection against famine; except for that, I know of nothing more eminently tasteless.'

See also: Poisons in food

Pregnancy

It is convenient to consider separately the various stages of giving birth to a healthy child.

Conception: The severe lack of food occurring during famine interferes with conception, as seen by the development of amenorrhoea. The lesser degrees of nutritional deficiency from which women suffer in various parts of the world do not appear to affect their ability to conceive. At the other end of the scale, however, obesity is known to reduce the chances of conception, and gynaecologists report that weight reduction often helps an overweight woman to conceive.

Pregnancy: The effects of inadequate nutrition do not seem to change the course of pregnancy, with the exception of osteomalacia which may occur from repeated pregnancies in women with a combined deficiency of calcium and vitamin D. On the other hand, poor diet during pregnancy may produce an infant of low birth weight, and thus with an increased risk of perinatal death.

No special dietary recommendations are needed during pregnancy, with perhaps two exceptions. It is important to avoid overweight, and it may be useful to give supplements of folic acid to avoid the small risk of developing megaloblastic anaemia. Otherwise, a diet containing foods of high nutrient density, such as milk, meat, fish, fruit and vegetables, with minimal amounts of foods of low nutrient density, such as sugar, confectionery, cakes and biscuits and alcoholic beverages, will ensure adequate supplies of essential nutrients while helping to prevent overweight.

If a woman has had a miscarriage in previous pregnancies, or if there is any other reason to suggest that the current pregnancy is threatened, some doctors prescribe vitamin E. However, several studies have demonstrated that this will not affect the course of the pregnancy.

Weight gain during pregnancy should be 1–2lb in the first 10 weeks, 6–10lb in the first 20 weeks, and a further 1lb or so a week up to the end of pregnancy. The total gain during the whole of the 40 weeks of pregnancy should be about 28lb.

If the gain is substantially more or substantially less than these figures, search must be made for the cause. The most likely cause of too rapid a gain is excessive food intake, and this should be dealt with during the pregnancy and not postponed until later, so risking the development of hypertension and other complications.

The nutrition of the developing foetus during pregnancy tends to take precedence over that of the mother, the baby being nourished if necessary at the expense of the mother's body. It is possible, however, that the risk of having a stillborn infant is increased if the nutrition of the mother is less than optimal. During the Second World War, there was a reduction in the number of stillbirths among the poorer women of the UK, and this has been put down to the improvement in their diets because of the policy of food rationing.

Childbirth: Chronic malnutrition in the mother from childhood may lead her to have anatomical inadequacies, such as a small pelvis, with consequent difficulty during childbirth and increased risk of damage to the infant. Obesity too is associated not only with difficulties in delivery for the mother, but also with increased risk to the infant.

Protein

The word 'protein' comes from a Greek word meaning basic or primary or fundamental. Proteins are essential components of all living matter. In earlier times, they were called proteids or albuminoids. Since all living organisms are undergoing 'wear and tear', and some are also growing, it is necessary that new proteins shall be constantly made available to them. In green plants, proteins are manufactured from nitrogen-containing and other materials from the soil, together with the carbon dioxide that their leaves take from the air. These substances are first used to build about 20 different amino-acids, which contain carbon, oxygen, hydrogen, nitrogen and sometimes sulphur. The amino-acid molecules act as building blocks, and the plant combines them in different proportions into much larger molecules that constitute the different proteins.

Animals cannot synthesize all the amino-acids as green plants can. Those that they cannot synthesize are called the essential amino-acids; animals, therefore, in order to build up their proteins, have to get proteins from plants, either directly by eating them, or indirectly by eating animals that have eaten plants. The food proteins thus obtained are digested into amino-acids. These are absorbed by the animal and are built into the particular proteins the animal requires by putting together the appropriate amino-acids in the appropriate proportions and in the appropriate order.

The proteins in the diet are digested in the alimentary canal by a series of protein-splitting (proteolytic) enzymes. These include pepsin in the gastric juice, trypsin from the pancreas, and several enzymes in the digestive juices secreted by the small intestine. The food proteins are thus broken down into smaller and smaller fragments, until they are almost totally converted into their constituent amino-acids. But it seems that, at least in some people, part of the original food proteins escapes digestion altogether, and may enter the blood more or less unchanged. Such people may have an allergy to one or more of the proteins in particular foods, such as strawberries, or shellfish, or even milk.

The proteins in foods differ in the extent to which they supply all or some of the essential amino-acids. It used to be the practice to divide the proteins nutritionally into first-class and second-class, depending on whether they were or were not well endowed with the essential amino-acids. This classification has now been abandoned. Firstly, it ignored the fact that people do not eat protein; they eat the foods that may (or may not) contain protein. Moreover, most people get protein from several sorts of food, and it often happens that the amino-acids from these different proteins supplement one another. For example, the proteins in wheat have only rather small quantities of the essential amino-acid lysine, so that bread alone is unlikely to be an adequate source of protein unless very large quantities are consumed. On the other hand, the proteins in pulses – peas and beans – have quite adequate amounts of lysine, but not much of another essential amino-acid, methionine; wheat proteins, however, have quite reasonable amounts of methionine. Thus, a diet that contains both wheat products and pulses could provide a good protein mixture with adequate amounts of all the essential amino-acids including lysine and methionine. The essential amino-acid in a protein that supplies the smallest proportion of the amount required is known as the limiting amino-acid.

A mistaken belief is that all animal foods provide more of the essential amino-acids than do any of the vegetable foods. Gelatin, which comes from animal sources, is in fact a very poor protein, whereas the proteins found in soya beans are of exceptionally high quality.

The elucidation of the arrangement of the amino-acids in different proteins is one of the most important recent advances in biochemistry. The first protein so analysed was insulin, and its structure – that is, the exact sequence of the amino-acids of which it was composed – was determined by Sanger in 1951. Insulin contains only 51 amino-acids, but today we know the sequence of some proteins that contain many hundreds of amino-acids; by 1982, the amino-acid sequence had been determined for well over 1,000 proteins.

The amino-acid sequences of the proteins in the body are fixed with absolute precision by the genes. A change in even a single amino-acid in the sequence, due to a defect in the corresponding gene, can severely affect the functioning of the protein. For instance, the replacement of just one amino-acid by another in the sequence of 580 that make up human haemoglobin causes the serious disease, sickle cell anaemia. Because it is a defect in the gene that leads to the amino-acid replacement, this disease and many others like it are hereditary.

The human body of normal weight contains on average something like 17% of protein. A man weighing 65kg (about 140lb) has about 11kg of protein in his body. Except in starvation, this amount will vary by less than 500g whether his diet is high in protein or fairly low in protein. There is no agreement as to what purpose is served by these few hundred grams. Some people believe that it represents some sort of reserve and may help the body in a way not easily detected, such as increasing its resistance to infection.

The question about how much protein is required in the diet has been debated for a century or more. The earliest research workers thought that an adult person needs at least 100g of protein a day, perhaps as much as 150g. On the other hand, in the early part of this century an American research worker, Russell H. Chittenden (1856–1943), thought this vastly excessive. From his own experiments, he decided that an intake of 40g a day was adequate, provided it was of good quality.

Although the current view is that a man certainly does not need as much as 100g a day, there is still no agreement as to whether 40g is enough. Those who believe that the requirement is as low as this rely mostly on the results of balance experiments. Subjects are given measured amounts of protein and the minimum quantity determined that will just enable the body to replace its normal breakdown and prevent loss of protein.

As well as the results of balance studies and of the experiments of Chittenden, the view that protein intake should not be too high has been supported by those who believe that an unnecessarily large amount of protein could put a strain on the kidneys, which have to get rid of the products of protein breakdown, such as urea. Not many nutritionists take this view today because we know that the kidneys have a considerable reserve that in health can cope with much more work than they normally have to do. Again, there are many populations, like the Masai of East Africa and the people who work on the ranches in South America and Australia, who live very healthy lives on foods providing 200g or more of protein a day.

Probably the majority of nutritionists accept that it is likely to be useful to take more protein than the minimal amount to ensure balance, so as to provide for any possible increase in protein requirements for common minor illnesses.

So far, we have been speaking of the protein requirements of adults. Clearly, more protein is required for a pregnant woman or for a nursing mother. A child, too, needs a higher proportion of protein in its food than an adult does; depending on its age and size, however, the absolute amount of protein required will not necessarily be greater. We have been assuming, too, that the protein in the diet is of reasonable value, i.e. it contains a reasonable proportion of the essential amino-acids.

Finally, it is wrong to refer to some foods, such as meat, fish, eggs and cheese, as if they *are* proteins. All of these foods contain other components in addition to protein. They all contain water, but even lean roast beef, for example, contains about 10% fat, and as a result there are just as many calories available from the fat as from the protein. Moreover, although in much smaller quantities, the meat provides significant amounts of several vitamins and mineral elements.

See also: Allergy; Amino-acids; Biological value of proteins; Dietary requirements; Gelatin; Nutrient balance tests

Protein-energy malnutrition (PEM)

Adults suffer rarely from protein deficiency, except in association with diseases in which there is faulty intestinal absorption. In children, on the other hand, diets deficient in protein, or in energy, or both, are a common feature of the poorer countries of the Third World, and this is a major cause of the high mortality among young children in many countries; as many as 50% of the children in some countries do not reach their fifth birthday.

A deficiency simply of food leads to marasmus, the condition lay people would call semi-starvation. The diet is inadequate in calories (energy), although it also clearly lacks protein and other nutrients. A deficiency that is more specifically one of protein is known as kwashiorkor; it is more likely to occur in countries where the staple food is low in protein, such as cassava or matoke (green bananas), rather than cereal.

There is, however, a wide range of intermediate deficiencies between those that show the characteristic feature of pure calorie deficiency, or of pure protein deficiency; the whole spectrum, which was originally given the name protein-calorie malnutrition, is now known as protein-energy malnutrition, or PEM. There seems to be no special reason, however, why the term 'malnutrition' is used rather than deficiency; it would be just as logical to speak of scurvy as 'vitamin C malnutrition', or beri-beri as 'thiamin malnutrition'.

PEM is seen usually in children between 2 years and 5 years, often following weaning. Marasmus used to be common in the industrial cities of Western countries up to the end of the nineteenth century. It is brought about by inadequate diets, and exacerbated by repeated infections caused by the lack of facilities for maintaining hygiene. Such infections, especially when associated with diarrhoea, both decrease the amount of food absorbed and increase the rate at which the body utilizes food. The child is fretful and restless, and cries a great deal. It is obviously shrunken, with virtually no fat under the skin, and with wasted muscles; this is most clearly seen on the buttocks. The child is considerably underweight and weak. Diarrhoea is a common factor.

Typically, kwashiorkor differs from marasmus in that the child is apathetic rather than fretful, and swollen with oedema rather than skinny. There are patches of pigmentation on the skin, often in a crazy paving pattern, but later there may be ulceration. The hair is sparse and soft; in black children it may show red patches. Deficiency of other nutrients may be evident, so that for example pellagra may be present.

Between these two extremes, children with a mixture of these features may be classified as having marasmic kwashiorkor. Moreover, in areas of the Third World where PEM is common, varying degrees of nutritional inadequacy may be seen, ranging from only low weight for age to the fully developed conditions described. However, an underweight child can be precipitated into severe and perhaps fatal marasmus or kwashiorkor because of a respiratory infection or gastroenteritis. This is even more likely because of the tendency of the mother to feed such a child on something like rice water with very little nutritive value.

The main cause of PEM is poverty. To this should be added ignorance, or rather misinformation. Custom often determines that the father is given what little meat or other protein-rich food is available, while the child (and the mother) may be given the water in which it was cooked. This distribution is based on the belief firstly that the father requires the meat because of his work, secondly that it is in any case unsuitable for the child. The high-pressure marketing of proprietary preparations may persuade the mother to give up breast-feeding, and then to feed the child with the preparation in over-diluted form because it is costly. Poverty is responsible not only for the poor diets; it is responsible also for the lack of facilities for adequate hygiene such as accessible running water, so that it becomes difficult if not impossible to avoid repeated infection.

The treatment of severe PEM should be carried out in hospital. It may require intravenous feeding, and the administration of antibiotics if infection is present.

After hospital treatment, or with less severe cases, a protein-rich diet should be given at home, possibly supplemented with vitamin and mineral preparations. Skimmed milk powder is a good basis for making up a more generous mixture, so as to ensure adequate energy intake. Unfortunately, when the child is at home, or is taken home from hospital, the conditions are likely to be such that malnutrition recurs.

The prevention of PEM is clearly a matter requiring the intervention of the authorities so as to ensure adequate and safe water supplies, good food production, and efforts to eliminate poverty. Only then is it logical to concentrate on nutrition education, especially for mothers.

See also: Oedema

Puberty

The age when puberty, the beginning of sexual maturity, is reached by girls is at the time when menstruation begins. This phenomenon, known as the menarche, is caused by the first ovulation, that is, the ripening of an ovum and its discharge from one of the ovaries. No such precise time occurs in boys, in whom puberty is a period lasting several months, during which the voice breaks and hair begins to be evident in the pubic region.

The corresponding changes occurring in girls are the development of the breasts and also the growth of pubic hair. These changes in both sexes are caused by the hormones produced by the ovaries and testes under the stimulus of hormones from the anterior pituitary gland situated at the base of the brain.

The onset of puberty in Western countries occurs in girls most commonly at the age of 12 or 13, and a year or so later in boys. However, there is considerable variation between individuals, and certainly it can occur earlier or later than these ages. During the past 100 years, the age of puberty has decreased by about two years; it is said that it takes place about three months earlier each decade. It is commonly believed that puberty in tropical countries occurs at younger ages than it does in temperate climates; the truth is that it occurs later in the tropics.

Why puberty has become earlier in the wealthier Western countries is not certain. One suggestion is that it is due to improved nutrition, and that this is shown by the fact that children are now taller and heavier than they were in earlier generations. In fact, the age of menarche is linked more closely to body weight than to the ages of girls.

A Swiss physician has suggested a more specific nutritional explanation, which is that the more rapid growth and earlier menarche is the result of an increase in sugar consumption during the past century. This suggestion is perhaps less implausible than appears, when one recalls that a high sugar intake can induce an increase in the amounts of at least two hormones in the body, insulin and cortisol, both of which interact with the sex hormones.

There is a spurt in the growth of the body during the three or four years around puberty. This amounts on average to about 5kg a year. This is equivalent to the retention of a little over 1kg a year of protein, about $2\frac{1}{2}$g a day. The protein has to be accompanied by fat and other constituents, building them all into additional body tissue. It is then not surprising that adolescence is accompanied by a noticeable increase in appetite. There is, however, no increased need for any specific foods or nutrients; the general rules governing the choice of a nutritious diet will ensure the nutritional requirement for the growth spurt of puberty as this is accompanied by increased food intake.

See also: Anthropometry

Pulses

Otherwise known as legumes, various pulses – beans, peas and lentils – are in many parts of the world an important food. This is especially true in India, China and many parts of Africa. Mostly it is only the seeds that are eaten; occasionally the pod too is eaten, as in green beans, runner beans and the variety of pea appropriately known as mange-tout.

The seeds have a high protein content. The protein is especially rich in lysine but poor in methionine; since the cereal proteins tend to be low in lysine but rich in methionine, the two sorts of foods complement each other, so that the combination of pulses and cereals provides protein of a high biological value.

If fresh peas, or beans in their pods, are consumed, they provide small to moderate amounts of vitamin C and carotene; when dried, however, the only vitamins retained in reasonable amounts are nicotinic acid and thiamin. Mostly, the pulses are eaten after they have been dried, when they can be stored for very long periods. They are then soaked in water before cooking.

The green gram or mung bean, which is an important crop in India and China, is often germinated by the Chinese, and the bean sprouts then provide a good source of vitamin C.

In some instances, the cooking of dried pulses is important not only because it makes them edible. Soya beans, and French or kidney beans, as well as several others, contain an anti-trypsin which inhibits the digestion of the protein in food. This substance is destroyed by cooking. Again, some raw pulses contain toxic substances called haemagglutinins (lectins), which result in the clumping of the red cells in the blood of those who eat the raw beans; these substances are also destroyed by cooking. It is important, however, that the cooking of pulses, especially during manufacturing processes such as canning, should not be excessively long or at excessively high temperatures, since this reduces the biological value of the protein by destroying some of the amino-acids, as well as destroying some of the vitamins.

Pulses are liable to cause flatulence; some people are more susceptible than others. People with indigestion are usually advised not to eat pulses. The flatulence is said to be due to the presence in pulses of two tetrasaccharides, stachyose and verbascose; each is made up of two molecules of galactose combined with one of glucose and one of fructose. They are not digested in the small intestine, so that they reach the colon and are attacked by the colonic bacteria, resulting in the production of gas.

Q

Quantities

It is not enough to say that for growth and health the body requires energy and nutrients; it is necessary to add that it requires them in the correct quantities. Thus, it reveals very little about a food to say that it contains protein, or vitamin A, without saying how much it contains. Further, in order to assess its nutritional value, it is necessary to know not only how much of the nutrient is contained in, say, an ounce or 100g of the food; it is necessary to know how much of the food is likely to be eaten. These examples will illustrate the importance of quantities in assessing the extent to which a food is making a contribution to a person's nutritional needs.

(1) Honey is widely supposed to be a particularly nutritious food. One reason for this is said to be that it provides a large range of nutrients, including iron, calcium and B vitamins. Ounce for ounce, honey contains less of these items than does unfortified white bread, which is considered to be a particularly non-nutritious food by most of those who praise honey.

(2) Parsley has a high concentration of vitamin C, and is therefore often quoted as an important source of this vitamin. One hundred grams has 150mg of vitamin C, compared with 100g of orange juice with 50mg. But 100g of parsley is in fact a vast quantity; it would be unlikely that people would eat as much as this in a year, but even if they did, they would get an average of rather less than $\frac{1}{2}$mg of vitamin C a day. The chief source of the vitamin in the British diet turns out to be potatoes, which supply an average of 13mg a day: this in spite of the fact that cooked potatoes contain on average only some 7mg of vitamin C in 100g.

(3) The milling of wheat to produce white flour of 70% extraction reduces the quantity of several nutrients present in the whole grain. But to say that calcium is reduced by 60%, or sodium by 78%, at best says little about the relevance to human nutrition; at worst it is misleading. For someone eating an average amount of bread, the quantity of calcium lost from the whole grain would reduce the daily intake of calcium by less than 20mg, out of the average consumption of 1,100mg and the daily requirement of

some 500mg. The loss of sodium is about 1mg a day out of an average intake of about 5,000mg. Thus, it does not help to express quantities of nutrients in percentages; what matters is the absolute amount of the nutrient in a realistic quantity of a food, so that it can be compared both with the absolute amount in the diet and the absolute amount needed.

(4) It is not realistic to say that pulses contain at least as much protein as does meat, although according to the reference books 100g of lentils contain 24g of protein and 100g of shoulder of lamb 16g. But no one eats either of these in the raw state; when they are cooked, the lentils take up a great deal of the water they lost when they were dried, and the lamb loses some of its fat and its water. The realistic figures are that, as eaten, 100g of lentils contain 7.5g of protein and the shoulder of lamb 20g.

R

Reducing sugar

This has nothing to do with weight reduction. It refers to the property of many sugars to react with a substance in a way that oxidizes the sugars while causing the opposite effect – reduction – on the substance. If glucose is heated with a solution containing, among other substances, some copper sulphate, the clear blue solution becomes cloudy with the formation of a red copper compound called cuprous oxide; the copper sulphate has become reduced. This is the basis of the common tests for glucose in the urine of diabetics.

Glucose and fructose, and all the other monosaccharides, are reducing sugars because they contain an aldehyde group or a ketone group; in the process of reducing the copper sulphate or some other substance, they become oxidized to acid groups. A disaccharide formed by the combination of two monosaccharide molecules might still be a reducing sugar if one or both of the reducing groups remain free; this is true of lactose or maltose. On the other hand, sucrose is formed by a combination of glucose and fructose through their reducing groups, so that sucrose itself is not a reducing sugar.

See also: **Carbohydrates**

Remissions and relapses

There are several diseases that characteristically fluctuate in intensity over a period. At times they diminish in intensity and may indeed produce no symptoms; at other times they increase in intensity, with exacerbation of symptoms. Examples of diseases with such periodicity, having alternating remissions and relapses, are muscular rheumatism, rheumatoid arthritis, multiple sclerosis and schizophrenia. Occasionally, especially with schizophrenia, there is ultimately complete spontaneous remission with no relapse.

For some of these conditions, orthodox medical treatment does not always have a certain cure, so that people who suffer from them understandably tend to seek unorthodox remedies. Since these may include preparations of vitamins or minerals or non-essential dietary items such as lecithin, pollen or royal jelly, they are of special interest to the nutritionist.

In assessing the efficacy of such remedies, it is useful to bear in mind the natural history of the illness being treated. It may be that the condition is one that improves spontaneously, that is, would have done so without treatment. If on the other hand it is one that shows periodicity, then the most likely time for the sufferer to seek unorthodox treatment will be when there is an exacerbation of symptoms. Thus, the most likely direction in which the disease now proceeds will be towards a remission, and this will often be taken as evidence of the efficacy of treatment. Relapse, with treatment again followed by improvement, will be seen to reinforce this conclusion. Alternatively, repeated relapse may persuade the patient that the treatment is in fact ineffective, but this is less likely to be publicized than the initial enthusiastic belief that megavitamin therapy, or massive doses of vitamin C, or pyridoxine, really have cured schizophrenia, or a cold, or arthritis.

See also: Arthritis

Respiratory quotient

When the body oxidizes (metabolizes) carbohydrate, or protein, or fat, or alcohol, it uses oxygen and produces carbon dixoide and water. Other substances are also produced from the protein, but these are excreted in the urine and not in the expired air. Because the four metabolized food components have different compositions, they produce different quantities of carbon dioxide for a given quantity of oxygen used. The ratio of the volume of carbon dioxide expired to that of the oxygen used is called the respiratory quotient or RQ. This quotient is 1.0 for carbohydrate and roughly 0.8 for protein, 0.7 for fat and 0.65 for alcohol.

The simplest example expressed in chemical terms is the oxidation of a carbohydrate such as glucose:

$$C_6H_{12}O_6 + 6O_2 = 6CO_2 + 6H_2O$$
glucose/oxygen/carbon dioxide/water
$$RQ = \frac{CO_2}{O_2} = \frac{6}{6} = 1.0$$

Another example is the oxidation of alcohol:

$C_2H_5OH + 3O_2 = 2CO_2 + 3H_2O$
alcohol/oxygen/carbon dioxide/water

$$RQ = \frac{CO_2}{O_2} = \frac{2}{3} = 0.67$$

See also: Metabolism

Rhodopsin

The retina of the eye contains a material known as rhodopsin or visual purple. It is a compound of protein with retinal, the aldehyde of retinol (vitamin A). The visual purple is contained in the tiny rods of the retina, which are mostly in the periphery of the retina. They are concerned with detecting dim light, but cannot detect different colours; these functions belong to the cones concentrated at the centre of the retina.

The sensitivity of the rods to dim light depends on how much visual purple is present. When the retina is exposed to bright light as strong as that of the daytime, or bright artificial light, the amount of visual purple in the rods is decreased because the light splits the retinal from the protein. In darkness or in dim light, the visual purple is slowly reconstituted so that the sensitivity of the rods increases; a dimly lit object thus gradually becomes visible.

In deficiency of vitamin A, there is an inadequate amount of retinal present to give the retina enough visual purple; the result is the inability to see dimly lit objects, even after a long time in the dark. This is the condition of night blindness, or nyctalopia.

See also: Vitamin A

Riboflavin

In the early days of the discovery of the vitamins, and subsequently their separation and identification, it soon became evident that 'water-soluble B' consisted of more than one substance. When extracts of liver or yeast were heated, the factor that protected against beri-beri was lost, but the remaining extract still retained its growth-promoting activity; the former factor was given the name vitamin B_1, and the latter vitamin B_2. But this vitamin B_2 also contained more than one factor and after much work the growth factor itself was isolated in 1933 from milk. It was first called lactoflavin, but then it was synthesized in 1935 and given the name riboflavin.

Riboflavin is a yellow fluorescent material which proved to be identical to a substance identified in 1932 as an essential component in the oxidation processes of most living cells. Deficiency in man is common, since it often occurs with deficiency of other vitamins of the B group. When pellagra is treated with pure nicotinic acid, for example, the subsequent improvement often stops short of complete cure, and signs of riboflavin deficiency remain.

The best sources of riboflavin are milk, liver, yeast extract and eggs. Unlike some of the other vitamins in the B complex, there is little in cereal grains, but large amounts in milk. It is not easily destroyed by heat, the only losses being the amounts dissolved in the cooking water that is not subsequently used. Riboflavin is sensitive to light, so that the amounts in milk will diminish if milk in transparent bottles is left on the doorstep in the sunshine.

The effects of riboflavin deficiency are seen in the eyes, on the skin, and on the tongue. There is reddening of the eyes; in particular, there is corneal vascularization, so that the cornea, which normally has no blood vessels, now has a ring of capillaries around its edge growing in from the conjunctiva. The skin at the angles of the nose and chin

---

RIBOFLAVIN IN FOODS
Recommended daily intake (RDI) for moderately active man – 1.6mg riboflavin

FOOD	PORTION	RIBOFLAVIN, mg
Milk	100ml	0.15
Beef	100g	0.2
Fish	100g	0.3
Liver	100g	2.5
Bread, wholemeal	30g	0.08
Bread, white	30g	0.03
Rice, lightly milled	100g	0.1
Rice, highly milled	100g	0.03
Yeast extract	5g	0.3

becomes greasy and inflamed; there is angular stomatitis in which the angles of the mouth are cracked and painful; cheilosis appears as reddened denuded patches on the lips; the skin on the external genitalia and adjoining areas of the thighs becomes inflamed and itchy and may resemble tinea or dhobi itch. The combination of the lesions around the mouth and on the genital organs is sometimes referred to as the oro-genital syndrome. The tongue is often red or magenta coloured, sometimes very smooth but sometimes fissured. There are no characteristic appearances that can with certainty distinguish an abnormal tongue due to nicotinic acid deficiency from that due to riboflavin deficiency, particularly because in practice pure deficiency of a single vitamin of the B group rarely occurs.

Deficiency of riboflavin never progresses much, so that it does not result in serious disability, let alone death. Improvement occurs within days following the administration of any rich source of riboflavin, such as yeast extract or the pure vitamin.

See also: Eye; Skin; Vitamin history

Rice

After wheat, rice is man's most important staple food. It is grown in the tropics and sub-tropics, mostly under water in paddy fields, although some rice is grown on dry land. Rice usually gives two crops a year; moreover, it is sometimes possible to cultivate fish in the paddy fields between a harvest of one crop and the planting of the next.

The rice grain has a structure similar to that of wheat. Removal of the husk by home pounding and sieving leaves much of the thiamin and other B vitamins on the grain, but a great part of the vitamins can be lost when the rice is washed. Repeated milling (polishing) in commercial mills also removes a great deal of the vitamins, and it is from diets containing a large proportion of highly-polished rice that beri-beri can arise.

On the other hand, if before milling the rice grain is soaked and boiled, a significant amount of the vitamin is transferred to the starchy inner part of the grain, the endosperm. At the same time it becomes more difficult for milling to remove some of the outer parts of the grain that are rich in the vitamins. This process, parboiling, is routine in some parts of the world, and is sufficient in itself to make beri-beri far less common there.

Rice contains less protein than does any other cereal, but it is of higher quality.

See also: Beri-beri; Cereals

Rickets

Babies and young children develop rickets if they do not get enough vitamin D from their diet or the sunshine. This is a disease that was very common in the big cities of the industrialized countries because of the narrow streets and the pollution of the air. Rickets was especially common in England, which, in the eighteenth century, was the first country to become industrialized. It is said that this is why the Germans called the disease *die englische Krankheit*, but a more likely reason (and for the English a more acceptable one) is that it was first properly described by two English doctors, Whistler in 1645 and Glisson in 1650.

Rickets tends to occur also in quite sunny countries, such as Pakistan, where many children are brought up in houses with high walls and courtyards, and are kept indoors for a great part of the time. It is also seen in some of the immigrants into the United Kingdom from Pakistan, and this is presumably due to two factors: one is that the babies do not necessarily get cod liver oil, and the second is that later they tend to be given chapatis made from unleavened flour, which reduces the absorption of calcium because of the phytate it contains.

Rickets usually occurs between 6 months and 3 years. The child at first looks very well-nourished, with a well-formed head. This was the sort of infant who often won prizes in baby competitions. It is in fact rather flabby and pale and fretful. The abdomen tends to be rather swollen, and the infant commonly has some respiratory infection. Teething and walking tend to be late.

The most characteristic changes are in the bones. The skull becomes hard and bony later than it does in a normal infant. Wrist and ankle bones are swollen, and there is also a swelling on each of the ribs alongside the breastbone. This is sometimes called 'the ricketty rosary'. There is bossing of the bones of the forehead. The breastbone is prominent, producing the so-called 'pigeon chest'. The arms and legs are deformed, and knock-knees or bow legs are a distinctive mark of the disease. The pelvis may become misshapen. Sometimes the infant suffers from convulsions because of a decreased amount of calcium in the blood.

Before these changes become obvious, they can be detected by an

X-ray examination. This shows well the swellings at the wrist and ankles, and the fact that the growing end of the bone is not being properly constructed. Instead of the sharp line indicating active laying down of mineral in the bone, there is a hazy and irregular zone between the shaft and the end near the joint. Even earlier than the bony abnormalities, the blood shows an increase in the activity of the enzyme alkaline phosphatase.

Rickets can be prevented by giving infants one of the many preparations containing vitamin D, preferably as a daily routine from soon after birth. If for any reason this is not possible, a single large dose could be given, and this could be enough to last for 3 months. It is also necessary to ensure adequate calcium in the diet, best provided by milk.

If the disease has already developed and is still active, adequate vitamin D will produce improvement in bone calcification. If the bony changes are not very severe, the structure of the bones may become normal as the child grows and new bone is deposited in a way that restores a normal shape. The pelvis, however, is the least likely part of the body to show a complete restoration of its shape, and girls who have had severe rickets when young may later suffer difficulty in childbirth.

See also: Bone; Glisson; Vitamin D; Whistler

Rubner, Max (1854–1932)

Many of the fundamental discoveries in energy metabolism were made by Max Rubner. It was he who demonstrated, among other matters, that the rate of resting metabolism is proportional to the surface area of the body, and the phenomenon of dietary thermogenesis, i.e. that the metabolism is increased after food is ingested. He also showed that the law of conservation of energy applied to living systems.

Rubner was born in Munich in 1854. In due course he became a pupil there of Carl Voit while Pettenkofer (1818–1901), Atwater and others worked there. In 1885 he was appointed Professor of Hygiene at Marburg. Here he built a calorimeter in which he could measure the heat production of a dog. Similarly, he used Voit's respiration apparatus so that he could also measure oxygen consumption. He was thus able to compare the measurements of energy

DIE GESETZE

DES

ENERGIEVERBRAUCHS

BEI DER

ERNÄHRUNG.

VON

PROF. DR. MAX RUBNER

GEHEIMER MEDICINALRATH,
DIRECTOR DER HYGIENISCHEN INSTITUTE DER UNIVERSITÄT ZU BERLIN.

LEIPZIG UND WIEN.

FRANZ DEUTICKE.

1902.

output by direct and indirect calorimetry, and found a difference of only 0.2%.

He moved to Berlin as Professor of Hygiene in 1891, where he later became Professor of Physiology.

Rubner believed that an adult man required 150g of protein a day, a figure much higher than that accepted today. Because of this, he persuaded the German authorities during the First World War to rear large herds of cattle, a policy that considerably reduced the total energy available to the German people compared with the amount that could be obtained by growing more cereal instead. It is said that this contributed to Germany's losing the war.

See also: Basal metabolism; du Bois; Energy; Protein

Rye

Rye grows in cold climates, such as those of Scandinavia, north Germany and Russia. In these areas wheat does not grow well, although newer varieties have encroached into some of them. Rye can be baked into bread because it contains gluten, although less than the amount in wheat; as a result, rye bread is heavier than wheat bread. By itself, it is also a dark bread, but rye flour is often mixed with wheat flour, giving a lighter colour to the loaf. Such a bread was quite commonly used in the UK until the middle of the eighteenth century, and is still available in many countries as well as in specialized bakeries in the UK. The rye and wheat were often grown together, the crop of mixed cereals being known as maslin. Maslin flour was the commonest form used for bread-making in Europe between the fourteenth and seventeenth centuries. Pumpernickel is made without wheat flour, and often has caramel added, so that it may be almost black. Rye alone or mixed with wheat flour is often used for making crispbreads.

Wholemeal rye flour contains somewhat less protein (about 8%) and more riboflavin and less nicotinic acid than wholemeal wheat flour; in other respects its nutrient content differs very little from that of wheat flour.

Rye can be infected with ergot, a rust or fungus, and the consumption of the infected grain produces ergotism. The symptoms include convulsions, hallucinations and intolerable itching; the last is responsible for the name St Anthony's Fire for the disease. It is likely that the 20 witches executed in Salem, Massachusetts, in 1692 were simply women suffering from ergotism.

See also: Cereals; Poisons in food

S

Sago

The trunk of several varieties of palm, but particularly a variety called
the sago palm, produces a pith that contains a high proportion of
starch. This is extracted by cutting the trunk into pieces, removing the
bark, and washing out the starch as a paste. The paste is dried and
used as sago meal. It has about 0.5% protein, even less fat, small
quantities of B vitamins, and about 90% of starch, with a small amount
of moisture. In some of the Pacific islands, it forms an important part
of the diet, taken in soups, pudding and biscuits. In Western countries
it is sometimes used for thickening soups, but mostly for making milk
puddings.

Sauerkraut

Sauerkraut is the German word for sour cabbage. It is made by
adding salt to shredded cabbage, after which lactic acid bacteria
from the air begin to grow and to ferment the small quantities of
sugar that are in the cabbage. The bacteria produce lactic acid and
some acetic acid, and these, together with the salt, preserve the
product.

Scurvy

Epidemic scurvy can still occur after disasters, or in a town or military
garrison besieged for any length of time. Occasionally, scurvy is seen
in Western countries in individual women, and especially men, who
are living alone. Usually they are poor or unwilling or unable to look
after themselves properly. They then tend to live on an easily prepared
diet that contains little or no fruit or vegetables. The disease is known
as bachelor's scurvy. Up to 30 or 40 years ago, scurvy was sometimes
caused by ill-considered dietary advice given by doctors to patients
with chronic dyspepsia, who were told to avoid eating fibrous and
acid foods; this was interpreted by the patients as vegetables and

fruits. The term 'iatrogenic scurvy' is used for this condition, 'iatrogenic' meaning doctor-induced.

A hundred years or so ago, scurvy in infants used to be fairly common, curiously enough in the babies of parents who were relatively well off. At the end of the last century, it became fashionable for mothers not to breast-feed their babies but to give them a diet mostly of manufactured baby foods that were increasingly available. Dependence upon such foods without the addition of fruit juices or vegetables resulted in infantile scurvy. This often showed itself by the baby lying with its legs apart and the knees slightly bent, in a way that somewhat resembles a frog. The posture and the extreme tenderness of the joints was due to haemorrhages of the bones and joints, especially in the legs.

Haemorrhaging is the main feature of scurvy. It may be seen as spots under the skin (petechiae) or bruises (ecchymoses). Bleeding of the gums also occurs if the teeth are present, and bleeding under the covering membrane of the bones (the periosteum) and in the joints. Large and sometimes fatal haemorrhage may also occur into the membrane covering the heart muscle (pericardium) or into the brain. The healing of wounds is delayed and old wounds may re-open. The gums are swollen and often infected (gingivitis).

The onset of the disease is insidious. As Stefansson, the explorer, wrote: 'It begins with laziness, gloom and irritability, showing itself in a tendency to condemnatory and uncalled-for argumentativeness.' As the signs of gingivitis and haemorrhage appear, the diagnosis becomes evident. If the necessary facilities are available, it may be worthwhile to measure the amount of vitamin in the white cells of the blood, which falls to zero or almost zero in developed scurvy.

When long sea voyages of discovery, piracy and naval warfare were common, scurvy was an almost inevitable outcome among the crew. At the end of the fifteenth century, Vasco da Gama (c. 1460–1521) is said to have lost more than half his men on his voyage around the Cape of Good Hope. A century later, Admiral Richard Hawkins (c. 1562–1622) wrote that, in his own experience, 10,000 seamen had died of the scurvy. After Lind published his *Treatise of the Scurvy* in 1753, the British Navy – 50 years later – introduced a compulsory issue of what was termed lime juice. It is likely that this was in fact lemon juice, but it accounts for the Americans giving the British the name 'Limey'.

See also: Lind; Vitamin C

Seaweed

Brown seaweed (kelp) enters the diet mostly in the form of alginates, which are used as emulsifiers and thickeners; red seaweeds serve as a source for Irish moss carageenin and agar, which have a similar purpose. However, in a few countries, kelp itself is consumed. In Japan in particular, and in China to a lesser extent, seaweed is eaten in soups or as part of other dishes; an example is small baskets made of woven strips of seaweed filled with chopped vegetables. It is also eaten, but to a decreasing extent, in Ireland and Western Scotland; in Wales, it is made into laver bread, as fried cakes with or without the addition of oatmeal.

See also: Agar; Alginates; Iodine

Selenium

This is one of the essential trace elements that have recently come under intense study. Experimentally, it can be shown to replace to some extent the vitamin E in the diet of animals, preventing some but not all the effects of deficiency of the vitamin. It has been suggested by Chinese research workers that deficiency of selenium is a cause of a particular type of heart disease called Keshan disease, mostly affecting children up to the age of 8 or 9 years. The disease is found in a wide band of Chinese territory that runs from the north-east coast down towards the south-western border of the country. Within this band the soil, and consequently any crop grown on it, is low in selenium. In addition, it has been reported that the incidence of the disease has been considerably diminished in areas where selenium was given to children, but was not diminished in other affected areas where the children were not treated.

A report from Finland suggests that selenium deficiency in Karelia, the eastern part of the country, may be a partial explanation for the exceptionally high prevalence of (adult) coronary heart disease in that area. The evidence rests partly on the low selenium content of the soil, and partly on the fact that there was a higher mortality from heart disease, and a greater incidence of non-fatal heart attacks, in persons with a low concentration of selenium in their blood. Apart from these studies, there is no evidence that dietary deficiency of selenium plays a part in causing cancer or any other condition.

The average British diet provides about 60µg of selenium a day.

See also: Mineral elements

Semolina

Particles of endosperm from hard (durum) wheat are called semolina. When it is cooked the particles swell up and become soft, but do not disintegrate, as does the endosperm of soft wheat because it is richer in protein. Semolina can be used either for making pasta, such as macaroni or spaghetti, or for making milk puddings like those made from other starchy foods such as sago, tapioca and rice.

See also: Wheat

Sesame seed oil

The sesame plant is an annual; the harvesting of the seeds takes place by cutting the whole plant, which is then dried and the seeds shaken out of the opened capsules. The seeds contain 40–50% of oil, but the low yield makes its production not very economical. The total world crop is thus small and has not increased in recent years. As with other oil seeds, the residue after pressing out the oil, the seedcake, is used for animal feed. The seeds themselves are used for decorating bread and bread rolls, and also for making one or two Mediterranean foods, such as tahini and halva.

See also: Oils

Skin

The skin is affected both by shortage of energy and by shortage of some specific nutrients, as well as by hypersensitivity (allergy) to particular foods.

Starvation is often accompanied by brown patches on the face and trunk, which have often been described as a feature of famine. Deficiency of protein, more frequently referred to as protein-energy malnutrition (PEM) or kwashiorkor, may also produce pigmented skin, especially on the arms and legs, accompanied by a crazy paving appearance that is almost characteristic of the disease.

Many people believe that an unduly dry skin is caused by an insufficiency of fat in the diet. This was a common complaint in the UK during food rationing in the last war and for some years after it, yet average fat intake was only slightly reduced from 37% of the dietary calories to 33%. Moreover, most countries in the Third World have diets that contain very much less fat, yet it is rare to find individuals there complaining of dry skin.

Another common belief is that brittle nails are caused by a dietary deficiency of calcium. This is nonsense, since nails contain almost no calcium. They are made up mostly of keratin, the protein that is also the major constituent of hair.

Deficiencies of particular vitamins are often associated with skin conditions, although there is now less certainty about the specificity of these features. For example, it used to be taught that deficiency of vitamin A produced follicular hyperkeratosis, otherwise known as toad skin or phrynoderma. The rough skin in this condition is caused by plugs in the hair follicles of keratin, the horny material of which hair is made and which forms the outermost layer of the skin. It is seen especially on the backs of the arms and front of the thighs. It is not, however, always seen in deficiency of vitamin A, and it is sometimes seen in individuals who are certainly not short of the vitamin.

Other vitamin deficiencies may produce abnormalities of the skin; the best known of these are pellagra, and deficiency of riboflavin, biotin, and the essential fatty acids.

Most skin conditions nevertheless have nothing to do with nutrition. It is true to say, however, that a generally poor state of health, including that due to poor nutrition, is associated with dull-looking hair and with white patches on the nails. Severe iron deficiency anaemia also affects the nails, producing a depression in the nail, which is the reason they are called 'spoon-shaped'. The medical name is koilonychia.

See also: Acne

Smoked foods

The preservation of foods, especially meat and fish, by hanging them in the smoke of a wood fire has a long history. The preservative action is a combination of drying the food, and adding to it a range of chemical substances contained in the smoke, notably aldehydes and phenols. In addition, the smoke tends to colour the food. The modern tendency is to hasten the process by soaking the food in brine with chemical preservatives and with dye; the traditional process is more elaborate and slower, and hence more costly.

See also: Food preservation

Smoking

There are two circumstances in which a connection has been reported between tobacco smoking and nutrition. One is that smoking reduces the concentration of vitamin C in the body. This effect does not appear to be considerable, and indeed some observers have failed to find it. The sum of the evidence does not suggest either that cigarette smokers need significantly more vitamin C than do those who do not smoke, nor that cigarette smokers run a high risk of developing scurvy.

The second interaction between smoking and nutrition is its undoubted effect on body weight. Many smokers have observed an increase in body weight, sometimes a large increase, when they have stopped smoking; among American businessmen, it was shown that those who gave up smoking gained more than 8lb in three years, compared with a slight loss in control subjects over the same period. Again, it is known that heavy cigarette smokers tend to weigh less for a given height than do non-smokers. In one study of men over 40, the non-smokers were on average about 14lb (6kg) heavier than the smokers.

The reasons for the effect of smoking on body weight are obscure. Nevertheless, there is some evidence that there are two possible explanations. One is that people eat more when they give up smoking, and especially as many former smokers take to eating confectionery, presumably as an alternative form of oral gratification. The second possible explanation is that smoking affects metabolism; it is accompanied for example by an increased blood concentration of adrenalin and insulin, both of which tend to speed up metabolism.

See also: Obesity

Sodium

There is more salt in the blood than there is of any other mineral substance; more strictly, there are more sodium ions plus chloride ions. They are equivalent to nearly 1g of sodium chloride in 100ml of blood, and are responsible for the greater part of the osmotic pressure of the blood and tissue fluid.

It has been suggested that the concentration of salt in the blood of different species of land animals reflects the concentrations in the world's oceans when that species left the sea for the land; the concentration of salt in the oceans has been steadily increasing over the millions of years since the land solidified and then cooled sufficiently for the water vapour to condense.

Human beings, and many species of animals, show a great desire for salt. It is often supposed that this drive to consume salt is an indication of the body's need, but there is considerable doubt whether it is not simply a drive for the taste of salt. Certainly salt, when it is available, is highly sought after, as can be demonstrated by history as well as by the wide use of the word in language. The Latin word for salt is *sal*, which gave rise to saline, salad, sauce, saucer, souse and sausage. Roman soldiers were paid in part by a sum of money with which to buy salt; the Latin is *salarius*, from which we derive the word salary. Like other highly prized commodities, such as sugar and tobacco, salt has often been taxed, making it a convenient source of revenue. Both the Americans and more recently Gandhi used the public resentment of a salt tax as part of their campaigning against the British.

Phrases such as 'the salt of the earth', and to be 'worth one's salt' also point to the high value placed upon it. To be seated 'above or below the salt' at a banquet was an indication of one's status, or at least the host's opinion of one's status. Most people find cereals not very palatable without salt, giving rise to such derogatory phrases as 'tasteless as bread without salt'; this suggests that it is not entirely coincidental that agriculture, beginning with the cultivation of cereals, had its origin in and around the salty soils of the Middle East.

Not only cereals but also other vegetable products usually have a very low ratio of sodium to potassium, compared with the ratio in most animal products. It is tempting to suppose that this is the reason why herbivorous animals avidly avail themselves of salt licks, and why people find not only cereals, but also potatoes and green vegetables, more palatable with added salt. However, it is not easy on these grounds to understand why some vegetarian Africans who find difficulty in obtaining salt are content to flavour their food with vegetable ash, which consists largely of potash (hence its name).

The amount of salt consumed by people varies considerably. The average in Western countries is around 15g a day, with a wide range, however, from about 2–3g to 20g or more. There is evidence that in adults the higher intakes occur in those who have had high intakes in infancy and childhood. Studies in America suggest that salt naturally present in food contributes about 3g, another 8g is added during the processing of foods, and 5g added by the consumer. Most of the salt in manufactured foods is in bread and other cereal products; next come processed meat, poultry and fish, and next cheese and other milk products. Its use as an additive to these foods is either for palatability or as a preservative.

The daily requirement for sodium can be met by 1–2g of salt a day in people in temperate climates, whose activity does not result in unusually great sweating. Salt requirements can be considerably increased in situations where perspiration is high. A deficiency of sodium usually accompanies a deficiency of body water, i.e. dehydration. Loss of salt through perspiration can be as much as 50g a day. The concentration of salt helps to determine the volume of the extra-cellular fluid, because it is largely responsible for its osmotic pressure, so that a fall in the concentration of salt reduces both the volume of the blood and the volume of the tissue fluid. This leads to a fall in blood pressure. Deficiency of salt, or more accurately of sodium, also results in apathy, loss of appetite, vomiting and muscle cramps.

Sodium deficiency can occur after severe vomiting and diarrhoea. The loss of sodium because of these conditions or because of excessive perspiration is accompanied by a reduction of the amount excreted in the urine, which may fall to zero.

Excessive sodium accumulates in the body only when the heart or the kidneys are diseased. One result is the associated accumulation of water in the extra-cellular fluid because of the increase in osmotic pressure. This may be sufficient to cause oedema, which may lead to swelling of the limbs, especially the legs.

There is now reasonable evidence to suggest that the effect of high salt consumption is to increase the risk of developing hypertension, i.e. high blood pressure. Partly the evidence comes from epidemiology. The average consumption of salt in Japan is about 20g a day; in southern Japan it is around 15g, but in northern Japan it is nearer 25g, with some individuals taking 50g a day. The incidence of strokes due to high blood pressure in Japan is among the highest in the world, and is more common in the north than in the south. In addition to such epidemiological evidence, there is also good evidence that a reduction in salt intake can reduce high blood pressure.

Widespread reduction of salt would probably require intervention by governments, such as limiting the amount added to bread, or at least making it compulsory for manufactured food items to be clearly labelled. Especially, manufacturers of baby foods and formulae should be required to limit the amount of salt, as indeed many are now doing voluntarily.

A restricted salt intake amounting to about 6g a day is not very difficult to achieve; it involves the avoidance of adding salt at the table and of obviously salty foods such as bacon or tinned fish or meats. A low sodium diet of 3g or so a day requires in addition the avoidance of all manufactured sauces as well as cakes and biscuits. A further reduction, to a very low sodium diet of about 1.5g of salt, which is necessary for heart or kidney failure and in severe hypertension, can be achieved only by the use of special foods such as salt-free bread and low sodium milk. Many patients find this diet extremely unappetizing, so that it is often taken for a few weeks and alternates with the low sodium diet with 3g a day.

Most salt is hygroscopic, that is, it picks up water. Such damp salt tends to become lumpy and not to flow freely. Free-flowing salt is made by adding what are called anticaking agents such as magnesium carbonate in amounts of around 1%.

In some countries, salt is used as a vehicle for supplying iodine. This is done to prevent the development of iodine deficiency goitre.

Some people prefer to use sea salt in their kitchens, in the belief that it supplies useful quantities of trace elements. Any iodine that sea salt contains disappears quite quickly on keeping, because it vaporizes; this is not true of iodized salt, in which the iodine is added as iodide.

Salt substitutes contain potassium salts, especially potassium chloride.

See also: Blood pressure; Osmotic pressure

Soft drinks

Most soft drinks are sweet; the only exception is soda water, made by forcing carbon dioxide into ordinary water. Fruit juices made simply by pressing the fruit are not classified as soft drinks. On the other hand, many soft drinks contain some fruit. The most straightforward is fruit squash, which is chiefly fruit juice with the addition of sugar (sucrose); UK legislation requires a minimum quantity of both fruit and sugar. Whole fruit drinks are made from comminuted fruit, which contains the finely macerated peel and pulp; because this peel adds considerably to the flavour, a lower minimum quantity of fruit is allowed. Drinks that contain no fruit must be labelled as having 'fruit flavour' or 'orangeade' or some other '-ade'.

It can be assumed that there is little or no vitamin C in fruit drinks, unless it is claimed on the label; the vitamin may be derived entirely from the fruit, or it may have been added.

The only sweetened soft drinks that may legally have less than the usual minimum of sucrose are glucose drinks and diabetic and low-calorie drinks, sweetened partly or entirely with saccharine, or some other permitted non-caloric sweetener.

Soft drinks may be sold in a concentrated form or ready to drink; the latter are frequently carbonated. The colour is likely to be added in whole or in part in the form of a permitted additive. Cola drinks usually have added colour, and contain caffeine and phosphoric acid as well as their characteristic flavours. The amount of caffeine in a can of cola drink is likely to be 40–70mg; this is about as much as in a cup of tea or a weak cup of coffee. The bitter taste of tonic water, bitter orange and bitter lemon derives from the addition of quinine.

The best known of the cola drinks, Coca-Cola, originally contained cocaine, as its name implies; it was added as an extract of leaves from the coca shrub, grown in South America. This practice, however, was abandoned in 1903.

Apart from the vitamin C that may be present, the chief nutritional component of soft drinks is sucrose or glucose. A glass of fruit drink or tonic water, about 200ml, contains about 15g or so of sucrose; a standard can of cola of 350ml contains about 35g. It may also be important to realize that fruit drinks and fruit-flavoured drinks, unlike fruit juices, do not contain significant quantities of the potassium that may be required by patients or convalescents as part of their treatment.

Sorbitol

A white powder with about half the sweetness of sucrose, sorbitol is used instead of sucrose by some diabetics. This is because it raises the concentration of blood glucose more slowly, and to a lesser extent, than does sucrose; as a consequence, it also results in a lower rise in blood insulin. Sorbitol is therefore used in the manufacture of marmalade, jam, chocolate and canned fruits for diabetics. These are sometimes also used by people taking a low-calorie diet, in the mistaken belief that, since these products are sometimes labelled 'free from added sugar', they must provide fewer calories than do the corresponding conventional foods. However, although absorbed more slowly, sorbitol is ultimately completely absorbed and releases the same amount of energy of some 4 kcal per gram as sucrose does.

Taken in large quantities, sorbitol can cause abdominal discomfort and diarrhoea. The amount that has this effect varies from person to person, but most people can tolerate up to 40g or so a day with no unpleasant symptoms. If small quantities are taken first, and the amount increased each day, larger quantities of 70g or more a day can be tolerated.

Experiments with rats have shown similar effects of dietary sorbitol, with similar adaptation to gradually increasing amounts that can reach 30% of the diet. After a few weeks there is considerable enlargement of the intestine, with thickening of the walls; this is especially true for the caecum, which undergoes a threefold increase in its weight. The cause of this appears to be a vast increase in the number of micro-organisms that inhabit the intestine, especially the caecum and colon.

Sorbitol is present in several fruits, including apples, plums and cherries; other fruits, including strawberries and raspberries, have none.

Commercially, sorbitol is made by hydrogenating glucose. Its chemical composition puts it into the class of polyols, together with mannitol. The first product of its metabolism in the body is fructose. For this reason, some physicians are doubtful whether it is an entirely safe substance to give to diabetics.

See also: Fructose

Soya

Soya bean is an important crop that originated in south-west Asia but now grows extensively in other warm countries, for example, in the southern United States. The bean has been used in China as a legume for thousands of years. It contains about 38% protein and 24% fat. In the West it is used as a flour, either of the whole bean or after some or most of the fat has been extracted.

The protein is of higher biological value than that from most vegetable sources. The oil, which is rich in polyunsaturated acids, is used for cooking but more particularly in the manufacture of margarine, and the oil cake is of importance for animal feed.

The flour is added to many cereal foods, infant foods and milk substitutes, and to sausage and other meat products.

In the countries of south-west Asia, various products have been made from the soya bean, and some of these are now known in Western countries. A more recent product is textured vegetable protein (TVP). Soya sauce is traditionally made by slow fermentation with the mould *Aspergillus oryzae*; now a quicker process is used involving acid hydrolysis and heating. Soya bean milk and bean curd are other products.

See also: Novel protein foods

Spinach

True spinach, *Spinacea oleracea*, is grown in most countries with a temperate climate. The leaves are widely believed to be especially useful nutritionally because they are rich in iron. It is by swallowing spinach that the famous cartoon character, Popeye, restored the miraculous strength needed to extricate himself or some other character from imminent danger. It is true that spinach, with 4mg/100g iron, contains more than do other edible leafy vegetables, such as cabbage with 0.5mg/100g. But the iron is very poorly available. In addition, spinach has rather a lot of oxalic acid, and this reduces the availability of calcium from foods eaten at the same time. The only nutrient present in quite high amounts is carotene.

In many countries, the leaves of other plants are eaten in the same way that spinach is eaten. One example is New Zealand spinach, which belongs to a different family. So do spinach beet, and chard or seakale beet, which are both related to beetroots and to sugar beet.

Starch

Starch is a carbohydrate, and the major store of energy in most plants. It is found mostly in the roots, tubers and seeds. Chemically, it is made up of large molecules composed of many units of glucose molecules joined together. There are two main forms of starch. In amylose, there are several hundred glucose units forming a straight chain. In amylopectin, which constitutes perhaps 80% of the total starch store, the glucose units form branched chains. The carbohydrate stored in animals, glycogen, resembles amylo-pectin in its chemical structure.

In the plant, the starch is present as granules, each with a thin, cellulose-like coating. When heated in water or steam, the granules swell and burst. The starch can now dissolve in water, and makes a sticky paste. Hydrolysis of the starch, either by the enzyme amylase or by continued boiling, especially with mild acid or alkali, produces dextrins and later maltose. The starchy foods used in the household, for example to thicken soups, come chiefly from maize (corn starch), but potato starch and arrowroot are sometimes used.

The starch in unripe bananas and apples is gradually converted into sugar during ripening; on the other hand, much of the sugar in peas and maize is converted to starch as the seeds continue to mature.

See also: Carbohydrates

Stark, William (1740–70)

The brevity of the life of William Stark was the result of an enthusiastic attempt to compare in himself the effects of different diets.

He studied medicine at St George's Hospital in London, with John Hunter as his teacher of anatomy. He took his MD in Leyden in 1766, and three years later, encouraged by Sir John Pringle (1707–82), began to experiment on himself. For 2 weeks he took only bread and water and lost $3\frac{1}{2}$lb in weight. He followed this with a diet of bread, water and sugar, and then a range of other diets. On some of these he felt well, for example on bread and milk; on the other hand, his diet of bread and olive oil caused considerable purgation, so that he maintained it for only a few days. In spite of the ill effects of several of these diets, he persisted in his experiments for a total of 8 months, keeping copious notes all the while. This dedication and enthusiasm, sadly, was ended by his death in February 1770, at the age of 29.

17

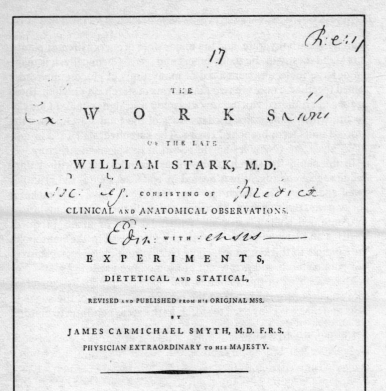

THE

WORK S

OF THE LATE

WILLIAM STARK, M.D.

CONSISTING OF

CLINICAL AND ANATOMICAL OBSERVATIONS,

WITH

EXPERIMENTS,

DIETETICAL AND STATICAL,

REVISED AND PUBLISHED FROM HIS ORIGINAL MSS.

BY

JAMES CARMICHAEL SMYTH, M.D. F.R.S,

PHYSICIAN EXTRAORDINARY TO HIS MAJESTY.

LONDON:

PRINTED FOR J. JOHNSON, No. 72, ST. PAUL's CHURCH-YARD.

M.DCC.LXXXVIII.

The records of Stark's experiments were published in 1788 by James Carmichael Smyth (1741–1821), under the title *The Work of the late William Stark MD consisting of Clinical and Anatomical Observations, with Experiments Dietetical and Statical.*

Stark himself was aware that his experiments had proved very little; the final words of his own notes read: '. . . these observations were made, not so much in hopes of determining anything on this subject, as of discovering how the land lay, and of enabling me to undertake some more accurate and decisive experiments.'

Sterols

The elaborate chemical structure of the sterols can exist in several forms, with small chemical groups attached to different parts of the skeletal molecule. This explains why there is a wide range of different sterols to be found in animal and in plant tissues. All have alcohol groups as part of their structure, so they are often found as esters with, for example, fatty acids.

Some of the sterols in the body are discussed elsewhere; these include cholesterol, vitamin D and bile salts.

The two most important sterols occurring in plants are ergosterol and phytosterol. Ergosterol is present in yeasts and fungi, and can be converted into vitamin D_2 (ergocalciferol) by irradiation with U V light. Phytosterol is found in many plant tissues. When it is present in the diet, it is not well absorbed into the blood; moreover, it reduces the absorption of the cholesterol that may also be present in the diet.

Stroke

When the blood supply to a part of the brain is cut off, the result is a stroke; another rather old-fashioned term is apoplexy. The interference with the blood supply can come about through one of three events: haemorrhage, thrombosis or embolism. The adjective cerebral attached to any of these terms indicates that the event is occurring in the brain. Doctors often use the term 'cerebrovascular accident' instead of 'stroke'.

Haemorrhage of one of the blood vessels supplying the brain is most often caused by an artery that is affected by atherosclerosis.

Thrombosis (clotting), too, is most likely to occur in such an artery. Finally, an embolism is produced when something is carried in the blood until it blocks one of the arteries; this also is most likely to be a piece of a plaque or a clot from an atherosclerotic artery, although it may also be air or some fat.

A high blood pressure (hypertension) is a major cause of a stroke. This is because it not only increases the chances of an artery leaking and thus causing the haemorrhage, but also increases the chances of atherosclerosis in any of the arteries in the body, including those of the brain.

The result of a stroke may be minimal, or more severe yet with rapid recovery, or more severe with permanent damage, or it may be rapidly fatal. The effects depend on which part of the brain is damaged and on the extent of the damage. Permanent damage of some sort is common; it affects either sensation or movement or both. The reason for this is that the cells of the nervous tissue soon die if their blood supply is cut off, and unlike the cells of most other tissues, the body is not able to replace dead nerve cells.

A common effect of a stroke is weakness or complete paralysis of a limb, or impairment of speech. Improvement occurs if part of the disability is caused by pressure upon some of the cells in the brain from inflammation surrounding the destroyed cells; as the inflammation disappears, the disability improves. Improvement can also occur, especially in movement, if unaffected adjoining muscles gradually take over some of the movements previously carried out by muscles that no longer have living brain cells to command them.

A raised blood pressure and thus a stroke are probably less likely in people who restrict their intake of salt. If raised blood pressure already exists, it can be alleviated or at least held in check by a low intake of salt. This will also reduce the chances of developing atherosclerosis. Other dietary measures that are widely recommended are the avoidance of overweight and the consumption of a diet low in saturated fat, although the last is not universally agreed.

See also: Blood pressure; Sodium

Strontium

This is not an essential element, but it is so close to calcium in its chemical behaviour that any strontium taken into the body is picked up by the bones; it also finds its way into the other tissues even though their concentration of calcium is much smaller. The radioactive form of strontium, ^{90}Sr or strontium-90, acquired some notoriety because it was released into the atmosphere during early nuclear explosions. The strontium was then picked up by plants, including grass, and thus by cattle, so that it found its way into milk along with the calcium. This phenomenon raised the anxiety of the public, since prolonged exposure to the radioactive strontium-90 could be carcinogenic. Fortunately, the body excretes strontium more readily than it excretes calcium, especially if calcium is taken in large amounts. Monitoring of the amount of strontium-90 in the atmosphere, and monitoring of milk, have shown a continuing fall since the early 1960s, and it is now considered by the authorities to pose no health problem.

Sucrose

This is the commonest sugar and is also known as table sugar, or cane sugar, or beet sugar, or most simply as 'sugar'. Nearly 99% of the sugar we consume is made from the sugar-cane or the sugar-beet, yet the name 'cane-sugar' is often used to mean sucrose, whatever its source. In spite of popular belief, there is no difference in taste or any other ordinarily recognizable property in the sucrose isolated from the cane or the beet. They each contain more than 99.9% pure sucrose; only the most sophisticated and sensitive analytical techniques can detect the difference because of the presence of substances characteristic of either the cane or the beet that are present in vanishingly small quantities.

The sugar-cane originated in India before the Christian era, and slowly spread westwards until it reached the Caribbean. Commercial production from sugar-beet began in 1828, and now accounts for about one-third of total world production.

The discovery that sugar-beet might be a source of sucrose was made by the German chemist Marggraf (1709–82) in 1747, but it was not until the Napoleonic wars that another German, Achard (1753–1821), working in France, demonstrated that it could be refined on a commercial scale. Its main advantage was that, unlike sugar-cane, beet could be grown in temperate climates, and France began producing beet sugar in 1811 so as to overcome the effects of the Allies' blockade in preventing the import of cane sugar.

About two-thirds of the sugar used in the UK is produced from the cane, and one-third from the beet. Very small quantities are also produced from the maple in New England and Canada, from the palm in India, and from millet in the southern United States. Other sources, in quite small quantities, are grapes, carob beans, dates and figs.

The preparation of sugar from the cane begins with cutting the canes, chopping them into pieces and washing the pieces with some water so as to extract the juice. This is filtered and heated with lime, a process that carries down a great part of the impurities from the solution. The clarified juice is then evaporated, first in open vessels and then in vacuum pans. When the sugar crystallizes, the resulting mass is centrifuged. This separates the raw sugar from the cane molasses (syrup). This procedure is repeated twice more, and the mass centrifuged each time, after which it is difficult for any more of the sugar to be crystallized. Each time this process occurs, some of the sugar is caramelized, so that the molasses produced becomes progressively darker.

The raw sugar is brownish in colour, and is usually exported to the country where it is to be refined. This is done by washing the sugar and then dissolving it in water, passing the solution over charcoal to decolorize it, and finally crystallizing and drying it. At this stage it is white.

Beet sugar is prepared in much the same way, except that the preparation is continuous from the cutting up of the beet through to the end of the refining process. For this reason, all raw sugar and molasses come from the cane and not from beet.

The composition of raw sugar and the various grades of molasses varies, depending on the particular plant making them; approximate analyses are given in the Table.

Production of sugar was low for a very long time, so that it was an expensive luxury until well into the eighteenth century. In the UK, average consumption was about 2kg a year until then; it rose slowly during the next 100 years, and much more rapidly when sugar duties were reduced and finally removed after about 1850. In most Western countries, average consumption stands at about 50kg a year. In the

UK it has fallen slightly since the early 1970s and is now somewhat less than 50kg.

The rapid rise in sugar consumption was due to many causes: the introduction of the sugar-beet, the improvement in yields and in the cost of refining, the improved incomes, and the advances in food technology that made it possible to manufacture inexpensive sugar-containing products, such as confectionery, soft drinks, cakes and biscuits. In addition, sugar is added to a large number of manufactured foods which would not be expected to contain it, such as canned vegetables, soups and sauces. About half of the sugar taken in the UK is in manufactured foods and drinks.

The varied uses of sucrose in food manufacture occur because it has several properties other than sweetness. It gives bulk to confectionery, acts as a preservative, gives 'mouth feel' to soft drinks, and forms a gel with pectin in the making of jams and jellies. For these and other reasons, sucrose cannot be entirely replaced by artificial sweeteners such as saccharin.

In the wealthy countries, there is little difference in sugar intake among people of different incomes. Not much is known, however, about other factors affecting distribution; the few data available in the UK indicate that intake increases with age, up to about 16 years, and then falls. At any particular age, consumption is higher among males. The highest average consumption therefore appears to be among teenage boys, and this is about twice the national average. On the other hand, there is probably a wider variation among individuals in sugar consumption than in any other dietary component except alcohol; some people take no more than 25g or so a day, while others take 350g or more.

The rise in sucrose consumption with increasing affluence has been accompanied by an almost equal fall in the consumption of starch. This is the greatest dietary change in the wealthier countries during the past 200 years or so, so the question arises whether this could have produced any change in the patterns of disease in the wealthier countries.

There is now little doubt that sucrose is a potent cause of dental decay. In addition, it is an important cause of obesity, since it often occurs in foods or drinks taken because of their taste rather than because they provide more energy.

It has also been suggested that a high intake of sucrose is the cause of coronary heart disease and diabetes. Part of the evidence for this is epidemiological, namely that the prevalence of these conditions in populations is on the whole proportional to their sugar consumption.

However, there is also evidence from experiments. In human subjects, diets with high sucrose raise the concentration of triglyceride and total cholesterol, and reduce the concentration of low density lipoprotein cholesterol. In a proportion of subjects, it also increases insulin and cortical hormone, reduces glucose tolerance, and increases the clotting capacity of the blood by increasing the 'stickiness' of the blood platelets. In experimental animals, it can be shown that sucrose also makes the tissues insensitive to the action of insulin, and produces changes in the retina and kidney characteristic of diabetes.

It is important to remember that there are two sorts of brown sugar. One sort is indeed raw (or unrefined) cane sugar; the other sort is white cane sugar or beet sugar, to which molasses or caramel has been added. The unrefined raw sugar is usually destined for the refineries, and thus has not been prepared with much care; it will then contain undesirable ingredients such as gum, bacteria, peices of string, dirt and sometimes sugar lice, so you really should not use it. Some raw sugar, however, is prepared very carefully so as to be quite suitable for consumption.

As to nutritional value, recent research shows that the darker raw sugars contain significant quantities of some of the trace elements. Thus, while it is still true that it is best not to take sugar, if you do take it, make sure it is clean dark raw sugar.

Raw beet sugar and semi-refined beet sugar are never made available, because they carry with them bitter materials from the beet.

There are several forms in which white sugar is presented. Sometimes the differences are in the sizes of the crystals, examples being granulated sugar with larger crystals and caster sugar with smaller crystals. Icing sugar is produced by finely grinding the sugar. Preserving sugar consists simply of the irregular pieces inadvertently formed when slabs

COMPOSITION OF SUGARS AND SYRUPS

Typical analyses in 100 grams

	WHITE	DEMERARA	MUSCOVADO	GOLDEN SYRUP	BLACK TREACLE
Energy, kcal	395	395	375	300	260
Calcium, mg	2	50	150	25	400
Iron, mg	Trace	0.9	5	1.5	9

of sugar are cut into cubes; these pieces have no preserving or other quality different from those of cubes or crystals of sugar.

See also: Appetite; Carbohydrates; Coronary heart disease; Dental decay; Diabetes

Sunflower seeds

Related to the common daisy, sunflowers are grown for their seeds in Eastern Europe, as well as in their original habitat in North America and Mexico. The seeds are eaten raw in Russia; otherwise they are fed to poultry or to cage birds. They yield an oil rich in polyunsaturated fatty acids; the amount produced commercially is similar to that of groundnut oil or cottonseed oil, and the residue provides a protein-rich oil cake for animal feed.

See also: Oils

Survival rations

People who have been cut off from normal supplies of food by ship-wreck or earthquake, or in battle, need to have access to emergency rations if possible. It cannot be stressed too much, however, that far more important than the supply of food is the supply of water. People can readily survive for weeks without food, but only for days without water. Even if all steps are taken to minimize water loss, at least one litre of water a day is required. If no water is available for drinking, the loss of 2 litres causes discomfort and reduces efficiency; the loss of 4 litres results in virtually complete inability to carry out even small tasks; the loss of 8 litres is fatal. Thus, even in the best circumstances, survival cannot be expected for more than one week or so; in adverse circumstances, death can occur within 2 or 3 days. Water loss can be reduced chiefly by avoiding as much as possible exposure to the sun, or exertion during the heat of the day. In addition, the food rations should contain as little salt as possible and should also be low in protein; these will minimize the volume of urine excreted.

It is not enough to rely on thirst; people can better gauge the adequacy of their water consumption by ensuring that they excrete reasonable amounts of urine.

If normal supplies of food are interrupted for only a few days, special measures are necessary only for military personnel, who may need to maintain their strength and stamina until such time as normal supplies are restored. However, apart from this particular instance, food itself does not have a high priority. It is likely to be more important to provide for such items as shelter from the sun, and perhaps for radio equipment.

The food rations do not have to provide adequate quantities of all the nutrients; deficiency of protein, mineral elements and vitamins will not occur during the 2 or 3 weeks for which it is reasonable to expect the food to last. There is no basis for the common belief that the provision of vitamin concentrates will substitute for the provision of food.

Carbohydrate and fat should constitute the major components of the food: toffees and other sweets are usually recommended, but biscuits and other sources of starch might be better than sucrose-rich items which might cause indigestion and hypoglycaemia.

See also: Expeditions; Water

Sweetening agents

The best-known material used for sweetening is sucrose, or ordinary table sugar. As well as being sweet and readily soluble in water, it has several other properties, such as preservative power and bulk, that contribute to its widespread use. However, there is a demand for alternatives to provide sweetness, either without the high energy that sucrose provides, or that are suitable for diabetics because they are metabolized differently, or in order to avoid its harmful effects on the teeth and perhaps on other organs.

These alternative sweetening agents thus fall into two main categories that can be called caloric and non-caloric. The former are mostly hydrogenated sugars such as sorbitol, xylitol, mannitol and isomalt. The non-caloric sweeteners are extremely sweet, and so are used in very small quantities. They do not therefore have the bulk and preservative qualities of sucrose. The best known of the non-caloric sweeteners is saccharin; others are cyclamate, aspartame, acesulfam-K and thaumatin. Apart from cyclamate, which was withdrawn in 1969, all of these are now permitted in the United Kingdom.

Saccharin was discovered in 1879; it is about 300 times as sweet as sucrose. It has a rather bitter aftertaste, noticed more by some people than by others. Its use in food manufacture is limited, in that it decomposes when heated, so that it cannot be used when the preparations have to be sterilized by heat. The relative sweetness of the other sweeteners varies from about 30 times to about 3,000 times that of sucrose.

The degree of sweetness of a sweetener is assessed by this comparison. However, it is not as simple as may appear. Clearly, it is impossible simply to taste a solution of sugar and a solution of the same strength of the sweetener and assess whether the latter is as sweet as the sugar solution, or not as sweet, or twice or 20 or 200 times as sweet. One way then is to make up various strengths of the sweetener and of sugar, and find the lowest concentration of each that has a detectable sweetness. This is a measure of the sweetness threshold. If one finds that the concentration of the sweetener that can just be detected is twice as great as that of the sugar, then one can say it has half the sweetness; if the concentration of the sweetener is one-hundredth of that of the sugar, then it is 100 times as sweet.

This is how the figures in the Table have been ascertained. But it ought to be said that somewhat different figures might be achieved if, for example, the solutions of sweetener and sugar were hot, or if a small amount of acid were present. Nevertheless, the figures do give a good guide to the manufacturer of the sweetener, who wants to know for example how much he should use to replace a particular amount of sugar.

RELATIVE SWEETNESS OF SWEETENING AGENTS

Threshold sweetness: Sucrose = 1.0

CALORIC SWEETENERS		NON-CALORIC SWEETENERS	
Glucose	0.5	Cyclamate	30
Sorbitol	0.5	Acesulfame-K	150
Mannitol	0.7	Aspartame	200
Xylitol	1.0	Saccharin	300
Fructose	1.7	Thaumatin	3,000

See also: Sucrose

Sweet potato (*Ipomoea batatas*)

In spite of its name and its appearance, the sweet potato is not a botanical relative of the ordinary potato, sometimes called the Irish potato. Nor, with the possible exception of some of the Pacific islands, does it ever contribute a significant amount of food to human diet. The sweet potato is grown mostly in the western tropics, but it can grow too in such climates as those of New Jersey in the US and Spain.

It contains rather less water than do yams and potatoes, and less protein than either of these crops. Its main solid constituent is starch, but it also contains some sugar which gives it its sweet taste. Sweet potatoes are usually cooked by boiling, but they are sometimes baked.

T

Tables of food composition

For several reasons, some obvious and some less obvious, it is necessary to know how much energy and how much of each of the nutrients are contained in the foods that people are eating. An obvious example is for a person who is being allowed to choose a calorie-restricted diet from a wide variety of foods, who will need to know the calorie value of each of the foods. But there are other reasons too:

(1) To decide whether the habitual diet of a patient is a possible cause of his illness.
(2) To ensure that a special diet prescribed for an individual is nutritionally adequate.
(3) In planning the supply of foods for a country during an emergency.
(4) In planning the supply of food to a hospital, school or other institution.

There are now reasonably accurate and reliable methods of measuring the energy value of food and its content of proteins, vitamins, mineral elements and fibre. As a result, it is possible to get lists of foods, together with information of their composition. The detail they give may vary from nothing except the calorie value, to details of the content of protein, fat, carbohydrate, fibre and perhaps 10 vitamins and 10 mineral elements.

In spite of the care, effort and precision with which the data have been compiled, it is essential to recognize that the figures printed in the various tables must not be used as exact representations of the particular item of diet that is being consumed. In the first place, no two samples of food have precisely the same composition; one tomato may have twice as much vitamin C as another even if they were bought together. Especially, samples of meat may vary enormously in their calorie value because of variation in the amount of fat they contain. Again, made-up dishes will vary greatly; the home cook will have her own recipe and will change it slightly from time to time; food manufacturers certainly change their recipes occasionally.

The amount of the vitamins differs greatly in different samples, and this is particularly true for the water-soluble vitamins in cooked foods.

COMPOSITION OF FOODS

Quantities in 100g (Typical values)

	Water, g	kcal	kJ	Protein, g	Fat, g	Carbohydrate, g	Sodium, mg	Calcium, mg	Iron, mg	Zinc, mg	Vitamin A, µg	Vitamin D, µg	Vitamin B₁, mg	Riboflavin, mg	Nicotinic acid, mg	Vitamin B₁₂, µg	Folic acid, µg	Vitamin C, mg
Fruits																		
Apple, eating, whole	85	45	190	0.3	—	12	2	4	0.3	0.1	5	0	0.04	0.02	0.1	0	5	6
Banana, skinned	70	80	340	1.1	0.3	20	1	7	0.4	0.2	35	0	0.04	0.07	0.8	0	20	10
Currants, dried	20	240	1,040	1.7	—	65	20	95	1.8	0.1	5	0	0.03	0.08	0.5	0	10	0
Orange, peeled	85	35	150	0.8	—	8	3	40	0.3	0.2	10	0	0.1	0.03	0.3	0	35	50
Vegetables																		
Cabbage, boiled	90	20	85	2.8	—	3	7	60	0.6	0.4	50[1]	0	0.03	0.03	0.5	0	35	20
Carrots, boiled	90	20	85	0.6	—	4	50	40	0.4	0.3	2,000[2]	0	0.05	0.04	0.5	0	25	5
Potatoes, new, boiled	80	75	320	1.6	—	18	40	5	0.4	0.3	—	0	0.02	0.03	1.6	0	13	17
main crop, boiled	80	80	340	1.4	—	20	3	4	0.3	0.2	—	—	0.08	0.03	1.1	0	14	5
Spinach, boiled	85	30	130	5.1	—	1	120	600	4.0	0.4	1,000	0	0.07	0.15	1.8	0	140	25
Tomato, raw	93	15	65	0.9	—	3	3	13	0.4	0.2	100	0	0.06	0.04	0.8	0	40	20

[1] Average: dark outer leaves may contain 50 times as much as the pale inner leaves
[2] Average: the deeper the colour, the more vitamin A (as carotene) is likely to be present
'0': no detectable amount of nutrient; '—': trace of nutrient present

COMPOSITION OF FOODS

Quantities in 100g (Typical values)

	Water, g	kcal	kJ	Protein, g	Fat, g	Carbohydrate, g	Sodium, mg	Calcium, mg	Iron, mg	Zinc, mg	Vitamin A, µg	Vitamin D, µg	Vitamin B₁, mg	Riboflavin, mg	Nicotinic acid, mg	Vitamin B₁₂, µg	Folic acid, µg	Vitamin C, mg
Meat, fish, eggs																		
Meat, medium lean, roast	52	290	1,200	27	20	0	80	10	1.3	2	—	—	0.1^1	0.25	10	0.2	5	0
Liver, ox, stewed	60	200	840	25	10	3	110	11	8	4	20,000	1.0	0.2	3.5	15	110	290	0
Fish, white, steamed	75	100	420	23	1	0	120	50	0.6	0.4	—	—	0.1	0.15	10	1	15	0
fatty	65	200	840	20	13	0	170	30	1	0.5	50	25	—	0.2	8	11	10	0
Egg	75	150	620	12	11	—	140	50	2	1.5	140	1.8	0.08	0.4	4	1.7	22	0
Bread, dairy products																		
Bread, white fortified	40	230	960	8	1.7	50	540	100	1.7	0.8	0	0	0.2	0.03	3	0	30	0
wholemeal	40	220	920	9	2.7	42	540	23	2.5	2	0	0	0.25	0.1	4	0	40	0
Cheese, Cheddar	35	400	1,650	26	35	0	600	800	0.4	4	350	0.3	0.04	0.5	6	1.5	20	0
cottage	80	100	420	14	4	1.5	450	60	0.1	0.5	35	0.02	0.02	0.2	3.5	0.5	10	0
Milk	88	65	270	3.3	3.8	4.7	50	120	0.05	0.35	35	0.02	0.04	0.2	0.8	0.3	9	1.5
Sundries																		
Chocolate, plain	2	520	2,200	5	29	65	10	40	2.4	0.2	7	0	0.07	0.1	1.2	0	10	0
Ice-cream	65	165	690	3.5	8.2	21	70	120	0.3	0.4	—	—	0.04	0.15	1	0	2	0
Honey	23	290	1,290	0.4	—	76	11	5	0.4	—	0	0	—	0.05	0.2	0	0	0

'0': no detectable amount of nutrient; '—': trace of nutrient present

[1] Values for beef and lamb; the value for pork is about 0.5mg

Cooking also influences the mineral content of foods; not only are some mineral salts leached out of the food, but calcium may be added, especially if the cooking is in hard water. Iron may be accidentally added through the use of utensils during cooking or in the preparation of the food by a food manufacturer. For these reasons, the analysts who compile the tables examine several samples of the same food and it is the average of the food values found which is printed in the food table.

Finally, when all these difficulties are recognized and care is taken to minimize them, it must be remembered that no one has ever analysed the precise apple or piece of bread you are about to eat. The food tables must therefore be used with respect; they should not be taken as assessing the composition of one food or of a whole diet with the degree of precision with which one can weigh or measure an article.

As an example, there are said to be 230 kilocalories in 100g of white bread. If the amount of bread consumed is not weighed but estimated to be 'about 1oz', say 25g, then the calculation would say that the bread has provided 58 kcal, but 'about 1oz' may have been 20g or even 35g. If so, the energy content was as low as 47 kcal or as high as 82 kcal. Moreover, these assumptions are made on the basis that the sample of bread really did contain 233 kcal per 100g. In fact, depending on the sample, it could easily have had 225 kcal or 245. Taking the lowest estimate of kcal and weight, and the highest estimate, the true statement of the energy from the bread is that it was between about 45 kcal and 86 kcal.

Since these uncertainties exist for other items of food and with each of the nutrients, it is unrealistic for people to calculate a 24-hour dietary intake to the nearest kcal, and gram or milligram of nutrient.

Tannin

The astringent quality sometimes noticed when one drinks strong, stale tea is due to a mixture of chemical substances called polyphenols; the older name is tannin or tannic acid. It is found in the leaves, or fruits, or bark, or other parts of many plants. Mostly, tannin gets into the body from tea and coffee. Traditionally the tanning of animal hides to produce leather was done with plant extracts, in England usually from oak galls or oak bark. However, today synthetic poly-phenols are increasingly used.

Tannin has the property of precipitating dissolved proteins and some other complex chemical substances, and is sometimes administered as an antidote to a person who has swallowed strychnine or atropine or some other alkaloid. It also reacts with iron, so that it may reduce the absorption of that mineral element that is present in the diet.

See also: Coffee; Tea

Tartaric acid

One of the acids found in fruit, tartaric acid occurs mostly in grapes and so in wine. Since it is not very soluble in dilute alcohol, it is one of the constituents of the insoluble materials appearing during the making of wine, or those gradually 'thrown' as a sediment in some old wines.

The acid is sometimes used in making up fruit-like flavours for adding to ice cream, soft drinks, sweets and desserts. Tartaric acid, or cream of tartar which is one of its acid salts, is often a constituent of baking powders. The other major constituent is usually bicarbonate of soda, and when the mixture is dissolved, the acid and the bicarbonate react to release carbon dioxide gas.

See also: Wine

Taste

The pure sensation of taste is evoked by the contact of food with the taste buds, special minute organs on the tongue and palate. Through this contact, the impulses that these constituents of the food evoke in the taste buds are transmitted by special nerves to the brain, which can recognize four primary tastes (sweet, sour (acid), salt and bitter). Different parts of the tongue are specially sensitive to particular tastes: the tip of the tongue is sensitive to salt and sweet, the back of the tongue to bitter, and the edges to sour and salt.

But the appreciation of the taste of a food is not confined to these primary sensations; to them are added sensations of smell, and it is these that make it possible to distinguish, say, the taste of chocolate from that of coffee. An attack of the common cold, or even pinching the nose, reduces the appreciation of such different flavours.

Finally, if we widen the term taste to include the total degree of attractiveness of a food, or of its lack of attractiveness, it is necessary to add its other qualities such as appearance and texture. When food manufacturers test their new products, it is this combination of qualities on which they pass judgement; the technical description for this combination is 'organoleptic'.

See also: Appetite

Tea (*Camellia sinensis*)

For some thousands of years, tea as a beverage has been popular in China. It was introduced into Europe as a luxury in the seventeenth century. From the late nineteenth century it became popular, especially in the United Kingdom, when it was discovered that the shrub could be grown in Sri Lanka (Ceylon) and India. A good crop requires a fertile soil, a high rainfall and a warm climate.

The shrubs grow to about 4 feet; this makes it easy for the young leaves to be picked from the top of the shoots. They are allowed to wither; soon fermentation (in fact oxidation) begins because of the action of the enzymes in the leaf. When fermentation is complete, the leaves are dried by heating and these constitute black tea. Green tea, favoured especially by the Chinese, is made by heating the leaves soon after picking; this destroys the enzymes, so that no fermentation takes place.

When the tea leaves are infused, caffeine and tannin are extracted. The caffeine, at one time called theine, is released more readily than the tannin, so that a freshly brewed cup of tea gives almost as much of a stimulus as that which has been infused for a long time, but has less astringency. An average cup contains between 50 and 80mg of caffeine. In addition, tea may contribute a significant amount of fluoride to the diet, since one cup provides around 0.25mg; the average British intake of 5–6 cups of tea a day would thus provide 1–2mg of fluoride, which would be sufficient to meet the daily requirements of an adult as assessed, for example, by the German Nutrition Society.

In China and many other countries, the tea is drunk with no additions except the occasional small quantity of flower petals such as jasmine. In Britain especially, tea is commonly drunk with the addition of milk, and often sugar too.

Tea taken with a meal or soon after can significantly reduce the absorption of iron present in some other foods, because it reacts with the tannin.

See also: Caffeine; Tannin

Thermogenesis

After foods have been eaten, there is a rise in the metabolic rate of the body, which was given the name of specific dynamic action (SDA). It is now more commonly called the thermic effect of food, or dietary induced thermogenesis (DIT). It used to be thought that it was caused only or largely by the protein in the food, but it appears that different foods do not greatly differ in their effect on the degree of increase in metabolism. Nor is this influenced much by the amount of food consumed. In the average person, the increase in metabolism over a 24-hour period amounts to between 5% and 10%.

It is not clearly understood why the consumption of food speeds metabolism, although several explanations have been suggested. One is the heat produced by the secretion of gastric and other digestive juices by the alimentary canal. A second is that digested food stimulates the manufacture of new protein. However, these and the other suggested explanations do not account for all the known features of the phenomenon.

See also: Brown adipose tissue; Energy

Thyroid gland

The thyroid gland is situated in the neck in front of the trachea or windpipe, and consists of two lobes joined by an isthmus. The normal adult gland weighs only 20–25g, but it contains about one-quarter of the total iodine in the body. It is of interest in relation to diet for two reasons. One reason is because of the effects of deficiency of iodine on the gland and on the rest of the body. The second reason is that the hormones produced by the gland have a profound effect upon the body's metabolism, so that it is necessary to consider the possible role of these hormones in the cause and treatment of obesity.

Deficiency of dietary iodine is the most important cause of simple goitre, in which the gland is enlarged, sometimes quite considerably. The amount of iodine in the gland diminishes, sometimes to as little as 1mg. Simple goitre occurs mostly in areas with a low iodine content in the soil and thus in the locally-grown crops. It is often found in mountainous areas, such as the Alps, the Himalayas, and the Andes. Nevertheless, it also occurs in non-mountainous areas where the soil is low in iodine, such as around the Great Lakes of North America. In the UK, it used to be common in Derbyshire, where the enlargement of the thyroid gland gave the name 'Derbyshire neck' to the condition. The prevalence of the disease in Derbyshire, the Alps and the United States and Canada is now less common, probably with the wider distribution of food through increased facilities for transporting and storing, as well as increasing affluence allowing a wider choice of food; nevertheless, it is said still to be present in 6% or more of the women in Derbyshire.

The availability of dietary iodine is affected by other mineral elements. Thus, goitre is more common in areas with hard water or with a high concentration of fluoride.

As well as shortage of iodine, simple goitre may be caused in part by the consumption of 'goitrogenic' foods containing goitre-producing substances. These are mostly brassica vegetables such as cabbage, turnips and mustard seed. They contain 'progoitrins' which are converted to 'goitrins' by an enzyme in the vegetables. Since this is destroyed by heat, the cooked freshly-picked vegetables are likely to be innocuous. One of the products of the action of the enzyme is thiocyanate, which is excreted in the urine. Measurement of this can thus be used as a measure of the goitrogens in the diet. It has been suggested that recent outbreaks of simple goitre in Zaïre were due to the consumption of cassava containing the goitrogen linamarin.

Simple goitre is more commonly seen in girls and women, especially during adolescence and pregnancy. The effects may be confined to enlargement of the gland, with no systemic effect, although if the enlargement is considerable it can cause discomfort or even difficulty in breathing, by pressing upon the trachea. On the other hand, the simple goitre may produce so little of the thyroid hormones that deficiency may occur as cretinism or myxoedema.

There are two hormones produced by the gland, both containing iodine; they are thyroxine and tri-iodothyronine. Because of the number of iodine atoms contained in these hormones, they are often referred to as T_4 and T_3. They have a considerable influence on basal metabolism and on growth.

Deficiency of these hormones, or of iodine, from birth, results in cretinism. This is characterized by a low metabolic rate and by retardation of physical and mental development. In adults, and rarely in infants and children, deficiency of hormones or iodine produces myxoedema. It is commoner in women than in men, and occurs mostly between the ages of 30 and 50. A person with myxoedema has puffiness under the skin, due to an accumulation of mucinous material. The temperature is below normal, the individual feels the cold and is excessively sleepy. The hair, including the eyebrows, tends to be thin. Treated early enough with thyroid hormone, or if necessary with iodine, both cretinism and myxoedema can be cured.

Because deficiency of thyroid hormones leads to diminished basal metabolism, it is often suggested that obesity should be treated with thyroxine. This can be justified only if the obese subject shows signs of deficiency such as those seen in myxoedema; if these are not present, treatment with thyroxine may produce the effects of hyperthyroidism, which include irritability, an excessively fast pulse, and tremor.

See also: Basal metabolism; Hormones; Iodine; Obesity

Tomatoes (*Lycopersicon esculentum*)

Like its relative the potato, the tomato is a native of the Andes, although it did not grow in such an extensive area. It was brought to Italy in the middle of the sixteenth century, where it was given the name *pomodoro* or golden apple. In England it was thought to be an aphrodisiac and was known as the love-apple, although it did not become popular there until the early nineteenth century. It is now grown in most parts of the world. In warmer climates it will fruit well outdoors, but in the cooler climates of northern Europe it is grown under glass.

The green part of the plant, like that of the potato, contains solanine, and so is poisonous. The typical fruit is spherical and red, but its colour can be yellow, white or green, and it can be oval, pear-shaped or ribbed.

Tomatoes are eaten raw, or cooked in one of several ways. A large proportion is canned, or made into tomato juice, ketchup or concentrate. Much of this processing is carried out in Italy, with strains of tomatoes especially grown for these purposes.

The nutrients in worthwhile amounts in the tomato are carotene (pro-vitamin A), which is part of the colouring materials of the skin, and vitamin C. There is very little protein or fat, and its energy content too is quite low.

Tonic

There is a widespread belief that there are foods or medicines that act as tonics in that they improve the body's functions and increase the sense of wellbeing. In the amounts in which it is present in tea or coffee, caffeine may be said to produce the latter effect. Apart perhaps from this effect of caffeine, it is difficult to find any substance that can produce general improvement in the way the body functions, without at the same time carrying with it the likelihood that it also produces undesirable side effects.

In the early part of this century, minute doses of arsenic were frequently prescribed as a tonic, as were valerian, gentian and glycerophosphates. Quinine, the bitter ingredient in tonic water, bitter orange and bitter lemon, is still found in some proprietary tonics. Today's more fashionable tonics, sometimes prescribed by doctors, often under pressure from patients, contain iron and vitamins, especially vitamins of the B group. None of these has any tonic action other than that of suggestion, which accounts also for the existence of preparations made more impressive by the addition of exotic colours and flavours.

See also: Health foods

Tyramine

Some foods, notably cheese, extracts of yeast and meat, and some wines, contain tyramine, an amine derived from the amino-acid tyrosine. Tyramine is normally destroyed quite rapidly in the body by an enzyme, monoamine oxidase (MAO). Some of the drugs prescribed for the treatment of depression work by inhibiting this enzyme, so they are called MAO inhibitors. If a patient taking such a drug eats one of the tyramine-containing foods, the amine is not destroyed and so accumulates. The effect is to increase blood pressure, sometimes quite considerably. This can produce severe headache, migraine, dizziness and occasionally cerebral haemorrhage. Because of the risk of these reactions, a patient taking MAO inhibitor drugs is always given a list of foods that must be avoided. It should be added that not all anti-depressant drugs are MAO inhibitors, and many doctors first prescribe those which are not, and the inhibitor only if the first drugs are not effective enough in that patient.

See also: Cheese

U

Unconventional foods

The solution of the present and continuing problem of food supplies is being sought both by an attempt to increase the production of conventional foods such as cereals, and also in the development of unconventional foods. In some ways, there have been spectacular increases in yields of crops, but the so-called green revolution has also raised problems.

The search for unconventional or non-traditional foods, and their exploitation, have also led to an alternation of optimistic forecast and pessimistic realization. The approach has been largely a search for edible items rich in protein. Two possible sources of such foods have been intensively investigated: the production of protein concentrates from material from higher plants, and the cultivation and harvesting of micro-organisms. Although these foods are rich in protein, they should not be called 'protein', because they contain other substances in addition. This is just as wrong as to call bread and potatoes carbohydrates; they have carbohydrate as a major constituent but they do contain other ingredients.

Both seeds and leaves have been used in the search for foods rich in protein. The seeds are those that are already known to be good sources of protein; the object is to concentrate these to an extent that produces materials that can be used as an alternative to other protein-rich foods such as meat. The seeds that have been used in these attempts have been mostly soya beans, but they include field beans and peas, sunflower seeds and rape seeds. Some seeds cannot be used because they contain toxic substances not easily removed, such as gossypol in cotton seeds. Many other seeds have toxic substances that present less of a hazard, because the toxin content may be reduced either by breeding or by relatively simple treatment. It is only soya beans that are free from these harmful constituents. On the other hand, all the seeds, including soya beans, may become contaminated with moulds that produce the poisonous aflatoxins, so that it is necessary carefully to select the harvested crops and to store them well.

Green leaves growing both on land and in water contain protein in amounts that can be extracted without too much difficulty. It has been said that alfalfa (lucerne) grown on an area half the size of Texas could produce enough protein to meet the requirements of the total world population. Nevertheless, the cost of harvesting, and especially of extraction and purification, is quite high; moreover, the protein is not of good quality and the products so far available are not very palatable. Again, toxic products are sometimes present. The cost could be partly offset by using the residues after pressing out the juice for animal feed, but the economic feasibility of this would depend on such factors as cost of transport and the price of other feeds for animals.

See also: Aflatoxins; Novel protein foods

Urine

The body has three major ways in which it discards its unwanted waste from food and drink. The food materials not digested and absorbed in the digestive tract, as well as other materials added to them in their passage through the intestinal tract, are excreted in the stools (faeces). Those materials that are absorbed but not wanted, together with waste products produced during metabolism, are cleared from the blood in one of two ways; the urine carries away dissolved solid waste products, and the expired air carries away carbon dioxide as a gas. However, in addition to these mechanisms that have the function of maintaining the constancy of the body's composition, there are other mechanisms by which materials are discarded, as it were fortuitously, only because they happen to be involved in carrying out some quite different function; an example of this is the loss of water in sweat, which occurs because this is one of the ways in which the body maintains a constant temperature.

Urine is derived from the blood. It is formed continuously in the kidney, and passes to the bladder; this is sometimes called the urinary bladder to distinguish it from the gall-bladder. Here it accumulates until the pressure rises to the point where one is conscious of a desire to urinate (micturate).

Urine formation takes place in very small units in the kidney called nephrons. Essentially, these consist of filter-like structures, in the cup of which there is suspended a skein of capillaries called the glomerulus Fluid leaves these capillaries just as tissue fluid leaves all capillaries; it contains therefore none of the blood cells or platelets or protein, but does contain all the substances that consist of small molecules, such as glucose, salt, urea and uric acid.

This filtrate passes down the tube of the nephron, which joins other tubes, until they eventually reach the ureter leading from the kidney to the bladder.

While still in the tubule of the nephron, considerable absorption of filtrate occurs. About 99% of the water is absorbed, so that the formation of one litre of urine in a day is accompanied by the filtration of 100 litres of blood, containing something like 100g of glucose, 400g of salt and a quantity of other substances. Of this, all of the glucose and most of the salts are re-absorbed. The absorption of these and some of the other materials helps to maintain the concentration of essential substances in the blood, and also to maintain its pH. On the other hand, most if not all of the unwanted materials in the blood, such as urea and uric acid, products of protein metabolism, remain in the fluid now being transformed to urine.

See also: Kidney

V

Vanaspati

Just as ghee (samna) is in effect butter without its water, so vanaspati is margarine without water. It is made, mostly in India, by hydrogenation of vegetable oils, but the admixture with water to make margarine is omitted. Vitamins A and D may be added, as they are to margarine in some countries.

See also: Margarine

Vegetables

A wide range of plants and parts of plants are included in this term: leaves such as cabbage and lettuce, fruits such as cucumbers, stalks such as celery, roots such as potatoes, parsnips and turnips, flowers such as cauliflowers. Apart from root vegetables, however, they have not been a very popular group of foods, except recently and in Western countries. During the Middle Ages, few vegetables were grown and eaten in Western countries; the occasional vegetable garden of the monasteries grew mostly herbs for flavouring and for medicinal use. Even among the poor in countries such as India, where a reasonable supply of leafy vegetables in the diet would prevent xerophthalmia and blindness from vitamin A deficiency in hundreds of thousands of children, they constitute only a small part of the diet, and then mostly from wild plants rather than from cultivated plants. Nor do the children of the affluent West take vegetables with the eagerness their parents would like. It is perhaps only when there is a range of other foods available, and sophisticated methods of preparing them, that leafy vegetables are routinely incorporated into the diet. It may be that, in poorer countries and less affluent times, for the same cost or the same effort, foods such as cereals are much more filling, that is, provide more energy more economically.

Green vegetables can make a significant contribution to the intake of vitamin A (as carotene), vitamin C, folic acid, vitamin K, vitamin E and fibre.

Vegetarianism

There are three main reasons that people give for deciding not to eat meat. One is that it inflicts unnecessary cruelty on animals. Second is the belief that it is healthier to eat a diet without meat. The third reason is that man is by nature a vegetarian, so that meat and other animal products are, for him, unnatural foods.

Another advantage claimed for vegetarianism is that only a small part of the feed for farm animals is from pasture; the rest is from cereals and other foods that could be used directly to feed at least five times as many people as are fed on the meat, milk and eggs produced when these foods are first fed to animals.

It is not possible to dispute the moral argument that it is cruel for people to rear animals for the express purpose of killing them for human food. On this view, milk and egg production too are no less cruel, in that most of the male calves and chicks are kept for only a short time and then killed. The health argument is not so easy to sustain, unless it is accepted that the fat in the farm animals now being produced is a cause of coronary disease and perhaps colonic cancer, and that the only way to avoid these conditions is by avoiding animal products in our diets.

The 'natural' argument, however, is misconceived. The vegetable foods eaten by our ancestors of 5 or 10 million years ago clearly did not contain the cereals and pulses that began to be cultivated by neolithic agricultural man 10,000 years ago. These foods are very much more concentrated than the leaves, fruits and roots our vegetarian ancestors ate, except for the few seeds and nuts they could find; in the terminology of some vegetarians, we must conclude that cereals and pulses are as 'unnatural' as are the meat and milk brought into man's diet by the domestication of animals during the same neolithic revolution. In order to get even as little as 2,000 kcal a day, our vegetarian primate ancestors would have needed to eat something between 2kg and 10kg of leaves, roots and fruits, which would have taken them most of the day to collect and consume.

There are several grades of abstention practised by people who consider themselves to be vegetarians. There are those who avoid meat, but do not avoid fish, eggs or milk. Others also exclude fish, or fish and eggs; these may be called ovo-lactovegetarians or lacto-vegetarians. Finally, there are those who take no food of animal origin; they may also avoid the non-food use of animal products, such as leather for their footwear. This last group is known as vegans.

Apart from the vegans, vegetarians have no nutritional problems. Like non-vegetarians, unless they choose in an eccentric fashion what they eat and how much, they are likely to get all the energy and nutrients they require, together with a higher quantity of fibre than do most of those who are not vegetarians. Vegans, on the other hand, have problems getting enough assimilable iron and calcium, and ordinarily their diet contains no vitamin B_{12}. This last fact explains why some have developed the neurological disorder, sub-acute combined degeneration of the cord, also seen in pernicious anaemia, and why a few have died. On the other hand, the megaloblastic anaemia of pernicious anaemia does not occur, because the diet is rich in folic acid. Nowadays, vegans are able to obtain vitamin B_{12} preparations from non-animal sources, made as a by-product in microbiological fermentation during the manufacture of antibiotics such as streptomycin.

See also: Neolithic revolution; Vitamin B_{12}

Vinegar

The oxidation of ordinary alcohol (ethyl alcohol or ethanol) produces acetic acid, the essential constituent of vinegar. Any source of alcohol can therefore be the material from which vinegar is made; these sources include wine, cider, fermented malted barley, or distilled spirits.

Vinegar contains 4% or more acetic acid; the particular colour and flavour of the product depend both on the raw material used and on any added substance. Thus, malt vinegar, which has a brown colour and a taste derived from the malt, is often improved by the addition of caramel and artificial flavours.

It is possible to make vinegar by the dilution of synthetic acetic acid; however, food regulations usually require labelling to indicate that the product has not been produced by brewing.

There is nothing about vinegar to support the popular view that it is useful in helping to reduce overweight.

See also: Cider vinegar

Vitamin A (Retinol)

The 'accessory food factor' reported by Hopkins in 1906 as being necessary for growth was later found to be present in the butter fat of milk, and called 'fat-soluble A'. When it was shown to be different from the fat-soluble dietary substance that prevented rickets, the growth factor was named vitamin A and the rickets-preventing factor vitamin D.

By 1930 it had been demonstrated that vitamin A could be replaced by carotene, an orange pigment found in green leaves, carrots and some other plant sources. The body converts the carotene into the vitamin in the wall of the intestine as it is being absorbed into the blood.

Because vitamin A itself and carotene each exist in more than one chemical form, and because they are not all equally active, it is now usual to give the name 'retinol' to the pure vitamin A. Thus the total vitamin A activity of a food, now called its retinol equivalent, is determined by how much it contains of retinol, materials chemically very close to retinol but not so active, and a range of carotenes also of varying activity. The most active form of carotene is beta-carotene, but even beta-carotene is not very efficiently converted into retinol. As a result, the vitamin A activity of the carotenes in foods is taken to be one-sixth of the total amount of carotenes they contain.

Retinol is found in rather few foods; these include liver, milk, butter and the yolks of eggs, and especially fish liver oils such as cod liver oil. Carotene is one of the pigments in all green leaves, and it occurs also in tomatoes and apricots; especially rich sources of carotene are carrots and red palm oil. Some part of the colouring matter of eggs and milk is also carotene.

If the intake of vitamin A is insufficient, the first effect is a diminution of night vision, or dark adaptation. Normally, if you sit in a dimly lit cinema, you are gradually able to see the people over whose legs you stumbled in taking your seat. The reason is that the eye's sensitivity to light depends on the amount of a substance in the retina called rhodopsin, visual purple; it is bleached in conditions of light, but regenerates in the dark, so leading to increased sensitivity. Since the manufacture of visual purple by the body needs vitamin A, a shortage of the vitamin leads to a shortage of visual purple and so to a decreased ability to adapt in dimly lit surroundings. This is called night blindness or nyctalopia.

Another effect of deficiency is on the skin, and the conjunctiva and cornea of the eye. The outer layers of the cells on the surface multiply and become flattened. In particular, the sebaceous glands of the skin become blocked with hard plugs of these cells, making the skin rough; this condition is known as follicular keratosis. It should be added that follicular keratosis sometimes occurs when there is no deficiency of vitamin A, and conversely may be absent when there is deficiency.

Meanwhile the eyes become dry, itchy and inflamed, and begin to grow opaque. This condition is known as xerophthalmia. The eyes may also become infected, so that the cornea may be totally destroyed and one or both eyes become blind; this is keratomalacia. Deficiency of vitamin A is the commonest cause of blindness in the Middle East and in India; it is said that 20,000 children go blind each year because of shortage of vitamin A. Moreover, it has been found that children with night blindness or other signs of deficiency of vitamin A have an abnormally high mortality, which is proportional to the severity of the deficiency. Yet all this could very easily be prevented if we could persuade the parents to see that their children eat some of the plentiful vegetables available in these countries.

Because deficiency of vitamin A reduces the resistance to infection of the soft covering tissues in some parts of the body, such as the respiratory tract, it was for some time called the anti-infective vitamin. It used to be fashionable to recommend people to take preparations of the vitamin in order to reduce their chances of getting coughs and colds. There is no evidence that this is effective. Westerners usually have a store of vitamin A in their livers sufficient to prevent deficiency for at least a year, even if during this time their diets contained virtually none.

Vitamin A as retinol is one of the few vitamins in which excess produces definite and severe effects. Sometimes children have been given large amounts by over-zealous parents, presumably in the belief that if a little is good, a lot is better. Hypervitaminosis A was first described, however, by Arctic explorers who ate the liver of polar bears; this may contain as much as 600mg of retinol in 100g of liver. The effects include loss of appetite, a dry, itchy skin often with peeling, intense headaches and an enlarged liver. This is the only known example of toxicity from excess vitamin from what may be considered, at least in the region of the Arctic, a normal food for man; it is avoided, however, by the indigenous Eskimos. Excessive intake of vitamin A or any other vitamin can otherwise occur only by the consumption of concentrated or synthetic preparations. Recovery is fairly rapid when intake is reduced.

Large amounts of carotene produce no effect other than an orange-yellow colour of the skin; before being visible in the skin, it may be seen in the palate. It can be distinguished from jaundice because the colour does not affect the eyes. The conversion of carotene into vitamin A is not fast enough to induce retinol toxicity; when the intake of excessive carotene is abandoned, the abnormal skin colour disappears.

VITAMIN A IN FOODS

Recommended daily intake (RDI) for moderately active man – 750 micrograms (μg) retinol equivalent (RE)

FOOD	PORTION	RE, μg
Milk	100ml	40
Cheese, Cheddar	25g	80
Butter	10g	80
Margarine	10g	90
Egg	60g (1 egg)	100
Liver, ox	100g	15,000
Cod liver oil	3ml	500
Halibut liver oil	0.05ml (1 drop)	600
Cabbage, dark leaves	100g	2,000
Carrot	100g	200

See also: Carotene; Rhodopsin

Vitamin B₁ (Thiamin)

Vitamin B₁ was purified in 1926 and synthesized 10 years later. Because of its role in preventing and curing most of the manifestations of beri-beri, including its neurological disorders, the vitamin was for a while called aneurine, analogous with the name of ascorbic acid for vitamin C. The current name, thiamin, derives from the fact that it is chemically an amine and also contains sulphur, the Greek word for which is *thios*.

Deficiency in animals such as rats and pigeons leads to a fall in appetite, loss of weight, and paralysis. In the body it takes part in a number of metabolic reactions; the best known of these is the completion of the oxidation of glucose, specially by the brain and nervous tissue. Deficiency of thiamin results in this process stopping at the point where the glucose has been partially oxidized to produce lactic acid and especially pyruvic acid, which then accumulate in the body. Because of its involvement in glucose oxidation, the requirements for thiamin are to some extent proportional to the amount of carbohydrate in the diet; rats fed a diet completely free from carbohydrate survive for long periods without thiamin.

The best food sources of thiamin are yeast, liver and the germs of cereals. Thus, the milling of cereals removes a great part of the thiamin. On the other hand, most foods contain at least modest amounts of the vitamin; the chief exceptions are sugar, fats and oils.

The vitamin is destroyed in the presence of the enzyme thiaminase, the anti-vitamin found in some species of raw fish. Since it is soluble in water and since its destruction is increased in alkaline conditions, the amount of the vitamin in cooked vegetables is best retained by not using soda, by using small amounts of water, and by not discarding the cooking water.

VITAMIN B₁ IN FOODS

Recommended daily intake (RDI) for moderately active man age 18–34 –1.2mg; age 35–64 – 1.1mg

FOOD	PORTION	THIAMIN, mg
Bread, wholemeal	30g	0.08
Bread, white fortified	30g	0.06
Rice, home milled	100g	0.4
parboiled	100g	0.3
polished	100g	0.1
Beef	100g	0.15
Pork	100g	1.0
Fish	100g	0.05
Milk	100ml	0.04
Egg	60g (1 egg)	0.05
Yeast, dried bakers'	5g	0.1
dried brewers'	5g	0.7
Liver	100g	0.2

See also: Beri-beri

Vitamin B$_6$ (Pyridoxine)

One of the vitamins in the B complex, vitamin B$_6$, exists in several forms. The basic substance is pyridoxine, which is chiefly the form in which the vitamin occurs in vegetable foods; in animal foods, it is present chiefly as pyridoxal and pyridoxamine. All of these varieties of vitamin B$_6$ are readily convertible to pyridoxal phosphate; this is the form in which it works in the body through being involved in many reactions as a co-enzyme, necessary especially for the action of the enzymes concerned with the metabolism of amino-acids and proteins.

Rich sources of vitamin B$_6$ include liver, whole cereals and bananas, but most foods contain some of the vitamin. As a result, primary dietary deficiency is rare. It occurred for a brief period in the 1950s when a new formula for babies was introduced, in which the vitamin B$_6$ originally present was inadvertently destroyed during manufacture. A small number of babies developed convulsions which, however, were rapidly cured by administering the vitamin.

Rarely, infants are found who need large amounts of the vitamin because of some congenital metabolic defect. In some diseases, administration of the vitamin may be necessary when some drugs have to be taken in unusually large amounts, such as isoniazid in the treatment of tuberculosis. Some women take vitamin B$_6$ for the treatment of morning sickness in pregnancy, or for the treatment of pre-menstrual tension; there is no satisfactory evidence that these conditions benefit from such treatment. On the other hand, very large doses of vitamin B$_6$, one of the examples of megavitamin theory in practice, have been known to produce lack of co-ordination in movement and impairment of sensation.

Vitamin B$_{12}$ (Cobalamin)

Pernicious anaemia, described first by Thomas Addison (1793–1860) in 1849, was, as its name implies, invariably fatal. The first effective treatment was described by Minot and Murphy in 1926, when they showed that the disease could be cured by the regular consumption of large amounts of liver. A further 22 years elapsed before the active substance was isolated from the liver in the minute amount of 20mg from one ton of liver. The reason for this long delay was that the testing of each of the many stages in separating the active material from the liver depended on testing the preparation on patients with the disease. Just as this laborious work was coming to fruition, the fortuitous discovery was made by another research worker that the principle active in curing pernicious anaemia was also active in promoting the growth of a particular strain of the micro-organism, *Lactobacillus lactis*. Soon after this the pure substance was isolated both in England and in the United States.

The active liver extract was found to contain the element cobalt, and because of its chemical structure was called cyanocobalamin. The 'cyano' part of the molecule was in fact introduced during the extraction process; although the vitamin exists in nature in several slightly different chemical forms, none of them has the cyano- group.

Vitamin B$_{12}$ is found only in foods from animal sources. The highest quantities are present in liver and kidney, and in herrings and sardines. Quite reasonable quantities are found in other fish, in meat and in milk. Ordinary vegetable foods contain none of the vitamin, but as it can be extracted from the mould *Streptomyces griseus* from which streptomycin is made, it is now available to vegans who take no food from animal sources.

Vitamin B$_{12}$ has two distinct functions. One is in cell division, and this shows itself especially in the rapidly dividing cells in the bone marrow that produce red blood cells. The second function is in the manufacture of the sheath that surrounds each nerve fibre; this consists of myelin, which is a complex phospholipid. With inadequate vitamin B$_{12}$ the integrity of the sheath is destroyed, and the effect is noticed especially in some of the nerve tracts in the spinal cord.

The blood picture of pernicious anaemia is described in the article on Anaemia. The disease of the spinal cord is called sub-acute combined degeneration of the cord (SACD). The features are impairment of both normal sensation and normal motor activity, i.e. movement. There is tingling and numbness especially of the limbs, and weakness and difficulty in walking. Occasionally there are also mental disturbances.

Dietary deficiency, that is, primary deficiency of vitamin B$_{12}$, is quite rare, although it has been reported in vegans, especially in the days before the availability of the preparation from streptomycin.

Pernicious anaemia is an example of a secondary deficiency. There is no shortage of vitamin B$_{12}$ in the diet, but the patient lacks the intrinsic factor in the stomach necessary to absorb the small amounts of vitamin B$_{12}$ in the diet. Since pure vitamin B$_{12}$ has become available, the problem of absorption from the gut can be overcome, either by injecting the very small amounts the body requires, or by giving, by mouth, much larger amounts than are present in foods.

Another example of a secondary vitamin B_{12} deficiency occurs, most commonly in Finland, through the consumption of raw fresh-water fish infested with the tapeworm *Diphyllobothrium latum*. The worm attaches itself to the intestinal wall and grows enormously; it can reach a length of 15m. It takes up vitamin B_{12} from the food of the host, who then develops megaloblastic anaemia.

The dietary requirements are very small indeed. In normal people, as little as 0.5µg a day is probably enough; to be certain of adequacy the British authorities recommend 2µg a day for adults. Patients diagnosed as having pernicious anaemia are given large doses of perhaps 1–2mg, at first twice a week and then smaller doses of perhaps 0.5–1mg at monthly intervals.

Vitamin B_{12} is clearly far more potent than any other vitamin. One ounce would be enough for the daily needs of the whole population of the UK.

When it was first isolated, it was believed that vitamin B_{12} was especially concerned with growth, and it was consequently prescribed by many doctors for babies and young children who appeared not to be thriving. There is no reason to suppose that the vitamin had any effect in accelerating their growth.

See also: Anaemia; Vegetarianism

Vitamin C (Ascorbic acid)

Although associated especially with oranges and lemons, vitamin C is found in varying amounts in almost every kind of food except sugar, confectionery, dried cereals and pulses; however, pulses and the seeds of cereals produce some of the vitamin when germinating.

Unlike most of the other vitamins, vitamin C is required by only a few species of animals. So far, the only mammals known to need it are human beings, primates, guinea pigs and the fruit-eating bat; a few species of birds also need vitamin C.

The vitamin as an interesting chemical substance was isolated from the adrenal gland in 1928 by the biochemist, Szent-Györgyi, but he did not recognize it as a vitamin. This recognition occurred in 1932, and its chemical composition was worked out in 1933. Vitamin C has a fairly simple formula, so it was soon synthesized, and it is now manufactured on a very large scale as ascorbic acid. This name was devised because it prevents scurvy; that is to say, it is anti-scorbutic. For a short time it was also called cevitamic acid.

Pure ascorbic acid is a white crystalline powder which is quite stable while it is dry. It readily dissolves in water, and it is reasonably stable in solution provided it is not neutralized or made alkaline, does not come into contact with metals, especially copper, and is not exposed to heat or light. On the other hand, boiling vegetables for some time, especially if bicarbonate of soda is used to preserve the green colour, can result in losses of three-quarters or more of the vitamin. This occurs partly by oxidation and partly by solution into the cooking water. Vegetables kept hot after cooking also rapidly suffer loss of the vitamin.

Vitamin C is especially concerned in the manufacture of collagen, the main substance in the cells of the matrix or 'framework' of the body, comprising the connective tissue that is made by specialized cells but lies outside of them. Thus, a deficiency of the vitamin results in blood being able to leak through the walls of the capillaries, and in the poor quality of scar tissue formed over wounds, so that they heal slowly and old healed wounds may actually break down. Deficiency also leads to badly constructed cartilage being formed in the growing bones, so that the bone formed later from this cartilage is not properly mineralized.

It is not known what special function vitamin C performs in the eye or in the adrenal cortex, both of which have high concentrations of the vitamin. Stress, such as cold, energetic physical exertion, or the presence of disease, is known to encourage the development of scurvy when the diet is deficient.

There is also a great deal of discussion about how much vitamin C is needed. The British authorities give the recommended daily allowance for an adult as 30mg. In the US, the latest recommendation is 45mg a day, but an earlier figure was 60mg. In the USSR, the recommendation is 100mg.

Dr Linus Pauling of the United States has suggested that the real requirements are very much higher, possible as high as 2–3g a day, which would be something like 60 or 100 times the amount considered adequate in the UK. Many people believe that, although not so much is required regularly, amounts of several hundreds of milligrams a day will help to prevent the common cold, and amounts of 1g or more a day, as recommended by Dr Pauling, would help to cure a cold. Moreover, other diseases are thought by Pauling and his followers to be prevented by the regular intake of 2–3g of vitamin C a day: these include cancer, coronary heart disease, and many infections in addition to colds.

On the other hand, there are some who believe that large amounts of ascorbic acid might be harmful. In particular, since one of the products of the metabolism of ascorbic acid is oxalic acid, it has been suggested that a continuing high intake might cause oxalate kidney stones. As to colds, a careful appraisal of all the evidence does suggest that moderate supplements, of the order of 100mg a day, might in some people reduce their severity, though not their frequency or duration.

VITAMIN C IN FOODS

Recommended daily intake (RDI) for moderately active man – 30mg

FOOD	PORTION	VITAMIN C, mg
Blackcurrants, raw	100g	200
Strawberries, raw	100g	60
Orange, weighed with skin	200g	80
Apple	120g	5
Cabbage, boiled	150g	30
Potatoes, new, boiled	100g	18
main crop, boiled	100g	9
Milk, pasteurized	100ml	2

See also: Lind; Megavitamin therapy

Vitamin D (Cholecalciferol)

Cod liver oil has been used in the treatment of rickets for at least 150 years. There was confusion, however, because of the contradictory claim that rickets could be cured by the apparently quite unrelated treatment of exposing the skin to sunlight. The role of cod liver oil was confirmed in 1918, when Mellanby showed that it could prevent or cure the disease experimentally produced by him in puppies. He also pointed out that the effect was due to a fat-soluble vitamin, which was soon shown to be different from vitamin A. One year later, it was definitely established by a German worker, Kurt Huldschinsky

(1883–?) that rickets could be cured by irradiation with ultra-violet rays.

We now know that vitamin D exists in two main forms. One is produced in the skin by the action of ultra-violet rays: this is called vitamin D_3 or cholecalciferol. The second main form is produced by ultra-violet rays acting upon ergosterol, which is found in yeast and fungi; this is vitamin D_2 or ergocalciferol. This hardly exists in nature, but it is manufactured for the special purpose of adding it to infant foods and other 'fortified' foods. What used to be called vitamin D_1 turned out to be a mixture of active and inactive substances, and the name is no longer used.

Vitamin D_3 is present in only a few foods; rich sources are fish liver oils, while fatty fish such as herring and salmon contain less of the vitamin, and butter and milk relatively small amounts. Many individuals, adults especially, can manage entirely without dietary supplies of vitamin D, since the amount they synthesize in the skin is usually quite adequate for their needs. Babies and young children on the other hand do need vitamin D in their diet, especially if kept mostly indoors and well-covered with clothes.

Vitamin D is sometimes classified as a hormone, since it is made in one organ of the body, the skin, and acts on other organs, the gut and the bones, which it reaches through the bloodstream. Most people get the major part of their vitamin D supply from this synthesis in the skin; the rest comes from the 'natural' vitamin D_3 in the diet and from vitamin D_2 added to some foods.

In the body, vitamin D is involved in the absorption of both calcium and phosphate from the intestine into the blood. In addition, vitamin D together with the parathyroid gland is responsible for regulating the balance between the calcium in the skeleton and the calcium concentration in the blood.

Neither vitamin D_2 nor vitamin D_3 is itself active in the body; they are first converted into the active form. This has the formidable name of 1,25-dihydroxycholecalciferol, which fortunately can be written as $1,25\text{-}(OH)_2D$. It is formed in two stages: the first is the formation of 25OH-D in the liver, and the second the formation of the fully active $1,25(OH)_2D$ in the kidney.

As with vitamin A, a high intake of vitamin D is harmful. Indeed, it is more likely to occur, since the gap between enough and too much vitamin D is quite narrow. The recommended allowance for an infant is $10\mu g$ a day, and $50\mu g$ a day can produce toxicity. The effects in an infant are loss of appetite, nausea, vomiting and a failure to grow. The child is irritable and, if the high intake persists, may fall into a coma and die. Postmortem examination reveals calcification of the soft tissues, including the kidney, lungs and arteries. A history of high intake that raises the suspicion of hypervitaminosis D can be confirmed by the discovery of a raised concentration of calcium in the plasma.

Soon after the Second World War, many paediatricians reported a condition among infants that was known as 'hypercalcaemia with failure to thrive'. It was suggested that this was caused by the over-enthusiastic addition of vitamin D by the manufacturers to a wide range of baby foods, including milk powders, cereals and canned meals. An infant fed on several proprietary preparations of this sort would not only be taking an excessive amount of vitamin as calculated from the amounts claimed on the labels; he would be taking more than this because of the understandable practice of the manufacturer in putting in more than claimed in order to ensure that storage of the food did not result in loss of vitamin D, bringing the content below the amount claimed. The manufacturers were asked by the Ministry of Food to reduce the quantity of the vitamin added to their preparations, and hypercalcaemia with failure to thrive virtually disappeared.

Fortunately, the treatment of hypervitaminosis once diagnosed, like the treatment of hypervitaminosis A, is simple, in that a cessation of the excessive intake leads to rapid recovery.

VITAMIN D IN FOODS

Recommended daily intake (RDI) for children 1–5 years – 10µg cholecalciferol

FOOD	PORTION	CHOLECALCIFEROL, µg
Herring	100g	20
Tuna, canned	50g	3
Egg	60g (1 egg)	1
Butter	10g	0.1
Margarine	10g	0.8
Milk	100ml	0.02
Cheese, Cheddar	25g	0.6
Cod liver oil	3ml	7

See also: Bone; Calcium; Hormones; Mellanby; Phosphorus

Vitamin E (Tocopherol)

Vitamin E is a fat-soluble vitamin that has attracted many enthusiastic believers in Western countries; it has, however, a minimum of proven usefulness.

It was shown in 1922 that laboratory rats could grow quite well when fed a diet of starch, lard, butter and yeast, but they failed to reproduce. They mated normally but, although pregnancy ensued, the foetuses died about two-thirds of the way through and were reabsorbed. Prolonged deprivation in the male led to sterility. The addition of vegetable oils reversed or prevented these effects of deficiency in the female and – if not too advanced – reversed them in the male. In due course, the principle responsible was isolated and called vitamin E. In other species of animals, lack of vitamin E produces quite different effects. In rabbits, it results in degeneration of muscles, i.e. a form of muscular dystrophy. Young chicks develop brain damage, and young turkeys develop haemorrhages and an excessive exudation of fluid into the tissues.

These effects of experimental deficiency are exacerbated if the diet contains a high proportion of polyunsaturated fat; conversely, the addition of small amounts of selenium is protective.

Dietary deficiency of vitamin E, that is, primary deficiency, is not seen in human subjects. The only conditions in which deficiency may occasionally occur are, in infants, premature birth and, in adults, inability to absorb fat properly. In both instances the red blood cells are usually fragile, although actual anaemia develops only in infants given iron or feeds rich in polyunsaturated fat at the same time.

It is generally believed that the reason that primary deficiency of vitamin E is not seen is explained by the wide distribution of the vitamin in foods, so that the human requirements, presumably small, are readily met. Nevertheless, the vitamin has been extensively used by the medical profession in the treatment of a variety of human diseases. These include threatened and habitual miscarriage, male infertility, muscular dystrophy and coronary heart disease. The evidence from carefully controlled tests shows that in all these conditions the consumption of vitamin E is quite ineffective. In addition to these treatments by doctors, many lay people take vitamin E in the unwarranted belief that it helps in athletic activities, reduces the effects of ageing such as wrinkles of the skin, and revives or improves sexual performance.

The chemical name for the most active form of vitamin E is alpha-tocopherol. Other tocopherols exist, with slightly different chemical formulae, as well as related substances called tocotrienols; they vary in activity from about one-half of that of alpha-tocopherol to no activity at all. As with vitamin A, it is usual to speak of the vitamin E equivalent of the combined activity of the substances found in a particular food. The pure substances exist as yellowish oils, and the quantities in foods are hardly affected by cooking.

Vitamin history

The vitamins were discovered by research workers who were independently pursuing two quite different lines of investigation. One was the attempt to discover the cause of beri-beri; the other was the attempt to discover what were the essential items needed in the diet of animals so that they could grow normally and remain healthy. The first line led to the discoveries by Eijkman in 1890 that beri-beri occurs in people with diets containing a high proportion of polished rice, and by Grijns in 1901 that it could be cured or prevented if this diet had the rice polishings added to it. Pursuing the second line of investigation, Lunin (1853–1937) had shown in 1881 that rats in the laboratory could not survive on a diet consisting only of protein, fat, carbohydrate and mineral salts. This work was followed in 1906 by the demonstration by Hopkins that the addition of small quantities of milk to such a diet was enough to make the rats thrive, and he suggested that this was because the milk provided essential 'accessory food factors'.

By 1912 it was clear that scurvy, beri-beri and pellagra and perhaps some other diseases in human beings, were due to the consumption of diets lacking in one or other of these substances. Attempts to identify the chemical nature of the 'accessory food factor' that prevented beri-beri revealed that it belonged to a group of substances called amines. In the belief that all these dietary essentials were likely to be amines, Funk in 1912 suggested that they be called 'vitamines', that is, vital amines. When this was later shown not to be so, the suggestion was made by Drummond in 1920 that the final 'e' should be dropped, so that the name became 'vitamin'.

The present names of the vitamins appear muddled and confusing, but the original intention seemed simple and logical. The discovery by Hopkins that rats would grow on a simple 'chemical' diet only if milk was added was followed by experiments of other research workers, which showed that continued growth required also the addition of yeast to the diet. Soon it became evident that these two foods owed their effects to a substance dissolved in the butterfat of milk, and another substance that could be extracted with water from the yeast. These materials were called 'fat-soluble A' and 'water-soluble B'; later they were called vitamine A and vitamine B. The next stage was to give the name vitamine C to the material in fruits and vegetables that was necessary to prevent scurvy. It then emerged that fat-soluble A had the property not only of promoting growth, but also of preventing rickets. When butterfat is heated, it loses its growth-promoting activity, but retains its anti-rickets activity; it therefore contains two separate substances. They were now called vitamin A and vitamin D, according to the new nomenclature adopted by Drummond.

Further confusion followed when it was found that the water-soluble material from yeast also had two different actions. One was to prevent beri-beri and the other to prevent pellagra; the substances responsible were then called vitamin B_1 and vitamin B_2. The latter remained when a water solution from yeast was heated, but this so-called vitamin B_2 itself soon turned out to comprise several vitamins; later, B_2 was used for the vitamin we now know as riboflavin. Sometimes a research worker would demonstrate that he could make an extract from yeast which prevented some hitherto unobserved condition in rats, or pigeons, and gave it a new name so that we soon had vitamin B_3 and B_4 and B_5. But with more and more refinement in the separation, purification and testing of these extracts from yeast, it transpired that some of them were in fact one or other of the substances that were already known. This is the reason why we have vitamins B_1, B_2, B_6 and B_{12}, but no B_3, B_4 or B_5, and no B_7, B_8, B_9, B_{10} or B_{11}.

In the meantime, research workers were separating and purifying the known vitamins, working out their chemical structure, and if possible actually synthesizing them in the laboratory. This was first done with vitamin C, the chemical constitution of which was worked out in 1932 and the vitamin itself synthesized in 1933. The next was vitamin B_1, and now the chemical structure of all the identified vitamins is known. With this knowledge, there was a move to give them names rather than letters; vitamin C has the name ascorbic acid; vitamin B_1 is thiamin; vitamin D is calciferol. But both the older names and the chemical names are still being used.

See also: Drummond; Eijkman; Funk; Grijns; Hopkins

Vitamin K

Like several of the other vitamins, vitamin K was discovered when animals were fed what was thought to be a complete diet. In 1934 it was reported that chicks on such a diet developed haemorrhages, and that this condition could be cured when lucerne (alfalfa) was fed, or a preparation of fishmeal. Within the next 5 years the protective substance was isolated and then synthesized. It turned out to be fat-soluble, and the Danish discoverer, Henrik Dam (1895–1976), gave it the name vitamin K, for *Koagulationsvitamin*, because of its role in blood-clotting. Lack of vitamin K leads to haemorrhages, which may be very severe.

Dietary lack in man is extremely rare. This is partly due to its wide distribution, because it occurs in most vegetable foods. Partly it is because some of the vitamin is synthesized by bacteria in the large intestine, and absorbed into the bloodstream. However, what is called secondary deficiency can occur, usually when there is some interference with the absorption of dietary fat and so an interference with the absorption of the fat-soluble vitamins including vitamin K. This most commonly occurs when there is a blockage of the bile duct, caused for example by gallstones, which causes obstructive jaundice. Since the bile salts are needed for fat absorption, the fat and the vitamin K in the diet are not well absorbed.

The patient may have to have the obstruction removed by surgery, so there is the danger that the possible deficiency of vitamin K will lead to uncontrollable bleeding. For this reason, the patient is injected with vitamin K before the operation. This is now easy to do because there are several substances available from drug manufacturers which have vitamin K activity, but which, unlike the natural vitamin K, are water-soluble.

Deliberate induction of some degree of vitamin K deficiency also occurs in medicine. In conditions where it is thought necessary to reduce the tendency of the blood to clot, for example in a patient who has survived an attack of coronary thrombosis, some physicians use anti-coagulant drugs, which counter the action of vitamin K. These substances include Warfarin, which is used to kill rats; it does this precisely because it causes deficiency of vitamin K and the animal dies through loss of blood from haemorrhage. The first antivitamin K to be discovered was isolated from spoiled sweet clover, when it was found that cattle given this in their feed developed a tendency to bleed. Further research established that the disease could be prevented or cured by administration of vitamin K. When anti-coagulants are used in medicine, the patient's blood is tested from time to time to see that the clotting property of the blood has not been too much reduced, which might then result in the unwanted occurrence of bleeding. If it is found that too much anti-coagulant has been used, the patient is given some vitamin K.

See also: Bile; Gall-bladder

Vitamin P

Sometimes called hesperidin, vitamin P is one of the non-existent vitamins. Its 'discovery' began with some research on guinea pigs in which scurvy was produced by a diet containing no vitamin C. The scurvy was accompanied, as always, by bleeding from the capillaries. The bleeding could be cured not only by giving the guinea pigs the missing vitamin C, but by giving them instead extracts made from cereals or from the pith of citrus fruits containing no vitamin C. The active substances were isolated and found to be pigments called flavones. These flavones are sometimes called bioflavinoids; the one from citrus fruits is citrin and the one from cereal is rutin. The name vitamin P refers to its early name, *Permeabilitätsvitamin.*

It is now accepted that the bioflavinoids are not dietary essentials; their action on the damaged capillaries in scurvy is a pharmacological one, and diets with all the essential nutrients but with no bioflavinoids do not produce any disability in any organism.

See also: Scurvy

Vitamins

The vitamins are food constituents of an organic nature (i.e. carbon compounds of varying complexity), essential for complete health. Diets lacking in particular vitamins may produce particular deficiency diseases, including scurvy, beri-beri and rickets. The nature of vitamins is best understood by recalling that all animals require very large numbers of different and inter-acting chemical substances in order to maintain a normal state of life. Most of these substances can be manu-factured from the major food constituents – protein, fat and carbohydrate – together with the mineral elements. The vitamins are those dozen or so different substances that cannot be manufactured in this way, so they have to be supplied by the food. The amounts needed by the human body are small; for an adult they vary from 30mg a day or so for vitamin C, down to 2 micrograms or less of vitamin B_{12}. Thus, 1g of vitamin C a day will be enough for more than 30 people, and 1g vitamin B_{12} a day enough for half a million people or more.

Not only are the amounts of the vitamins required to prevent deficiency small, but even the amounts required to improve manifest deficiency disease are not very much greater. Deficiency of vitamin B_1 will not occur if the average daily intake is just over 1mg, but a patient suffering from the heart failure of beri-beri, who untreated would be likely to die within 24 hours, after one dose of only 10mg of the vitamin would feel well enough to get up and walk out of the hospital.

It is the considerable potency of the vitamins, and the apparently miraculous effects they sometimes have in correcting the serious consequences of deficiency, that have created the quite unrealistic concepts in the minds of lay people of what vitamins can do. One concept is that, if deficiency of a vitamin leads to impairment of a function such as night vision, then large amounts of that vitamin will in a normal person lead to a supernormal ability to see in the dark. This accounts for much of the consumption of vitamin concentrates and pills, taken in order to improve digestion and cure constipation (vitamin B_1) or make a child grow taller than his genetic potential will allow (vitamin B_{12}) or prevent colds (vitamin A or vitamin C) or improve libido or sexual potency (vitamin E). Indeed, great amounts of vitamins are taken simply as a tonic by people who are not ill.

A second erroneous concept is that any substance that can produce important effects can be claimed as a vitamin. Thus, a material produced from apricot stones, unjustifiably claimed to cure cancer, was given the name vitamin B_{17}, with the alternative name of Laetrile; the use of the term vitamin implies that all those who do not get this substance will suffer from some disability and ultimately develop cancer.

Such concepts are manifestly unacceptable if one remembers that vitamins are substances required for complete health in all members of a species, and that inadequacy produces specific symptoms and signs of deficiency. Moreover, an intake greater than the amount needed to prevent these effects does not improve normal bodily function to superior levels; rare instances in which a clinical condition can demonstrably be improved by very large intakes of vitamins are doubtless due to some pharmacological action different from their action as dietary components. On the other hand, large doses of some vitamins, including vitamins A, B_6 and D, can be harmful. Another point is that each of the vitamins occurs in several foods, some indeed in most foods; there is no vitamin found uniquely in one food, and especially not uniquely in a product such as apricot stones, which is not an ordinary item of diet.

Not all species need the same vitamins. Some may be able to manufacture in their own bodies essential materials that other species cannot manufacture and have to have in their diets. Vitamin C is needed in the diet by human beings, primates and guinea pigs, but it is not needed in the diet eaten by most other species of animals; for these, therefore, it is not a vitamin.

Although there are diseases that are linked with deficiency of particular vitamins, such as pellagra and nicotinic acid, or beri-beri and thiamin, it is in practice rare to find deficiencies of single vitamins. This is because the foods lacking in a poor diet will usually be sources of more than one essential nutrient.

Finally, the question is often raised about the pronunciation of the word vitamin. Most lay people say 'vitamin' with the 'i' as in 'hit'; most nutritionists say 'vitamin' with the 'i' as in 'vital'. The latter is probably what Casimir Funk intended, because he thought they were all vital amines. On the other hand, Sir Frederick Gowland Hopkins, who was awarded the Nobel Prize for his part in discovering them, pronounced the word with the short 'i'.

See also: Health foods; Laetrile; Nutrition education

Voit, Carl von (1831–1908)

Voit was born in Bavaria and lived there for most of his life. In 1854 he graduated in medicine in Munich, where he studied under Liebig and Pettenkofer (1818–1901). He helped to lay the foundations of the modern knowledge of metabolism and nutrition, and introduced the technique of balance studies, working first with dogs. In the late 1850s, with the help of Pettenkofer, he devised a metabolism unit large enough to enclose a man, where he confirmed the theoretical studies that maintained that protein requirements were not affected by muscular exercise. This contradicted the views of his teacher, Liebig, who in 1870 publicly acknowledged that he had been wrong.

HANDBUCH DER PHYSIOLOGIE

DES

GESAMMT-STOFFWECHSELS

UND DER

FORTPFLANZUNG.

ERSTER THEIL.

PHYSIOLOGIE DES ALLGEMEINEN STOFFWECHSELS

UND DER

ERNÄHRUNG

VON

C. von Voit in München.

LEIPZIG,
VERLAG VON F. C. W. VOGEL.
1881.

Voit also calculated the caloric value of fat and carbohydrate, as well as that of protein. He assessed the caloric requirement of adults, and pointed out that it was affected by clothing and atmospheric temperature, but much more by work. He measured the food intake of the local population, and also calculated it in terms of protein, fat and carbohydrate.

See also: Basal metabolism; Energy content of food; Nutrient balance tests; Protein

W

Water

Most chemical reactions do not occur without moisture. Absolutely dry iron, in a dry atmosphere, does not rust. A mixture of dry bicarbonate of soda and tartaric acid remains unchanged; moistened, however, the mixture releases carbon dioxide gas and so can be used as baking powder in order to make the dough rise.

Water is thus essential so as to permit the body, with the aid of its many enzymes, to carry out the huge number of chemical reactions that make up its activity as a living organism, i.e. its metabolism. The body composition of the average adult man includes 60% as water, amounting to about 40 litres. About 25 litres are inside the cells, and about 15 litres outside the cells in the so-called extra-cellular fluid; of this, about 12 litres is in tissue fluid and 3 litres in the blood plasma.

It is important that these quantities of water do not change very much, because this would affect the balance of the metabolic reactions. An adult losing 4 litres of water is very thirsty, with skin dry, pinched and inelastic. Hallucinations may occur with this degree of loss, and when the loss reaches 8 litres or 10 litres, death ensues.

The constancy of the volume of body water is maintained in spite of the constant loss from the lungs, in the stools, from the skin as visible or invisible perspiration, and in the urine. Water is replaced from three sources: the oxidation of food (metabolic water), the water in solid foods, and chiefly the water taken in drinks.

The amount lost from the lungs is about 500ml a day, and from the stools about 150ml; these values do not vary much in health. The amount lost in perspiration is rarely less than 500ml a day, but can vary considerably, depending on the environmental temperature and on physical activity; it is not, however, affected by the amount of water consumed. The amount lost in the urine is the amount needed to preserve the balance between intake and output.

The input of water from the metabolism of food is also not determined by the amount needed to produce a balance of input and output. This is also largely true of the amount taken in from solid foods, although one can imagine a thirsty person eating an apple or other juicy fruit for its water rather than as a food. Chiefly, however, it is water taken as drinks that contributes mostly to ensuring an adequate intake. Much of what is drunk is determined by custom, or because it contains a desirable component such as caffeine or alcohol or some attractive flavour.

In normal circumstances, water intake is more than enough to meet minimal water output, and the fine balance of input and output is brought about by precise regulation of urine volume. If, however, output tends to exceed input, a sensation of thirst constitutes a stimulus to increase input, so that this acts as a rough control in the maintenance of water balance.

Where no fluid is taken, urinary excretion falls. There is, however, a minimal level of excretion which includes the amount that has to be lost through the kidney in order to excrete the urea and other products of metabolism, even if nothing is being eaten. This 'obligatory water' amounts to some 250–300ml a day; together with the amount lost from the lungs and stools and through the skin, a body cannot help losing about 1.5 litres a day, even in a temperate environment and with little physical exertion. Since a deficit of 8 litres can be fatal, it is clear that people cannot survive without water for more than some 5 or 6 days; if they are having to exert themselves, or are in a hot environment, survival can be as little as 2–3 days.

See also: **Kidney; Mineral waters; Urine**

Weaning

For physiological reasons, the transition to solid foods, from feeding an infant with milk at the breast or from a bottle, need not take place until the baby is 6 months old or so. There is a tendency, however, especially in prosperous countries, to wean infants at quite an early age; in one study in the UK, 40% of 4-week-old infants were already being given solid foods, and by 4 months the figure was 90%. Two common reasons given for early weaning are that it is a way of ensuring good nutrition, and that it lessens the rejection of unaccustomed foods when they are introduced later. It is doubtful if this latter objection is well-founded. As for nutrition, breast milk or a good brand of a dried milk preparation can provide entirely adequately for the needs of an infant up to at least 6 months; the introduction of solid food much before that may help the infant to become overweight, especially with the common practice of using sugar-sweetened cereals as one of the first weaning foods.

Ideally, the weaning from the breast or artificial milks should not be spread over more than 2 or 3 weeks. It is not necessary to begin by the introduction of a cereal, and in any case this should not form a substantial part of the new diet. More stress should be laid on fish, meat, eggs, vegetables and fruit; provided they are chopped or cut up fairly small, it is not necessary that they be sieved. It is also better to persevere in trying to give these foods without the addition of sugar, which mothers often use in order to trick the child into eating un-accustomed food. Similarly, drinks of plain water are better than sugar-sweetened drinks. These practices gradually increase the development of a sweet tooth, which is difficult to abolish later.

Since the mother usually tastes any new food that she is going to give to her baby, some manufacturers of proprietary baby foods tend to add salt and sugar, and also colour and flavour to make the food more 'appetizing'. Most manufacturers, however, do not now add salt, and some do not add sugar or monosodium glutamate. Nevertheless, some mothers still mistakenly 'improve' the baby's food with additions of this sort.

See also: Anthropometry; Milk

West Indian cherry

There is a remarkably high quantity of vitamin C in the West Indian cherry or acerola. Without its stones, 100g of the fruit contains 1,000mg of the vitamin. This may be compared with the 5mg in the same amount of ordinary cherries, 25mg in raspberries and 50mg in oranges and in strawberries. The West Indian cherry plant grows in tropical and semi-tropical regions of America.

Wheat

It seems that the present varieties of the cultivated cereal are derived from a hybrid wild wheat that originated in the Middle East some 10,000 years ago. Although there are now said to be 30,000 varieties or more of the cultivated wheat, almost all belong to two types of the genus *Triticum*: *T. durum* and *T. aestiva* (or *vulgare*). The many varieties of the latter provide the wheat for bread-making; *T. durum* is a specially hard wheat which is used for making macaroni and other pasta.

The wheat grain (wheat berry) consists of three major parts. These are the bran, constituting about 12% of the weight of the grain, the germ, about 3% and the endosperm, about 85%. Milling may be considered as roughly separating these three fractions; in the production of white flour, the bran and the germ are removed together with some of the outer layers of the endosperm, leaving about 72% of the original grain. It is possible to remove more, or less, of the grain, and the proportion that remains in the resulting flour is known as the extraction rate. Thus, flour made from the whole of the wheat berry, including the bran and the germ, would result in a flour of 100% extraction, also known as wholewheat flour. However, flour of, say, 85% extraction is not necessarily made by removing 15% consisting only of the bran and germ. If the miller wished, it could be made by putting together any combination of the fractions produced with the highly complex milling machinery which mills and sieves in several stages of the process; so long as this added up to 85% of the original wheat, it could be called 85% extraction flour.

The composition of the various parts, and so their nutrient content, varies considerably. The bran contains a high proportion of indigestible material, or roughage, now more commonly called dietary fibre. It also contains 25–30% of starch, and some protein. The germ contains nearly 10% of fat and 25% of protein; it is particularly rich in vitamin E and some of the B vitamins. The endosperm contains a high proportion of starch, but also about 10% of protein.

See also: Cereals

Whistler, Daniel (1619–84)

Daniel Whistler studied first at Oxford University and then qualified in medicine at Leyden University in Holland. His MD thesis of 1645 was his only publication. It was entitled *De morbo puerili Anglorum; quem patrio idiomate indiginae vocant The Rickets* ('On the disease of English children; which the natives colloquially call The Rickets'). It is likely that his thesis was not a very original work, being based largely on the observations of Glisson and other physicians.

Many people today, incidentally, must feel grateful to 'the natives' for calling the disease rickets rather than the name favoured by Whistler – paedosplanchosteoclases.

The publication of the thesis predates Glisson's *De rachitide* by five years, and thus remains the first published work to deal with rickets as a clinical entity. It was also only the second book to deal with a single disease, the first being that by Caius on the 'sweating sickness', published in 1552.

Whistler became Treasurer of the Royal College of Physicians in 1682, and its President in the following year. However, he neglected his duties both as Treasurer and as President and allowed the affairs of the College, especially in relation to its property, to fall into muddle and confusion.

See also: Glisson; Rickets

Wild rice

Because it is a native of the United States, wild rice is also known as American wild rice; another name is Indian rice. Although the plant is an aquatic grass, it is in fact not closely related to ordinary rice. Mostly, it is used as a feed for waterfowl, although it is also harvested by American Indians for their own consumption. Some finds its way into food stores, but only in small quantities because, since its yield is small, it is quite expensive. It is bought either as a special delicacy, or because it is supposed to have superior nutritional virtues. It is somewhat richer in protein than is ordinary rice, but no different in other respects; since it is consumed in such small quantities, however, its nutritional composition will in any case contribute very little to the nutrient content of the total diet.

Wine

Although it is possible to make wine from any fruit, and even many vegetables, wine usually refers to the product of fermentation of the grape. From the point of view of the nutritionist, there are not many essential features in the making and composition of wine; the consumer, however, has much more interest in the variations within these general features.

The vine and the making of wine from grapes have been known since at least biblical times. They may have originated in Persia, but most of the countries in or bordering the Mediterranean region have for millennia cultivated the vine. The Romans spread it into the Alps, France and Germany, and it soon reached England. Reasonable quantities of English wine were available from the early eighth century, especially as vines were planted in church gardens almost as soon as the building of the church began. English wine was commonly made until the middle of the thirteenth century; later, French wine became more readily available, so that the vineyards of England began to be used for other crops. Today, wines are made in many other parts of the world, notably North Africa, South Africa, Australia, South America, and in New York State and California in the United States.

The wine is made from grape juice which contains the sugar and the yeast necessary for producing the alcoholic fermentation. The yeast is the *ellipsoides* variety of *Saccharomyces cerevisiae*, which is normally present on the skin of the grape, so that it is present in the juice (the must) when the grapes are pressed. Bacteria do not readily grow in the must because it is acid and contains a fair amount of sugar; although the sugar is gradually used in the fermentation, bacterial growth continues to be inhibited because of the production of CO_2, which keeps the product anaerobic.

Fermentation ceases either when the sugar is exhausted, or when the concentration of alcohol stops the growth and activity of the yeast. This occurs when the content of alcohol reaches about 10g/100ml; stronger wines, such as sherry and port with 15–20% alcohol, are produced by the addition of brandy or pure alcohol when fermentation has stopped.

Red wine is made by pressing the skins of black grapes so that their pigment is released into the must. White wine is made either from white grapes, or from black grapes without expressing their skin pigment.

Sparkling wines are made either by preventing the escape of the CO_2 produced during fermentation, as in the champagne process, or by passing CO_2 into the wine after the wine-making has been completed.

The nutritional contributions of wine are its energy and its iron. The energy is derived from both the sugar and the alcohol, and in a table wine amounts to some 70–80 kcal/100ml, which is about the quantity in a full wineglass. There is a variable amount of iron, on average between 0.5mg/100ml and 1.0mg; there is no worthwhile quantity of any other nutrient.

See also: Ageing; Alcohol; Fermentation

X

Xylitol

Like sorbitol, xylitol is a white powder that is chemically an alcohol derived from a sugar, in this instance a 5-carbon sugar called xylose. Xylose in turn is the unit sugar that forms the polymer, xylan, the major fibrous material forming the cell walls of wood. In the body, xylitol gives rise to ribose. It is about as sweet as sucrose, but not fermented by the acid-producing bacteria in the mouth. Consequently it does not cause dental decay, and is used as a sugar substitute in the manufacture of sweets and chewing gum.

See also: Sweetening agents

Y

Yams

Most yams are grown in the tropics; the two main areas of cultivation are in the wet regions of West Africa, and in and around Indonesia. They are often planted in mounds or ridges of earth, rather like potatoes, and can be harvested after 8–12 months. The tubers can be stored for several months on racks, or hung up in barns. They are eaten boiled and mashed, or roasted or fried. Nutritionally, they provide mostly starch; they have a little protein, about as much as in potatoes, but they have less of the B vitamins and vitamin C.

In America, the term yam is often used to mean the sweet potato.

See also: Potatoes

Yeast

The uses of yeast in brewing and in the baking of bread were probably both discovered by accident. It seems possible that the first relevant observation was that fruits that were allowed to become overripe were found to have the qualities we now associate with fermentation and with the manufacture of wine. That dough would rise ('prove') could similarly have been an accidental discovery. If these suggestions are accepted, both examples of fermentation would have been caused by adventitious inoculation of the dough or the grape juice by yeast spores present in the air, on the skin of the fruit, or on the hands of those working with the fruit or the flour.

In bread-making, some yeast could have been transferred by putting aside a batch of the dough and adding this when another batch was being made. The process could be repeated indefinitely unless the dough became infected with an organism that produced unwanted or unpleasant effects on the dough. This method is still used in some remote rural areas.

An alternative source of yeast might have been the discovery that the scum rising to the surface during the fermentation of fruits or grain could be skimmed off and used for proving the dough.

Yeast itself has played an important part in the early discovery of the vitamins of the B group, their separation and their identification. It was used in the early treatment of some of the deficiencies of these vitamins, such as beri-beri, pellagra or riboflavin deficiency. More recently, it has found use also as part of the treatment of diseases in which the role of diet is less certain; these include the burning feet syndrome, a condition first described by prisoners-of-war held by the Japanese, and nutritional amblyopia, with loss especially of central vision.

Yeast and preparations of yeast are still taken by many persons as a tonic, or as a general nutritional supplement. Usually it is dried brewers' yeast; more commonly, yeast extracts such as Marmite are taken. These are made by allowing a concentrated suspension of yeast cells in water to digest themselves, i.e. autolyse. This is extracted with water, and salt and perhaps other substances added.

Apart from the absence of vitamin B_{12}, yeast is a good source of the B vitamins. There is little difference between bakers' yeast and brewers' yeast, except that the latter contains more thiamin. However, the amount of thiamin in yeast extract gradually diminishes as it is stored. Since most of the available yeast extracts contain a great deal of salt, the amounts likely to be consumed will not provide much of the vitamins. The salt content may amount to 10%, and some paediatricians doubt therefore whether yeast extract is a desirable preparation to give to babies and young children.

The yeasts used for baking and brewing are strains of *Saccharomyces cerevisiae*, of the variety *ellipsoides*.

NUTRIENT COMPOSITION OF YEAST

(quantities in 5g – about 1 tsp)

	DRIED BAKERS' YEAST	YEAST EXTRACT (*Marmite*)
Energy (kcal)	9	9
Protein (g)	1.8	2.0
Available carbohydrate (g)	0.2	0.1
Fibre (g)	1.1	—
Thiamin (mg)	0.12	0.15
Riboflavin (mg)	0.2	0.5
Nicotinic acid (mg)	1.8	3.0

During the Second World War and after, efforts were made to produce a yeast, *Torula utilis* (now known as *Candida utilis*), which could be used as a source of inexpensive protein for animal feed, or more directly as a dietary supplement for human beings. It can be grown quite readily on a wide variety of carbohydrate-rich waste products, such as those produced during sugar refining. It was soon found, however, that it was not economically feasible to produce it for animal feed, and that it was not acceptable as a regular item of food for people. It was one of the early examples of the uselessness of producing a food for inclusion as a normal item in human diet, however desirable in terms of nutrient content, if it is not sufficiently palatable: a lesson that still has not been fully learned.

See also: **Baking; Beer; Fermentation; Novel protein foods; Vitamin history**

Yoghurt

Yoghurt is made by fermenting milk with bacteria that produce lactic acid from the lactose the milk contains. One result is that the milk curdles. In Western countries, it is common to use skimmed or partly skimmed milk, sometimes with added dried skimmed milk powder. More recently, preparations of yoghurt to which sugar and fruit have been added have been made commercially available.

The bacteria used commercially to produce yoghurt are most commonly a mixture of *Lactobacillus bulgaricus* and *Streptococcus acidophilus*. Because the milk is usually boiled before the culture of bacteria is added and because the *acidophilus* bacteria tend to grow much faster than do any chance pathogenic organisms that may reach the milk, yoghurt is usually a safe product, even in countries with poor hygiene.

At the beginning of this century, the suggestion was made by the distinguished bacteriologist, Metchnikoff (1845–1916), that the consumption of yoghurt would lead to improved health and in particular would prolong life. This was brought about, it was supposed, by the replacement of the usual bacteria in the gut, which produced toxic substances, by beneficial lactic acid bacteria. In fact, this replacement either does not occur, or, if it does, occurs for only a short time. Nor is there any evidence whatever that yoghurt improves health in any other way. The nutritional value of yoghurt is no less and no more than that of the milk and possible additional substances from which it is made.

Similar preparations are made from the milk of other animals. Koumiss is made in Russia from mares' milk; the organisms that sour the milk produce not only lactic acid but also a modest amount of alcohol. Kefir is made in the Caucasus from cows' milk, but yeast as well as *Lactobacillus* is used in its fermentation; again, a small quantity of alcohol results.

See also: Longevity; Milk

Z

Zein

The major protein of maize (corn), the Latin name of which is *Zea mais*, is characterized by having a particularly low biological value. This is not only because it has a low proportion of lysine, a property that it shares with the proteins of other cereals, but also because it has a low proportion of another essential amino-acid, tryptophan, and possibly of a third, iso-leucine.

See also: Biological value of proteins; Milk

Zinc

Zinc is an essential trace element. Zinc deficiency in human beings has been recognized only since the early 1960s. It was reported among adolescents in Egypt and in Iran, where it is responsible for retarded mental and physical development and delayed puberty. It can be rapidly improved by the administration of zinc. The cause of the deficiency is not quite clear, but it seems to be linked with the consumption of unleavened bread made with high-extraction flour. This contains a high proportion of phytate, some of which would combine with zinc, as well as with other cations, such as calcium and iron, and so reduce the amount that can be absorbed by the intestine.

There is evidence too that the high consumption of bran and other sources of dietary fibre that some authorities have encouraged in Western countries may produce a decrease of the availability of zinc and other elements to an extent that may be deleterious.

Zinc is necessary for the action of several enzymes, including carbonic anhydrase, needed for the release of carbon dioxide from the venous blood passing through the lungs; it is also needed for the function of alkaline phosphatase and several other enzymes concerned with the synthesis of nucleic acids and protein. The total amount in the body is similar to that of iron, about 20g. The average Western diet contains about 10–15mg a day; the United States authorities recommend a daily intake of 15mg for an adult.

EQUIVALENTS

1 litre (l) = 1000 millilitres (or cubic centimetres)
1 millilitre (ml or cc) = 1000 microlitres (mcl)

1 kilogram (kg) = 1000 grams
1 gram (g) = 1000 milligrams
1 milligram (mg) = 1000 micrograms (μg or mcg)

INDEX

Abderhalden, *see* Funk, 170

Absorption, 9
of agar, 15; of alcohol, 17; and availability, 38; of biotin, *see* Avidin, 38; of calcium, *see* Oxalic acid, 275; *see* Phytic acid, 287; and digestibility, 121; faulty, *see* PEM, 304; of filtrate, *see* Urine, 358; of glucose, 180; in gluten sensitivity, 182; of iron, 206; of phytosterol, 335; of protein in pulses, 307; of starch-rich foods, *see* Cooking, 98

Absorption of fat, 10
bile in, 51; in coeliac disease, 95; *see* Fat, 142; gall-bladder in, 174; in gluten sensitivity, 182; lecithin in, 215; and lipoprotein, 220; lymph vessels in, 226; *see* Phosphorus, 286

Accelerated freeze drying, *see* Food preservation, 164

Accessory food factors, *see* Vitamin history, 374

Accum, *see* Food Adulteration, 158

Acerola, *see* West Indian cherry, 384

Acesulfam-K as sweetening agent, 343

Acetic acid, *see* Cider vinegar, 89; in food preservation, 163; *see* Vinegar, 361

Acetoacetic acid, in acidosis, 11; in ketosis, 209

Acetone, *see* Ketosis, 209

Achard, *see* Sucrose, 337

Achlorhydria, *see* Anaemia, 25

Acid fermentation, *see* Food preservation, 163

Acidity and acidosis, 10; *see* pH, 284

Acidosis, 10
see Buffer, 64; and ketosis, 209

Acne, 11
see Puberty, 306

Acrolein, *see* Oils, 270

Activated dough development, *see* Bread, 60

Acute, 12
gastritis, 175; inflammation, 199

Adaptation, to calcium reduction, 70; to dark, *see* Dark adaptation, 313

Addiction, 12
alcohol, 16; caffeine, 67

Additives, *see* Food additives, 154

Adipocytes, *see* Body fat, 55

Adolescence, *see* Anorexia nervosa, 28; *see* Puberty, 306

Adrenal glands, 13
cortisol from, *see* Cholesterol, 87; vitamin C and, 368

Adrenaline, from adrenal medulla, 13; in breakdown of body fat, 55; increase in smoking, 326; from phenylalanine, *see* Amino-acids, 23

Adrenal medulla, 13

Adulteration, *see* Food adulteration, 157; *see* Food and Drink Act, 158

Aerated bread, 59

Aerobic/Anaerobic, 14
see Acidosis, 10; bacteria, 39; fermentation, 145; intestinal bacteria, 201; metabolism, *see* Glycogen, 182; oxidation,276

AFD, *see* Food preservation, 164

Aflatoxins, 14
in food spoilage, 168; in fungi, 170; in groundnuts, 187; *see* Poisons in food, 291

Agar, 15
as emulsfier and stabilizer, 130; *see* Fibre, 148; *see* Seaweed, 323

Agar-agar, 15

Ageing, 15

Agene in ageing flour, 15; *see* Mellanby, 238

Alanine, *see* Amino-acids (Table), 23

Albumen, 16